Infections of the Gastrointestinal Tract

Microbiology, Pathophysiology, and Clinical Features

CURRENT TOPICS IN INFECTIOUS DISEASE

Series Editors:

William B. Greenough III
Chief, Infectious Disease Division
The Johns Hopkins University
School of Medicine
Baltimore, Maryland

Thomas C. Merigan
Head, Division of Infectious Disease
Stanford University Medical Center
Stanford, California

The Atypical Mycobacteria and Human Mycobacteriosis

John S. Chapman

Infections of the Gastrointestinal Tract: Microbiology,
Pathophysiology, and Clinical Features

Herbert L. DuPont and Larry K. Pickering

Coccidioidomycosis: A Text

Edited by David A. Stevens

Infections of the Gastrointestinal Tract

Microbiology, Pathophysiology, and Clinical Features

Herbert L. DuPont

Professor of Medicine
Director, Program in Infectious Diseases and Clinical Microbiology
The University of Texas Health Science Center Medical School
Houston, Texas

and

Larry K. Pickering

Associate Professor of Pediatrics
Director, Pediatric Infectious Diseases
Program in Infectious Diseases and Clinical Microbiology
The University of Texas Health Science Center Medical School
Houston, Texas

PLENUM MEDICAL BOOK COMPANY
NEW YORK AND LONDON

Library of Congress Cataloging in Publication Data

DuPont, Herbert L
Infections of the gastrointestinal tract.

(Topics in infectious disease)
Includes index.
1. Diarrhea. 2. Gastrointestinal system—Infections. I. Pickering, Larry K.,
joint author. II. Title. III. Series. [DNLM: 1. Gastrointestinal diseases. WI100
D938i]
RC862.D5D86   616.3'427   80-20352
ISBN 0-306-40409-5

To
Peggy and Mimi

Preface

Enteric infection has played an important role in the majority of the world's populations, including children (particularly those under four years of age), the aged, the malnourished, military populations, and persons from industrialized regions traveling to developing areas. The magnitude of the problem has been profound in areas of the world with reduced economic development, where there exists a greater reservoir of enteropathogens and a larger susceptible population with nutritional deficits. Morbidity from enteric infection in developing areas exceeds that seen in industrialized countries by severalfold, with the problem being most serious in infants who are bottle-fed and other infants and young children soon after being weaned from the breast ("weanling diarrhea"). Of greater significance than the inverse relationship of diarrhea morbidity with levels of industrial development is the relationship of death from intestinal infection and socioeconomic advancement. Mortality rate from diarrhea is *10 to 100 times* greater in developing areas. In many parts of the third world, diarrhea, resultant dehydration, and associated malnutrition are the leading causes of death in infants and young children and account for as great as one-third of pediatric deaths.

Control and prevention of diarrhea, our ultimate goals, will be possible one day through a variety of social, economic, educational, and medical interventions. Ultimately, widespread dissemination of safe and adequate water sources and implementation of sanitary systems for disposal of excreta and waste must be made available. These will be expensive, and, although prerequisites for control of enteric infection, they will not be sufficient in and of themselves. Improvement in personal and public hygiene and increasing levels of nutrition are necessary. Whether these will be possible without a more equitable distribution of wealth is unknown. Immediate areas for development include education (nutritional and psychological) about the importance of breast-feeding, principles of personal and food hygiene, institution of programs for oral fluid therapy, and specific therapy where applicable. Chemo- and immunoprophylaxis will be important supporting control measures for certain special high-risk groups but will not be useful to the overall control of diarrhea.

Over the past several years, laboratory techniques have become available so that the research laboratory has been increasingly able to detect enteropathogens in diarrheal stools. In the early 1970s, an etiologic agent could be detected in stool specimens of only 10 to 15% of persons with acute diarrhea. Through the application of tissue culture techniques, the use of refined cultural and serological procedures, and by employing the electron microscope, the yield of enteropathogen detection has been increased to 60% of those with an acute diarrheal syndrome. As soon as these laboratory assays are further developed and become applicable for routine use in hospital and clinical laboratories, remaining questions about the relative importance of the agents and their epidemiology and immunology will be forthcoming. In *Infections of the Gastrointestinal Tract*, we have attempted to review information which has accumulated about the etiology, epidemiology, pathophysiology, diagnosis, and eventual control of the infectious enteric diseases. We look forward expectantly to future developments in this important area of public health. The chapters on etiologic syndromes are arranged to reflect historical development in the field. We are fast approaching the day when knowledge of pathophysiology will allow us to organize the topic anatomically and functionally.

Herbert L. DuPont
Larry K. Pickering

Houston

Acknowledgments

Volunteer studies reported were conducted at the University of Maryland. The following federal grants or contracts supported investigations outlined: U.S. Army Medical Research and Development Command DA 49-193-MD-2867 and DA 17-67-C-7057; National Institute of Allergy and Infectious Diseases (National Institutes of Health) AI 12699 and AI 72534; and Center for Disease Control CDC-200-77-0702. Collaborators directing studies cited were Dolores G. Evans, Ph.D., Doyle J. Evans, Jr., Ph.D., Samuel B. Formal, Ph.D., Eugene J. Gangarosa, M.D., Richard B. Hornick, M.D., Jorge Olarte, D.Sc., Merrill J. Snyder, Ph.D., and Theodore E. Woodward, M.D. Editorial suggestions were made by Doyle J. Evans, Jr., Ph.D., William B. Greenough III, M.D., Thomas C. Merigan, Jr., M.D., and John J. Vollet III, Ph.D. Photographs were prepared by Hanna West and Patricia Byers, and Kathy Boyle typed the manuscript.

Contents

1

Immune Mechanisms in Infectious Diarrhea

INTRODUCTION

The most important factors that determine the occurrence and severity of diarrheal disease include a safe environment, consisting of an efficient water source and sewage removal system; adequate personal and food hygiene; and good standards of nutrition. Despite the presence of these factors, the human body is exposed continually to pathogenic and non-pathogenic microorganisms, toxic substances, and chemicals which would be damaging or fatal if not efficiently excluded by the gastrointestinal tract. Once organisms are swallowed, the occurrence of a diarrheal syndrome will depend upon the pathogenic potential of the agent (virulence), the number of viable cells or viruses ingested, and the status of host defense factors.

Host defense factors can be divided into those operating nonspecifically against a broad range of agents and those with an immunologic basis directed against components of a specific microbe to which the host has been exposed previously.

NONSPECIFIC GASTROINTESTINAL IMMUNE MECHANISMS

Gastric Trap

Once enteric pathogens are ingested, they are trapped temporarily in the strongly acidic environment of the stomach. Gastric acid is responsible for reducing the number of viable bacteria which reach the small intestine, since nearly all bacterial pathogens are highly susceptible to a low pH.[1] Without an adequate concentration of gastric acid, such as occurs in patients with achlorhydria, there is an increased proliferation of nonpathogenic bacteria in the upper gut,[2] and diarrheal disease is far more common.[3-8] In studies designed to produce clinical cholera in healthy adult male volunteers, the importance of gastric acidity to the pathogenesis of disease was demonstrated.[9] Although cholera did not predictably develop when as many as 10^8–10^{10} viable bacteria were ingested, when gastric acidity was buffered with orally administered sodium bicarbonate, the illness occurred in many men after receiving an inoculum of 10^4 *Vibrio cholerae*. The number of viable bacteria necessary to produce illness when the organisms were placed directly into the duodenum, bypassing the stomach, was even further reduced. In these volunteer studies conducted by Hornick and his colleagues, many of the men who developed cholera were shown to have a reduced capacity to decrease gastric pH 15 to 30 min after receiving the bicarbonate. Additional studies were conducted on patients with naturally occurring cholera, and it was discovered that many of the patients had achlorhydria,[3,10] which offers additional indirect evidence of the importance of gastric acidity in the pathogenesis of clinical cholera. Gastric acidity undoubtedly plays a predisposing role in other forms of diarrhea, including salmonellosis, [4-8] shigellosis,[11] giardiasis, [12-14] and strongyloidiasis.[15,16]

Many of the earlier studies attempting to link defects of hydrochloric acid secretion with acquisition of diarrhea probably overdiagnosed hypochlorhydria because of a general lack of methodologic principles.[17] However, it is reasonable to assume that a major reason why diarrhea so commonly occurs in the aged, those with prior gastric resection, and perhaps even in infants with malnutrition is a relative lack of gastric acidity mechanisms. The role of other gastric factors such as speed of stomach emptying and a protective barrier effect by mucus in resistance to intestinal infection is largely unstudied.

Intestinal Motility Patterns

While stomach acidity generally assures that material reaching the small bowel will contain small numbers of bacteria, motility of the upper gut will determine if local bacterial propagation is to occur.[18,19] Any disease or disorder which restricts propulsive movement by the upper gut appears to be associated with an overgrowth of enteric bacteria, leading to malabsorption and a fermentative type of diarrhea. Such disorders which influence motility include intestinal scleroderma, small-intestinal diverticulosis, diabetes mellitus with visceral neuropathy, gastrointestinal strictures or fistulas, Billroth II anastomosis with blind loop following gastrectomy, and tropical and nontropical sprue.

Slowing of intestinal motility by opiates, ganglionic blockers, or ligation allows bacteria to localize and multiply. To produce an intestinal infection in experimental animals, it is usually necessary to restrict intestinal movement patterns with drugs to allow enteropathogens to multiply and interact with the gut mucosa. Increased intestinal transit during intestinal infection may reflect to some degree attempts by the body to rid itself of bacteria and toxins. The mild diarrhea (one to two unformed stools) which is common among persons from one part of the world or country who travel to another probably reflects the body's attempt to expel foreign microbes or substances. Evidence has been offered to suggest that the time of contact between the epithelial lining of the gut and an invasive bacterial pathogen such as a *Shigella* or *Salmonella* strain is instrumental to the evolution of disease.[20,21] In fact, antidiarrheal compounds which directly inhibit motility may worsen clinical disease. Table 1.1 demonstrates the results seen in one study investigating the influence of antimicrobial therapy and antidiarrheal therapy on shigellosis. Note that the shortest duration of diarrhea was seen for those patients with bacillary dysentery who received the antimicrobial agent. Diarrhea persisted an average of two days less for the group receiving the antimotility drug when compared to the placebo group; however, the number of fever hours was significantly greater, and the antidiarrheal compound appeared to interfere with the beneficial effect of the antibiotic in view of the failure to eradicate pathogen excretion from among those taking both the antimotility and antimicrobial agents. We have seen a number of adults with shigellosis or salmonellosis who progressed to toxic dilatation of the colon requiring colectomy while receiving antimotility drugs for symptomatic relief of diarrhea due to *Salmonella* or *Shigella* strains.

TABLE 1.1
Effect of Lomotil and Oxolinic Acid on the Course of Bacillary Dysentery[a]

| Treatment group | | Number of subjects | Mean duration of diarrhea (days) | Mean duration of fever (hr) | Bacteriologic response[b] |
Antimicrobial agent	Antidiarrheal compound				
Oxolinic acid	Lomotil	6	7	16	1 (17%)
Oxolinic acid	Placebo	6	3	18	4 (67%)
Placebo	Lomotil	7	7	48	0
Placebo	Placebo	6	9	21	0

[a]Adapted from DuPont and Hornick.[21]
[b]Negative stool cultures within five days of treatment.

Intestinal Microflora

The indigenous bacterial flora of the intestine exerts a homeostatic influence on the gut by deterring potential pathogens. The autochthonous flora is remarkably stable in terms of predominant strains and level of growth. The resident bacteria elaborate antibacterial catabolites, including lactic acid and short-chain volatile fatty acids. The effects of these fermentative products are a reduced Eh and pH which reach antibacterial concentrations.[22] This natural defense is enhanced in breast-fed infants by means of increased metabolism of the anaerobic saccharolytic lactobacilli with production of acids which prohibit growth of certain bacteria. Alteration of intestinal flora by antimicrobial therapy increases susceptibility of animals[22,23] and humans[24] to progressive salmonellosis. Antibiotics not only decrease the infectious dose of *Salmonella* but prolong the fecal excretion of the infecting strain[25,26] and may on occasion convert an asymptomatic carrier state into a bacteremic illness[27] by reducing the intestinal flora and allowing the infecting strain to proliferate. The importance of intestinal flora to recovery from and prevention of other forms of enteric infection is unknown, although bacterial catabolites are known to be inhibitory to *Shigella* strains[28] and other gram-negative bacilli.[29] In addition to the local antibacterial effect of floral catabolites, there may occur an inhibition of hostile bacteria by the intestinal tract through other nonspecific factors such as lack of space and nutrients which are utilized by those bacteria proliferating locally,[30,31] colicinogenic strains of *Escherichia coli*,[32] or hydrogen sulfide in the gut[33] which may be inhibitory to bacterial growth.

IMMUNOLOGIC MECHANISMS IN ENTERIC INFECTION

Secretory Immune System

The importance of local immunity to invading pathogens was established in the first part of this century by Besredka[34,35] when he demonstrated in rabbits that immunity to the dysentery bacillus could be produced by the oral administration of killed bacteria. This immunity required an interaction between the organisms and the intestinal mucosa and was independent of serum antibody. The concept that antibody content of external secretions was a direct reflection of antibody content of serum was further questioned by Walsh and Cannon[36] in 1938 when they showed that antibody in the nasal cavity was produced locally. In the

1960s, IgA was shown to be the predominant class of immunoglobin in external secretions.[37,38] Since then, several discoveries have enabled the separation of the secretory from the humoral immune system: (1) IgA in external secretions has a structure significantly different from IgA in serum[39,40]; (2) the ratio of IgG to IgA in external secretions differs from that in serum[41-43]; and (3) the secretory system contains immunoglobulin classes other than IgA which are produced locally.[44-47]

The demonstration that IgA is the predominant immunoglobulin in external secretions was the basis for the theory that a distinct secretory or mucosal immune system was operative which was not merely a reflection of the systemic immune system. In humans, the IgG/IgA ratio in external secretions is 1:1 to 1:3, as opposed to the serum ratio of 5:1. The IgM, IgE, and IgG in external secretions also have been shown to be produced locally in the lamina propria of normal mucous membranes.

Serum and secretory IgA are structurally different. The IgA found in human serum exists as a monomer with 10–15% in polymeric form, while the IgA in external secretions exists mainly as a dimer. Two antigenically different subclasses of IgA can be identified in serum and external secretions. IgA1 accounts for about 90% of the total IgA in serum, whereas IgA2 comprises as much as 60% of the total IgA in external secretions. Secretory IgA consists of an IgA dimer, a molecule of secretory component (also called ''T'' component or ''transport piece''), and a molecule of J chain which functions *in vivo* by inducing polymerization of the subunits of IgA and IgM. The stabilization of IgA in secretions by the secretory component is probably responsible for the greater resistance of the secretory IgA molecule to the proteolytic action of enzymes in the unfavorable milieu of the gastrointestinal secretions.[48-50] The IgM present in secretions also has been shown to have secretory component bound to it, but IgG and IgE do not.

The site of synthesis of IgA is primarily in submucosal plasma cells. By immunofluorescence it has been demonstrated in rabbits that Peyer's patches contain an enriched source of precursors for IgA-producing cells.[51] In humans, the lamina propria of the gastrointestinal tract contains 20 IgA-producing cells per IgG-producing cell in close contact with the overlying epithelium. This is in contrast to an IgG/IgA ratio of peripheral lymph node and spleen cells of 3:1. The majority of IgA in the secretions of the gastrointestinal tract results from local synthesis in the lamina propria. The J chain also is produced by the submucosal plasma cells and may be the limiting factor in determining the proportion of monomer to dimer secreted by a given cell. The secretory component is an antigenically distinct glycoprotein which is produced locally in glandular epithelium and serves as a specific receptor on the intestinal epithelium which mediates transport of dimeric IgA and IgM across the epithelial surfaces. Gut-associated plasma cells produce IgM, of which 70% in secretions contains covalently bound secretory component. The IgE in external secretions does not possess secretory component and is similar to IgE in serum, indicating that a major portion of serum IgE is derived from submucosal plasma cells. The route of IgE transport into secretions is unknown. IgG in normal external secretions comes from both local synthesis and transudation from serum, but the route across the epithelium is unknown. With inflammation, transudation of IgG from serum, in addition to an invasion of the mucosa by IgG-producing plasma cells, occurs.

Antibody in stool of patients with diarrheal disease was first described by Davies[52] in 1922. In 1947, Burrows and associates[53] used the term "coproantibody" for antibody of intestinal origin. It is now known that IgA antibody is readily found in many biological secretions, including saliva, lacrimal fluid, urine, intestinal juice, respiratory secretions, and colostrum. Numerous studies have shown that locally produced antibody shows specificity against bacteria and viruses. The antimicrobial activity of IgA may not be defined by conventional immunologic principles where well-characterized opsonization and complement-dependent antibacterial mechanisms are operative.[54-56] IgA may be active in the absence of complement,[50,56] activity may be enhanced by lysozyme and complement,[57] or an antibacterial influence may occur by fixing late-acting components of complement.[58] In certain cases IgA may serve as an opsonin.[59]

In intestinal infection, coproantibody appears earlier than serum antibody,[52] and there probably is a better correlation between levels of coproantibody and protective immunity than with serum antibody and resistance to enteric infection.[60] Presence of viable enteropathogens in the gut in the absence of intestinal antibody is the general prerequisite for active infection or intestinal carriage of the microbe.[61] In experimental cholera, the intestinal antibody appears to prevent adherence of the vibrios to the mucosal surface,[55,62] analogous to the finding of antibody and the lack of adherence of oral streptococci to buccal mucosal cells.[63]

That the autochthonous flora is remarkably stable has been cited as evidence for the lack of common development in the intestine of antibacterial antibody to these bacteria.[64-66] It is likely that local antibacterial immunity is operative against the effects of invasive or mucosa-associated bacteria and that low-grade pathogens (i.e., intestinal flora) either are restricted to the lumen of the gut where immunologic interaction is prevented or display a low degree of antigenicity.[67] In children with protein–calorie malnutrition, IgA levels are depressed, with return to normal during hospital treatment.[8] This probaly helps to explain the propensity of these children to develop recurrent gastroenteritis.

Cell-Mediated Immunity

Investigations into the area of cell-mediated immunity (CMI) by secretory surfaces generally have involved the lungs and have demonstrated that the epithelial surfaces develop a CMI response which is independent of systemic immunity and that the nature of the immune response depends upon whether an immunogen is applied orally or parenterally.[69-71] This local CMI response, however, is not completely restricted to the site of immune induction but also occurs at distant surfaces such as the breast, where migration of lymphoid precursors provides immunity to suckling newborns.[72-74] Colostrum contains antibody to naturally occurring enteric microorganisms and T lymphocytes that respond to the capsular K1 antigen of *E. coli*.[75] Orally administered antigen stimulates a greater local CMI response than antigen administered parenterally.[69-71,76] It has been shown that lymphocytes committed to CMI are present in gut-associated lymphoid tissue (GALT)—tonsils, Peyer's patches, appendix, sacculus rotundus (in some species), and lamina propria. These immunocomponent cells in GALT are capable of responding to antigens present within the intestinal lumen.[77] These events are similar to those which occur within an antigen-stimulated lymph node. Peyer's patches contain the precursors of IgA-secreting plasma cells that ultimately populate the intestinal lamina propria and epithelium.[51] Studies suggest that the tissue environment is not important in terminal differentiation of plasma cells to produce IgA, since the cells are precommitted to produce IgA before they leave Peyer's patches.[51] They do not begin this activity until they travel through the mesenteric lymph nodes and enter the systemic circulation by way of the common thoracic duct, where they become part of the circulating lymphatic pool.[51,78-83] Transfer of thoracic duct lymph from immune donors has been associated with production of specific antibody in the gut of recipients not exposed to the antigen.[81] Many of these cells then return from the circulating pool to the lamina propria and epithelial areas of the intestine, avoiding significant accumulation within peripheral lymph nodes or spleen.[82] These cells are said to have "homed" to the intestine and are fully differentiated IgA-producing lymphocytes or plasma cells. Although intestinal antigen does not appear necessary for localization of IgA-containing cells in the gut, it does exert a significant influence on distribution of antibody-producing cells, since antibody usually concentrates at or distal to an antigen-boosted site.[81] GALT also contains T lymphocytes[82,84-86] with a migratory pattern thought to be similar to that described for B cells.[82] Using antisera specific for T lymphocytes, analysis of various types of GALT indicates that 13–28% of Peyer's patches, 58% of mesenteric lymph node cells, and 11% of the lymphocytes in the intestinal mucosa are thymus-derived.[86-87]

BREAST MILK AND GASTROINTESTINAL IMMUNITY

Several studies suggest that breast-fed infants are protected against gastroenteritis.[88-94] In populations where breast-feeding is prevalent, diarrhea is unusual during the first several months of life but becomes quite common during the second half of the first year and during the second year. This increase in illness after termination of breast-feeding has been referred to as weanling diarrhea.[95] Diarrhea does occur among breast-fed children, however, but to a lesser degree. Resistance to diarrhea among breast-fed infants relates to a complex set of factors. Undoubtedly, the passive transfer of antibodies directed against potential pathogens is important. Many nonspecific factors are operative as well. In areas where diarrhea is hyperendemic, as in many developing countries, a major value of breast-feeding is to improve cleanliness and decrease the opportunity of exposure to enteropathogens contaminating poorly prepared milk.[95] Cow's milk given to infants fed by bottle has a higher content of protein and phosphorus, with resultant lower buffering capacity, and high levels of caseinogen which tends to produce curdling or clotting, leading to uneven exposure to the intestinal mucosa.

Host Resistance Factors in Human Milk

Human colostrum and milk have been shown to possess both nonspecific and specific resistance factors. Nonspecific factors such as high lactose concentration, [90,93] a carbohydrate growth factor necessary for the growth of *Lactobacillus bifidus,* low bulk, and low buffering capacity contribute to the acidification of the infant gut and the establishment of a *Lactobacillus* flora.[96-98] This acid environment inhibits *in vitro* growth of *Shigella, E. coli,* and yeast.[33,39] Infants fed proprietary formulas develop mixed intestinal flora, including high counts of *E. coli.*[100,101] Other components of breast milk, such as lactoferrin, lysozyme, and lactoperoxidase, have been shown *in vitro* to possess antiinfective properties. Secretory IgA antibodies are important components of the immune system; however, the clinical importance of a variety of additional other factors remains to be delineated.

Antibodies

It is not a new observation that human colostrum and milk contain antibodies to bacteria and viruses.[102] Human milk has been demonstrated to contain antibodies to *Clostridium tetani, Corynebacterium diphtheriae,* coxsackie viruses B1, B5, and B9, enteropathogenic serotypes of *E. coli,* echoviruses, polioviruses 1, 2, and 3, *Salmonella, Shigella,* staphylolysin, *Streptococcus pneumoniae,* streptolysin, and rotavirus.[103,104]

The fate of ingested antibody in milk is not completely known, although the site of action appears to be confined to the gastrointestinal tract, since significant quantities of immunoglobulin cannot be absorbed from the infant gastrointestinal tract.[105,106] The major immunoglobulin in human milk is secretory IgA, which is resistant to acid conditions and to proteolytic activity of gut enzymes. Secretory IgA has been shown to survive passage through the gastrointestinal tract of infants.[107,108] Milk antibody is protected by the buffering action of milk and by dilution of acid which occurs during feeding. The pH of stomach secretions of full-term newborn infants falls to levels of 1–2 within 6 hr of birth[109-111] but increases following feeding.[112] This secretion of gastric acid does not appear to respond to increased endogenously produced gastrin[113] or exogenously administered pentagastrin,[114] indicating that newborn parietal cells are relatively unresponsive.

Colostrum and milk contain antibodies to naturally occurring enteric microorganisms. These antibodies probably play a role in passive immunization of infants, limiting disease production by intestinal bacteria, viruses, and other antigens. It has been shown that immunization of pregnant women with typhoid vaccine was associated with the subsequent occurrence of high-titer typhoid antibody in colostrum and in stool of their infants.[115] Infants fed human milk containing high titers of *E. coli* antibodies had such antibodies in their stools,[108,116,117] whereas infants fed cow's milk had an insignificant amount of *E. coli* antibody in stools. The colostrum of pregnant women orally immunized with an *E. coli* 083 strain during the last month of gestation contained IgA-producing plasma cells which were able to synthesize antibodies to *E. coli* lipopolysaccharide. Parenteral immunization of pregnant women with the same killed antigen produced antibody in serum but not in colostrum. A correlation exists between levels of antibody in stool of infants and the corresponding mother's milk.[108] Hanson and associates[118] demonstrated that secretory IgA, active against both somatic and capsular antigens of *E. coli,* could be detected in maternal milk. The high ratio of milk to serum IgA and the observation that the IgA content did not decline throughout the duration of a feeding suggest that the breast can synthesize and store immunoglobulins.

The actual functions of secretory antibodies of breast milk in the gastrointestinal tract for control of pathogens and prevention of antigen penetration have been postulated to be either direct killing of microorganisms, opsonization of bacteria allowing cellular destruction, or interference with adherence and proliferation. Adinolfi and associates[57] showed that secretory IgA antibodies against *E. coli* could cause bacterial lysis in the presence of lysozyme and components of complement. It has been shown that IgA antibodies cannot fix complement by the classic activation pathway[119]; however, they may activate complement by the alternative pathway.[120] This mechanism may not be important, since breast milk contains small amounts of complement.

A reduction in number of coliform bacteria in stool of breast-fed infants correlates with the presence of high agglutinating and bactericidal titers against specific *E. coli* in stool.[116] The concentration of coproantibodies appears to parallel the antibody titers in maternal colostrum. There is evidence to suggest that secretory IgA can opsonize.[59] The significance of bacterial lysis and opsonization of bacteria as a primary mechanism of secretory immunologic defense is unknown.

The importance of antibodies in breast milk in preventing adherence or attachment and proliferation in the gastrointestinal tract has been evaluated following the demonstration that colonization of epithelial cells by streptococci is interfered with by secretory IgA from the parotid gland.[63] Interference of *V. cholerae* adherence to the intestinal mucosa by antibody was demonstrated.[62] Local antibodies can inhibit absorption of soluble protein antigens by decreasing their adherence to intestinal cellular surfaces.[120,121] Secretory IgA prepared from colostrum was shown to agglutinate a number of common enteric bacteria.[122] Agglutinating activity was unaffected by trypsin or acid but was abolished by pepsin. The importance of colostral antibodies in combating intestinal adherence or attachment of *E. coli* has been demonstrated in piglets suckled by dams that had been vaccinated with K88 antigen, surface fimbriae which facilitate intestinal colonization of *E. coli*. They were significantly more resistant to death caused by neonatal diarrhea after challenge with a large dose of K88-positive enterotoxigenic strain of *E. coli* than piglets suckled from control dams.[123] These studies suggest that secretory immunoglobulins in breast milk can prevent attachment and subsequent proliferation of bacteria within the gastrointestinal tract.

Although information is available to indicate that breast milk antibodies are directed against bacterial surface antigens and enterotoxins, similar protective factors in breast milk directed toward enteropathogenic viruses are less well established. Antibody in colostrum and milk will prevent or inhibit replication of poliovirus within the gastrointestinal tract of newborns.[124,125] The milk antibody in this case can be shown to have the same neutralizing effects on viruses as serum antibody. Specific antibodies against respiratory syncytial virus[126] and nonspecific antiviral inhibitors[127,128] have been demonstrated in human colostrum. Studies of infection in calves,[129] lambs,[130] and swine[131] indicate that immunity of the gastrointestinal tract to viral infection is not related to serum antibodies but to the presence of secretory antibodies produced locally or ingested in colostrum or breast milk. In ewes and sows, rotavirus and transmission gastroenteritis virus antibodies are produced in the milk by oral or intramammary immunization but not by intramuscular immunization.[130,132]

Protection of infants against human rotavirus infection does not appear to be associated with the presence of maternal serum antibody.[133] It was shown, however, that during an epidemic of diarrhea due to rotavirus in a maternity ward, there was a lower incidence of infection among breast-fed infants. The presence of rotavirus antibodies in breast milk has been sought by several investigators using different assay procedures. Using immunofluorescence, Schoub and associates[134] did not find rotavirus IgA antibodies in human colostrum or milk specimens despite their presence in sera. Yolken *et al.*[104,135] have applied the enzyme-linked immunosorbent assay (ELISA) technique to demonstrate rotavirus antibodies in breast milk samples. Differences in technique and populations may be responsible for disparity in these reports. The specific degree of protection afforded by these specific antibodies is unknown.

Cells

The cellular component of human colostrum consists of approximately 55% polymorphonuclear leukocytes, 40% mononuclear phagocytes, and 5% lymphocytes.[103,136,137] The cell number decreases from 5000 cells/mm^3 on days 1 and 2 to 2000 cells/mm^3 on days 3–5. A progressive decrease is seen in transitional and mature milk. These cells do not represent a random collection of leukocytes but are a selected population of cells accumulated in response to sensitizing events within the intestine and respiratory tract. The colostral lymphocytes are immunologically reactive and correspond to mitogens, recall antigens, and allogeneic cells in mixed-lymphocyte reaction and can synthesize immunoglobulins, predominantly of the IgA class.[73,75,138-140] These antibody-forming cells appear to be selected to form antibody against enteric pathogens.[138] T cells identified by anti-T sera and sheep erythrocyte rosette formation constitute approximately 35–50% of the lymphocyte population.[73,74,140]

The phagocytic cells in breast milk have been shown to adhere to glass and to phagocytize and kill bacteria and fungi,[137,141] although this ability appears to be reduced compared to peripheral-blood phagocytic cells.[141] Human colostral monocyte macrophages in combination with antibody have been shown to destroy cells infected with *Herpes simplex* virus while demonstrating very low spontaneous (non-antibody-mediated) cytotoxicity.[142] The role of this mechanism in controlling enteric pathogens is unknown.

IMMUNOLOGIC CONTROL OF ENTERIC INFECTION

It is generally agreed that parenterally administered antigen does not induce mucosal immunity, although serum antibody may contribute to the level of gut immunoglobulins, particularly in inflammatory bowel disease. Any successful approach to local gastrointestinal protection against clini-

TABLE 1.2
Enteropathogens, Population at Risk, and Potential Control Using Immunoprophylaxis

Agent	Population at risk	Vaccine available[a]	Major obstacles
Vibrio cholerae	Persons living in areas of disease endemicity; during an epidemic	Killed whole-cell preparation given parenterally	Current vaccine only partially effective; role of antitoxin immunity is unresolved
Enterotoxigenic *Escherchia coli*	Persons traveling from low-risk to high-risk areas	No	Optimal immunizing agent must be established employing antigen(s) (surface fimbriae, enterotoxin, somatic) or antibody to these immunogens
Salmonella typhi	Persons living in areas of disease endemicity; during an epidemic	Killed whole-cell preparation given parenterally	Current vaccine only partially effective
Shigella strains	Institutionalized or confined populations	No	Multiple serotypes of *Shigella* are responsible for disease; there is a lack of a suitable vaccine candidate
Rotavirus	Infants and children	No	Antigenic properties of strains from varying geographic locations need to be determined; an efficient means of virus propagation is needed

[a]See individual chapters for information on vaccine development.

cal disease must therefore rely upon orally administered antigens as a basis for triggering local immune response. An excellent example of this mechanism was reported by Ogra and associates.[143,144] Studying patients with double-barreled colostomies, they demonstrated secretory IgA antibodies against poliovirus in secretions from portions of the intestine directly exposed to the virus rather than from unexposed sites elsewhere in the gastrointestinal tract. Although mucosal immunization can be accomplished by oral inoculation, it may be that parenteral priming followed by local boosting will prove to be the optimal approach to produce protective immunity to enteric infection.[81] Parenteral priming may prepare the entire gut for a secondary response to a local booster, and separate intracellular and intercellular immunologic events might be stimulated. Table 1.2 lists enteropathogens where immunologic control may be possible. Specific details of vaccine candidates and the nature of immunity can be found in the chapter corresponding to the specific enteric infection.

REFERENCES

1. Bartle, H. J., Harkins, M. J. The gastric secretion: Its bactericidal value to man. *Am. J. Med. Sci.* **169**:373–388, 1925.
2. Giannella, R. A., Broitman, S. A., Zamcheck, N. Gastric acid barrier to ingested microorganisms in man: Studies *in vivo* and *in vitro*. *Gut* **13**:251–256, 1972.
3. Gitelson, S. Gastrectomy, achlorhydria and cholera. *Isr. J. Med. Sci.* **7**:663–667, 1971.
4. Waddell, W. R., Kunz, L. J. Association of salmonella enteritis with operation on the stomach. *N. Engl. J. Med.* **255**:555–559, 1956.
5. Close, A. S., Smith, M. B., Koch, M. L., *et al.* An analysis of ten cases of salmonella infection on a general surgical service. *Arch. Surg.* **80**:972–976, 1960.
6. Nordbring, F. Contraction of salmonella gastroenteritis following previous operation on the stomach. *Acta Med. Scand.* **171**:783–790, 1962.
7. Giannella, R. A., Broitman, S. A., Zamcheck, N. Salmonella enteritis: I. Role of reduced gastric secretion in pathogenesis. *Am. J. Dig. Dis.* **16**:1000–1006, 1971.
8. Giannella, R. A., Broitman, S. A., Zamcheck, N. Salmonella enteritis: II. Fulminant diarrhea in and effects on the small intestine. *Am. J. Dig. Dis.* **16**:1007–1013, 1971.
9. Hornick, R. B., Music, S. I., Wenzel, R., *et al.* The Broad Street pump revisited: Response of volunteers to ingested cholera vibrios. *Bull. N.Y. Acad. Med.* **47**:1181–1191, 1971.
10. Sack, G. H., Jr., Hennessey, K. N., Mitra, R. C., *et al.* Gastric acidity in cholera (abstract). *Clin. Res.* **18**:682, 1970.
11. DuPont, H. L., Hornick, R. B., Snyder, M. J., *et al.* Immunity in shigellosis: I. Response of man to attenuated strains of shigella. *J. Infect. Dis.* **125**:5–11, 1972.
12. Haas, J., Bucken, E. W. Zum Krankheitswert der Lamblien-Infektion. *Dtsch. Med. Wochenschr.* **92**:1869–1871, 1967.
13. Yardley, J. H., Takano, J., Hendrix, T. R. Epithelial and other mucosal lesions of the jejunum in giardiasis: Jejunal biopsy studies. *Bull. Johns Hopkins Hosp.* **115**:389–406, 1964.

14. Hoskins, L. C., Winawer, S. J., Broitman, S. A., *et al.* Clinical giardiasis and intestinal malabsorption. *Gastroenterology* **53**:265–279, 1967.

15. Levin, A. L. The problem of eradication of *Strongyloides intestinalis. Am. J. Trop. Med. Hyg.* **10**:353–363, 1930.

16. Jones, C. A. Clinical studies in human strongyloidiasis. *Gastroenterology* **16**:743–756, 1950.

17. Callender, S. T., Retief, F. P., Witts, L. J. The augmented histamine test with special reference to achlorhydria. *Gut* **1**:326–336, 1960.

18. Dack, G. M., Petran, E. Bacterial activity in different levels of intestine and in isolated segments of small and large bowel in monkeys and dogs. *J. Infect. Dis.* **54**:204–220, 1934.

19. Dixon, J. M. The fate of bacteria in the small intestine. *J. Pathol. Bacteriol.* **79**:131–140, 1960.

20. Sprinz, H. Pathogenesis of intestinal infections. *Arch. Pathol.* **87**:556–562, 1969.

21. DuPont, H. L., Hornick, R. B. Adverse effect of Lomotil therapy in shigellosis. *J. Am. Med. Assoc.* **226**:1525–1528, 1973.

22. Meynell, G. G. Antibacterial mechanisms of the mouse gut: II. The role of Eh and volatile fatty acids in the normal gut. *Br. J. Exp. Pathol.* **44**:209–219, 1963.

23. Bohnhoff, M., Miller, C. P. Enhanced susceptibility to *Salmonella* infection in streptomycin-treated mice. *J. Infect. Dis.* **111**:117–127, 1962.

24. Hornick, R. B., Griesman, S. E., Woodward, T. E., *et al.* Typhoid fever: Pathogenesis and immunologic control. *N. Engl. J. Med.* **283**:686–691, 739–746, 1970.

25. Aserkoff, B., Bennett, J. V. Effect of antibiotic therapy in acute salmonellosis on the fecal excretion of salmonellae. *N. Engl. J. Med.* **281**:636–640, 1969.

26. Macdonald, W. B., Friday, F., McEacharn, M. The effect of chloramphenicol in salmonella enteritis of infancy. *Arch. Dis. Child.* **29**:238–241, 1954.

27. Rosenthal, S. L. Exacerbation of salmonella enteritis due to ampicillin. *N. Engl. J. Med.* **280**:147–148, 1969.

28. Hentges, D. J. Inhibition of *Shigella flexneri* by the normal intestinal flora: II. Mechanisms of inhibition by coliform organisms. *J. Bacteriol.* **97**:513–517, 1969.

29. Freter, R. Interactions between mechanisms controlling the intestinal microflora. *Am. J. Clin. Nutr.* **27**:1409–1416, 1974.

30. Sprunt, K., Leidy, G. A., Redman, W. Prevention of bacterial overgrowth. *J. Infect. Dis.* **123**:1–10, 1971.

31. Freter, R., Abrams, G. D. Function of various intestinal bacteria in converting germ-free mice to the normal state. *Infect. Immun.* **6**:119–126, 1972.

32. Fredericq, P., Levine, M. Antibiotic interrelationships among the enteric group of bacteria. *J. Bacteriol.* **54**:785–792, 1947.

33. Bergeim, O. Toxicity of intestinal volatile fatty acids for yeast and *Escherichia coli. J. Infect. Dis.* **66**:222–234, 1940.

34. Besredka, A. On the mechanism of dysenteric infection, antidysenteric vaccine per os, and the nature of antidysenteric immunity. *Ann. Inst. Pasteur Paris* **33**:301, 1919.

35. Besredka, A. *Local Immunization: Specific Dressings,* H. Plotz (trans.–ed.). Williams & Wilkins, Baltimore, 1927, 181 pp.

36. Walsh, T. E., Cannon, P. R. Immunization of the respiratory tract: A comparative study of the antibody content of the respiratory and other tissues following active, passive and regional immunization. *J. Immunol.* **35**:31–46, 1938.

37. Hanson, L. A. Comparative immunological studies of the immune globulins of human milk and of blood serum. *Int. Arch. Allergy Appl. Immunol.* **18**:241–267, 1961.

38. Tomasi, T. B., Jr., Zigelbaum, S. The selective occurrence of gamma-$_1$A globulins in certain body fluids. *J. Clin. Invest.* **42**:1552–1560, 1963.

39. Tomasi, T. B., Jr., Tan, E. M., Solomon, A., *et al.* Characteristics of an immune system common to certain external secretions. *J. Exp. Med.* **121**:101–124, 1965.

40. Deutsch, H. F. Molecular transformation of a gamma 1-globulin of human serum. *J. Mol. Biol.* **7**:662–671, 1963.

41. Claman, H. N., Merrill, D. A., Hartley, T. F. Salivary immunoglobulins: Normal adult values and dissociation between serum and salivary levels. *J. Allergy* **40**:151–159, 1967.

42. Tomasi, T. B., Jr., Bienenstock, J. Secretory immunoglobulins. *Adv. Immunol.* **9**:1–96, 1968.

43. Waldman, R. H., Cruz, J. M., Rowe, D. S. Immunoglobulin levels and antibody to *Candida albicans* in human cervicovaginal secretions. *Clin. Exp. Immunol.* **10**:427–434, 1972.

44. Stobo, J. D., Tomasi, T. B., Jr. A low molecular weight immunoglobulin antigenically related to 19 S IgM. *J. Clin. Invest.* **46**:1329–1337, 1967.

45. Brandtzaeg, P., Fjellanger, I., Gjeruldsen, S. T. Localization of immunoglobulins in human nasal mucosa. *Immunochemistry* **4**:57–60, 1967.

46. Brandtzaeg, P., Fjellanger, I., Gjeruldsen, S. T. Human secretory immunoglobulins: I. Salivary secretions from individuals with normal or low levels of serum immunoglobulins. *Scand. J. Haematol. Suppl.* **12**:3–83, 1970.

47. Turner, M. W., Johansson, S. G. O., Barratt, T. M., *et al.* Studies on the levels of immunoglobulins in normal human urine with particular reference to IgE. *Int. Arch. Allergy Appl. Immunol.* **37**:409–417, 1970.

48. Cederblad, G., Johansson, B. G., Rymo, L. Reduction and proteolytic degradation of immunoglobulin A from human colostrum. *Acta Chem. Scand.* **20**:2349–2357, 1966.

49. Shim, B. S., Kang, Y. S., Kim, W. J., *et al.* Self-protective activity of colostral IgA against tryptic digestion. *Nature* **222**:787–788, 1969.

50. Brown, W. R., Newcomb, R. W., Ishizaka, K. Proteolytic degradation of exocrine and serum immunoglobulins. *J. Clin. Invest.* **49**:1374–1380, 1970.

51. Craig, S. W., Cebra, J. J. Peyer's patches: An enriched source of precursors for IgA-producing immunocytes in the rabbit. *J. Exp. Med.* **134**:188–200, 1971.

52. Davies, A. An investigation into the serological properties of dysentery stools. *Lancet* **2**:1009–1012, 1922.

53. Burrows, W., Elliott, M. E., Havens, I. Studies on immunity to Asiatic cholera: IV. The excretion of coproantibody in experimental enteric cholera in the guinea pig. *J. Infect. Dis.* **81**:261–281, 1947.

54. Chaicumpa, W., Rowley, D. Experimental cholera in infant mice: Protective effects of antibody. *J. Infect. Dis.* **125**:480–485, 1972.

55. Fubara, E. S., Freter, R. Protection against enteric bacterial infection by secretory IgA antibodies. *J. Immunol.* **111**:395–403, 1973.

56. Dowdle, W. R., Coleman, M. T., Schoenbaum, S. C., *et al.* Studies on inactivated influenza vaccines: III. Effect of subcutaneous dosage on antibody levels in nasal secretions and protection against natural challenge. In D. H. Dayton (ed.), *Conference on Secretory Immunologic System.* National Institutes of Health, Bethesda, Md., 1971, pp. 113–127.

57. Adinolfi, M., Glynn, A. A., Lindsay, M., *et al.* Serological properties of gamma-A antibodies to *Escherichia coli* present in human colostrum. *Immunology* **10**:517–526, 1966.

58. Ellman, L., Green, I., Frank, M. M. Immune function in C_4 deficient guinea pigs. Demonstration of an alternate pathway for activation of the complement sequence (abstract). *Clin. Res.* **19**:440, 1971.

59. Wernet, P., Breu, H., Knop, J., *et al.* Antibacterial action of specific IgA and transport IgM, IgA, and IgG from serum into the small intestine. *J. Infect. Dis.* **124**:223–226, 1971.

60. Freter, R., De, S. P., Mondal, A., *et al.* Coproantibody and serum antibody in cholera patients. *J. Infect. Dis.* **115:**83–87, 1965.
61. Ganguly, R., Ogra, P. L., Regas, S., *et al.* Rubella immunization of volunteers via the respiratory tract. *Infect. Immun.* **8:**497–502, 1973.
62. Freter, R. Intestinal immunity: Studies of the mechanism of action of intestinal antibody in experimental cholera. *Tex. Rep. Biol. Med. Suppl.* **27:**299–316, 1969.
63. Williams, R. C., Gibbons, R. J. Inhibition of bacterial adherence by secretory immunoglobulin A: A mechanism of antigen disposal. *Science* **177:**697–699, 1972.
64. Carter, P. B., Pollard, M. Host responses to "normal" microbial flora in germ-free mice. *J. Reticuloendothel. Soc.* **9:**580–587, 1971.
65. Berg, R. D., Savage, D. C. Immunological responses and microorganisms indigenous to the gastrointestinal tract. *Am. J. Clin. Nutr.* **25:**1364–1371, 1972.
66. Foo, M. C., Lee, A. Immunological response of mice to members of the autochthonous intestinal microflora. *Infect. Immun.* **6:**525–532, 1972.
67. Shedlofsky, S., Freter, R. Synergism between ecologic and immunologic control mechanisms of intestinal flora. *J. Infect. Dis.* **129:**296–303, 1974.
68. Sirisinha, S., Suskind, R., Edelman, R., *et al.* Secretory and serum IgA in children with protein–calorie malnutrition. *Pediatrics* **55:**166–170, 1975.
69. Henney, C. S., Waldman, R. H. Cell-mediated immunity shown by lymphocytes from the respiratory tract. *Science* **169:**696–697, 1970.
70. Galindo, B., Myrvik, Q. N. Migratory response of granulomatous alveolar cells from BCG-sensitized rabbits. *J. Immunol.* **105:**227–237, 1970.
71. Waldman, R. H., Spencer, C. S., Johnson, J. E., III. Respiratory and systemic cellular and humoral immune responses to influenza virus vaccine administered parenterally or by nose drops. *Cell. Immunol.* **3:**294–300, 1972.
72. Roux, M. E., McWilliams, M., Phillips-Quagliata, J. M., et al. Origin of IgA-secreting plasma cells in the mammary gland. *J. Exp. Med.* **146:**1311–1322, 1977.
73. Diaz-Jouanen, E., Williams, R. C., Jr. T and B lymphocytes in human colostrum. *Clin. Immunol. Immunopathol.* **3:**248–255, 1974.
74. Parmely, M. J., Reath, D. B., Beer, A. E., et al. Cellular immune responses of human milk T lymphocytes to certain environmental antigens. *Transplant. Proc.* **9:**1477–1483, 1977.
75. Parmely, M. J., Beer, A. E., Billingham, R. E. *In vitro* studies on the T lymphocyte population of human milk. *J. Exp. Med.* **144:**358–370, 1976.
76. Barclay, W. R., Busey, W. M., Dalgard, D. W., *et al.* Protection of monkeys against airborne tuberculosis by aerosol vaccination with Bacillus Calmette–Guérin. *Am. Rev. Respir. Dis.* **107:**351–358, 1973.
77. Müller-Schoop, J. W., Good, R. A. Functional studies of Peyer's patches: Evidence for their participation in intestinal immune response. *J. Immunol.* **114:**1757–1760, 1975.
78. Gowans, J. L., Knight, E. J. The route of re-circulation of lymphocytes in the rat. *Proc. R. Soc. London Ser. B* **159:**257–282, 1964.
79. Griscelli, C., Vassalli, P., McCluskey, R. T. The distribution of large dividing lymph node cells in syngeneic recipient rats after intravenous injection. *J. Exp. Med.* **130:**1427–1451, 1969.
80. Hall, J. G., Parry, D. M., Smith, M. E. The distribution and differentiation of lymph-borne immunoblasts after intravenous injection into syngeneic recipients. *Cell Tissue Kinet.* **5:**269–281, 1972.
81. Pierce, N. F., Gowans, J. L. Cellular kinetics of the intestinal immune response to cholera toxoid in rats. *J. Exp. Med.* **142:**1550–1563, 1975.
82. Guy-Grand, D., Griscelli, C., Vassalli, P. The gut associated lymphoid system: Nature and properties of the large dividing cells. *Eur. J. Immunol.* **4:**435–443, 1974.
83. Lamm, M. E. Cellular aspects of immunoglobulin A. *Adv. Immunol.* **22:**223–290, 1976.

84. Raff, M. C., Owen, J. J. T. Thymus-derived lymphocytes: Their distribution and role in the development of peripheral lymphoid tissues of the mouse. *Eur. J. Immunol.* **1**:27–30, 1971.

85. McWilliams, M., Phillips-Quagliata, J. M., Lamm, M. E. Characteristics of mesenteric lymph node cells homing to gut-associated lymphoid tissue in syngeneic mice. *J. Immunol.* **115**:54–58, 1975.

86. Rudzik, O., Clancy, R. L., Perey, D. Y. E., *et al.* The distribution of a rabbit thymic antigen and membrane immunoglobulins in lymphoid tissue, with special reference to mucosal lymphocytes. *J. Immunol.* **114**:1–4, 1975.

87. Wilson, B. S., Teodorescu, M., Dray, S. Enumeration and isolation of rabbit T and B lymphocytes by using antibody-coated erythrocytes. *J. Immunol.* **116**:1306–1312, 1976.

88. Mata, L. J., Urrutia, J. J., Fernandez, R., *et al.*, *Shigella* infection in breast-fed Guatemalan Indian neonates. *Am. J. Dis. Child.* **117**:142–146, 1969.

89. Jelliffe, D. B., Jelliffe, E. F. Current concepts in nutrition: "Breast is best": Modern meaning. *N. Engl. J. Med.* **297**:912–915, 1977.

90. Bullen, C. L. Willis, A. T. Resistance of the breast-fed infant to gastroenteritis. *Br. Med. J.* **3**:338–343, 1971.

91. Mata, L. J., Urrutia, J. J., Gordon, J. E. Diarrhoeal disease in a cohort of Guatemalan village children observed from birth to age two years. *Trop. Geogr. Med.* **19**:247–257, 1967.

92. Alexander, M. B. Infantile diarrhoea and vomiting. A review of 456 infants treated in a hospital unit for enteritis. *Br. Med. J.* **2**:973–978, 1948.

93. Ross, C. A. C., Dawes, E. A. Resistance of the breast-fed infant to gastroenteritis. *Lancet* **1**:994–998, 1954.

94. Hinton, N. A., MacGregor, R. R. A study of infections due to pathogenic serogroups of *Escherichia coli. Can. Med. Assoc. J.* **79**:359–364, 1958.

95. Gordon, J. E., Chitkara, I. D., Wyon, J. B. Weanling diarrhea. *Am. J. Med. Sci.* **245**:345–377, 1963.

96. Bullen, C. L., Tearle, P. V., Stewart, M. G. The effect of "humanised" milks and supplemented breast feeding on the faecal flora of infants. *J. Med. Microbiol.* **10**:403–413, 1977.

97. Jelliffe, D. B., Jelliffe, E. F. P. Symposium: The uniqueness of human milk: Introduction. *Am. J. Clin. Nutr.* **24**:968–969, 1971.

98. Bullen, C. L., Tearle, P. V., Willis, A. T. Bifidobacteria in the intestinal tract of infants: An *in vivo* study. *J. Med. Microbiol.* **9**:325–333, 1976.

99. Hentges, D. J. Influence of pH on the inhibitory activity of formic and acetic acids for Shigella. *J. Bacteriol.* **93**:2029–2030, 1967.

100. Haenel, H. Some rules in the ecology of the intestinal microflora of man. *J. Appl. Bacteriol.* **24**:242, 1961.

101. Smith, H. W., Crabb, W. E. The faecal bacterial flora of animals and man: Its development in the young. *J. Pathol. Bacteriol.* **82**:53–66, 1961.

102. Vahlquist, B. The transfer of antibodies from mother to offspring. *Adv. Pediatr.* **10**:305–338, 1958.

103. Goldman, A. S., Smith, C. W. Host resistance factors in human milk. *J. Pediatr.* **82**:1082–1090, 1973.

104. Yolken, R. H., Wyatt, R. G., Zissis, G., *et al.* Epidemiology of human rotavirus types 1 and 2 as studied by enzyme-linked immunosorbent assay. *N. Engl. J. Med.* **299**:1156–1161, 1978.

105. Ammann, A. J., Stiehm, E. R. Immune globulin levels in colostrum and breast milk, and serum from formula- and breast-fed newborns. *Proc. Soc. Exp. Biol. Med.* **122**:1098–1100. 1966.

106. Nordbring, F. The failure of newborn premature infants to absorb antibodies from heterologous colostrum. *Acta Paediatr. Scand.* **46**:569–578, 1957.

107. Hodes, H. L., Berger, R., Ainbender, E., *et al.* Proof that colostrum polio antibody is different from serum antibody (abstract). *J. Pediatr.* **65**:1017–1018, 1964.

108. Kenny, J. F., Boesman, M. I., Michaels, R. H. Bacterial and viral coproantibodies in breast-fed infants. *Pediatrics* **39**:202–213, 1967.

109. Hess, A. F. The gastric secretion of infants at birth. *Am. J. Dis. Child.* **6**:264–276, 1913.

110. Avery, G. B., Randolph, J. G., Weaver, T. Gastric acidity in the first day of life. *Pediatrics* **37**:1005–1007, 1966.

111. Kopel, F. B., Barbero, G. J. Gastric acid secretion in infancy and childhood (abstract). *Gastroenterology* **52**:1101, 1967.

112. Barbero, G. J., Runge, G., Fischer, D., *et al.* Investigations on the bacterial flora, pH, and sugar content in the intestinal tract of infants. *J. Pediatr.* **40**:152–163, 1952.

113. Euler, A. R., Byrne, W. J., Cousins, L. M., *et al.* Increased serum gastrin concentration and gastric acid hyposecretion in the immediate newborn period. *Gastroenterology* **72**:1271–1273, 1977.

114. Euler, A. R., Byrne, W. J., Meis, P. J., *et al.* Basal and pentagastrin-stimulated acid secretion in newborn human infants. *Pediatr. Res.* **13**:36–37, 1979.

115. Schubert, J., Grünberg, A. Zur Frage der Übertragung von Immun-Antikörpern von der Mutter auf das Kind. *Schweiz. Med. Wochenschr.* **79**:1007–1010, 1949.

116. Michael, J. G., Ringenback, R., Hottenstein, S. The antimicrobial activity of human colostral antibody in the newborn. *J. Infect. Dis.* **124**:445–448, 1971.

117. Gindrat, J. J. Gothefors, L., Hanson, L. A., *et al.* Antibodies in human milk against *E. coli* of the serogroups most commonly found in neonatal infections. *Acta Paediatr. Scand.* **61**:587–590, 1972.

118. Hanson, L. A., Carlsson, B., Ahlstedt, S., *et al.* Immune defense factors in human milk. *Mod. Probl. Paediatr.* **15**:63, 1975.

119. Burdon, D. W. The bactericidal action of immunoglobulin A. *J. Med. Microbiol.* **6**:131–139, 1973.

120. Walker, W. A., Isselbacher, K. J., Bloch, K. J. Intestinal uptake of macromolecules: Effect of oral immunization. *Science* **177**:608–610, 1972.

121. Walker, W. A., Wu, M., Isselbacher, K. J., *et al.* Intestinal uptake of macromolecules: III. Studies on the mechanism by which immunization interferes with antigen uptake. *J. Immunol.* **115**:854–861, 1975.

122. McClelland, D. B., Samson, R. R., Parkin, D. M., *et al.* Bacterial agglutination studies with secretory IgA prepared from human gastrointestinal secretions and colostrum. *Gut* **13**:450–458, 1972.

123. Rutter, J. M., Jones, G. W., Brown, G. T. H., *et al.* Antibacterial activity in colostrum and milk associated with protection of piglets against enteric disease caused by K88-positive *Escherichia coli. Infect. Immun.* **13**:667–676, 1976.

124. Warren, R. J., Lepow, M. L., Bartsch, G. E., *et al.* The relationship of maternal antibody, breast feeding, and age to the susceptibility of newborn infants to infection with attenuated polioviruses. *Pediatrics* **34**:4–13, 1964.

125. Gonzaga, A. J., Warren, R. J., Robbins, F. C. Attenuated poliovirus infection in infants fed colostrum from poliomyelitis immune cows. *Pediatrics* **32**:1039–1043, 1963.

126. Downham, M. A., Scott, R., Sims, D. G., *et al.* Breast-feeding protects against respiratory syncytial virus infections. *Br. Med. J.* **2**:274–276, 1976.

127. Falkler, W. A., Jr., Diwan, A. R., Halstead, S. B. A lipid inhibitor of dengue virus in human colostrum and milk; with a note on the absence of antidengue secretory antibody. *Arch. Virol.* **47**:3–10, 1975.

128. Matthews, T. H., Nair, C. D., Lawrence, M. K., *et al.* Antiviral activity in milk of possible clinical importance. Lancet **2**:1387–1389, 1976.
129. Woode, G. N., Jones, J., Bridger, J. L. Levels of colostral antibodies against neonatal calf diarrhoea virus. *Vet. Rec.* **97**:148–149, 1975.
130. Snodgrass, D. R., Wells, P. W. Rotavirus infection in lambs: Studies on passive protection. *Arch. Virol.* **52**:201–205, 1976.
131. Abou-Youssef, M. H., Ristic, M. Protective effect of immunoglobulins in serum and milk of sows exposed to transmissible gastroenteritis virus. *Can. J. Comp. Med.* **39**:41–45, 1975.
132. Bohl, E. H., Saif, L. J. Passive immunity in transmissible gastroenteritis of swine: Immunoglobulin characteristics of antibodies in milk after inoculating virus by different routes. *Infect. Immun.* **11**:23–32, 1975.
133. Totterdell, B. M., Chrystie, I. L., Banatvala, J. E. Rotavirus infections in a maternity unit. *Arch. Dis. Child.* **51**:924–928, 1976.
134. Schoub, B. D., Prozesky, O. W., Lecatsas, G., *et al.* The role of breast-feeding in the prevention of rotavirus infection. *J. Med. Microbiol.* **11**:25–31, 1978.
135. Yolken, R. H., Wyatt, R. G., Mata, L., *et al.* Secretory antibody directed against rotavirus in human milk: Measurement by means of enzyme linked immunosorbent assay. *J. Pediatr.* **93**:916–921, 1978.
136. Gothefors, L., Winberg, J. Symposium on breast-feeding: Host resistance factors. *J. Trop. Pediatr.* **21**:260–263, 1975.
137. Ho, P. C., Lawton, J. W. Human colostral cells: Phagocytosis and killing of *E. coli* and *C. albicans. J. Pediatr.* **93**:910–915, 1978.
138. Ahlstedt, S., Carlsson, B., Hanson, L. A., et al. Antibody production by human colostral cells: I. Immunoglobulin class, specificity and quantity. *Scand. J. Immunol.* **4**:535–539, 1975.
139. Smith, J. W., Schultz, R. D. Mitogen- and antigen-responsive milk lymphocytes. *Cell. Immunol.* **29**:165–173, 1977.
140. Ogra, S. S., Ogra, P. L. Immunologic aspects of human colostrum and milk: II. Characteristics of lymphocyte reactivity and distribution of E-rosette forming cells at different times after the onset of lactation. *J. Pediatr.* **92**:550–555, 1978.
141. Pickering, L. K., Cleary, T. G., Kohl, S., *et al.* Polymorphonuclear leukocytes of human colostrum. I. Oxidative metabolism and kinetics of killing radiolabeled *S. aureus. J. Infect. Dis.* (in press).
142. Kohl, S., Malloy, M. M., Pickering, L. K., *et al.* Human colostral cytotoxicity: I. Antibody-dependent cellular cytotoxicity against *Herpes simplex* viral infected cells mediated by colostral cells. *J. Clin. Lab. Immunol.* **1**:221–224, 1978.
143. Ogra, P. L., Karzon, D. T., Righthand, F., *et al.* Immunoglobulin response in serum and secretions after immunization with live and inactivated poliovaccine and natural infection. *N. Engl. J. Med.* **279**:893–900, 1968.
144. Ogra, P. L., Karzon, D. T. The role of immunoglobulins in the mechanism of mucosal immunity to viral infection. *Pediatr. Clin. North Am.* **17**:385–400, 1970.

2

Amebiasis

INTRODUCTION

Amebiasis is a ubiquitous disease which is a particularly important problem in developing tropical countries. The causative agent, *Entamoeba histolytica*, was first described in 1875 by Lösch, a Russian physician in St. Petersburg.[1] He described the organisms in detail and called them *Amebae coli*. In a careful pathologic and clinical review in 1891, Councilman and Lefleur[2] described amebic dysentery as a distinct entity characterized by ulceration of the colon wherein the ulcers were undermined without products of inflammation. They furthermore indicated that liver abscess often complicated intestinal disease with occasional extension of the abscess to the lung. The true pathogenic potential of *E. histolytica* for humans was established in 1911–1913 by a series of studies of experimental infection induced in volunteers.[3,4] Filipino prison volunteers who ingested *E. histolytica* cysts developed dysentery, and stools were shown to contain the amebae. In 1919, the four species of commensal amebae were distinguished from *E. histolytica*.[5]

A symbiotic relationship between *E. histolytica* and certain bacterial species important to the development of pathogenicity was realized soon after the discovery of the agent.[2,4,6] Westphal[6] swallowed *E. histolytica* which had been obtained from a person convalescing from amebiasis and was free from symptoms for a period of eight months. He then ingested a stool filtrate devoid of the protozoan and developed dysentery after 23 days. He attributed the disease to the enhancing influence of the bacteria. Baetjer and Sellards[7] demonstrated that if animals were inoculated with amebae and streptococci, the incubation period was reduced when compared to administration of amebae alone. Boeck and Drbohlav[8] first cultivated *E. histolytica* in an artificial medium and showed the enhanced virulence of these cultures when combined with bacterial flora obtained from patients with intestinal amebiasis. Spector[9] and Deschiens[10] confirmed that bacteria enhanced the pathogenicity of *E. histolytica* in experimental infection employing a feline model. In 1914, Izar described a complement-fixation test for detecting antibody to *E. histolytica* (cited in Reference 11) which began the development of serodiagnosis of amebiasis.

EPIDEMIOLOGY

The distribution of *E. histolytica* is worldwide. Intestinal carriage is common, with 5–20% of asymptomatic persons having cysts in stools.[12] Intestinal carriage of *E. histolytica* cysts is about 5% for the population of the United States.[13,14] The incidence of amebic dysentery is higher in warm and humid areas of the world. The age groups with the highest incidence of infection and clinical symptomatology are the third through fifth decades,[15] although persons of all ages are susceptible, including infants and the elderly. Females are as likely to be infected with *E. histolytica* as males,[16] but amebic dysentery (bloody, mucoid stools) and liver abscess forms of the disease are more common in males.[15,17]

The manner in which *E. histolytica* cysts pass from the colon of an infected person to a susceptible individual is often dependent upon the level of economic development and hygienic practices of the region. The most common mode of spread of *E. histolytica* in the United States is undoubtedly person-to-person. Studies of the transmission of *E. histolytica* were performed by Ivanhoe[18] in a residential institution for children in New Orleans. She demonstrated that *E. histolytica* cysts were distributed throughout the environment: under the fingernails of children, on soiled underclothing, on a laundry chute, in sand of a playpen, and in the water of a wading pool. Control measures which were successful included the disinfection of the general area with steam and the treatment of the children with amebicidal drugs. In areas of disease hyperendemicity, flies and cockroaches may be responsible for spread of the infecting cysts. The housefly has been shown to be an efficient carrier of *E. histolytica* cysts[19]; cysts may remain viable for up to two days in the droppings of these household insects.[5,15] Other mammals such as dogs, monkeys, rats, and pigs may become infected and serve on occasion as reservoirs for human illness. Venereal transmission of *E. histolytica* occurs among both heterosexual and homosexual persons.[20]

Environmental errors which lead to acquisition of infection are ingestion of cysts in untreated (unfiltered) water, preparation of food by carriers of *E. histolytica,* or use of human excreta for fertilizing purposes in growing of fresh vegetables. Four general factors contribute to the incidence of amebiasis in a given area: climate, race, sex, and diet. Amebiasis is a particularly important problem in tropical and subtropical areas. Removal of infected individuals to temperate zones has been followed by an amelioration of their symptoms.[11] Persons living in areas of hyperendemicity frequently excrete the protozoan in stool but appear to be resistant to clinical disease. The nature of the food ingested is important to susceptibility where nutritionally incomplete diets or those rich in carbohydrates may be predisposing factors.[11] If diet is important, aside from reflecting regional differences where the disease is endemic, it probably enhances susceptibility by leading to an alteration of intestinal flora.

Earlier reports of outbreaks of amebiasis in the United States demonstrated that water supplies might become contaminated when plumbing defects led to the contamination of drinking water with sewage.[21-23] Such an occurrence in large cities of the world is probably unusual with improved sewage removal procedures. A number of important control measures have limited the disease rates in industrialized countries: installation of plants for filtration and chemical treatment of water supplies; widespread distribution of toilet facilities; improved food preparation, production, packaging, distribution, and preservation, including the removal of infected persons from public eating establishments; modern plumbing; prevention of insects from gaining access to food by screens; insecticides; and air conditioning.

For more than 20 years, an average of 3500 cases of amebiasis has been reported annually in the United States.[24] The frequency of liver abscess development in patients with amebiasis in between 1 and 3%.[25,26] The incidence of liver abscess does not always appear to reflect the frequency of occurrence of intestinal disease.[27]

PATHOGENESIS

E. histolytica undergoes three distinct stages in its life cycle: trophozoite, precyst, and cyst (Table 2.1). The trophozoites vary in size and are characteristically found in stool of patients with dysentery or diarrhea. The precyst stage is intermediate between the trophozoite and cyst stages. Precysts are smaller than trophozoites and are infrequently identified in stool. The cyst is more resistant to environmental stresses and is the infective stage. Cysts are found more frequently in formed stools.

The exact mechanisms of disease pathogenesis in amebiasis are unknown. Whether the *E. histolytica* trophozoite enters the colonic mucosal cells by cytolysis secondary to enzyme production, whether the pseudopodia play a role in producing attachment and/or injury, or if a defect in the existing mucosal barrier is a prerequisite is unestablished. As is the case for the causative agents of shigellosis and salmonellosis, it may be

TABLE 2.1
Characteristics of the Stages of Entamoeba Histolytica

Stage	Size	Characteristics of stool	Comments
Trophozoite	12–50 μm	Bloody, mucoid	Does not survive outside body; not important in transmission
Precyst	10–20 μm	Loose to partially formed	Rarely seen
Cyst	10–20 μm	Formed	Survives outside body; is the infective stage

that both invasiveness and toxin production are important virulence properties of *E. histolytica*. Jarumilinta and Kradolfer[28] noted that *E. histolytica* produced a leukotoxin, while Eaton *et al.*[29] and Knight *et al.*[30] further characterized the cytolytic effects of the protozoan. The importance of toxin production in amebiasis is unknown, and it is not known whether quantitative or qualitative differences in enterotoxicity or cytotoxicity correlate with virulence among strains of *E. histolytica*.[31]

The occurrence of colonic lesions from invasion by trophozoites within 24–90 hr after ingestion of cysts suggests that the amebae are able to cross the mucosal barrier without awaiting surface abrasions.[32] Colonic ulcerations classically are diamond- or flask-shaped with undermined edges where the ulcers are narrower at the surface and wider in the submucosa. These ulcers are a few millimeters to several centimeters in diameter and usually contain a yellow exudate. The mucosa between ulcerations may show hyperemia, although often it is normal, in contrast to bacillary dysentery, where the colitis is diffuse. The intestinal lesions may vary widely, showing frank ulceration, pustule formation, superficial erosions in an area of mucosal hyperemia, general hyperemia, and normal appearance. Submucosal hemorrhages may be present, giving the appearance of dark red patches with irregular margins. If the disease progresses, shaggy mucosal sloughs may be produced or even tubular mucosal casts may be passed. Spontaneous healing generally occurs, although occasionally lesions extend to muscular layers of the gut, and perforation may occur. Since there is minimal inflammation, fibrosis and scarring are not part of the healing process. Amebae are not pyogenic, and much of the cellular reaction consists of lymphocytes. The parasite can be found in tissue without associated inflammatory cells.[33] Polymorphonuclear leukocytes may be present in small numbers,[2,33,34] yet when they are prevalent, secondary bacterial infection should be suspected.[33] In certain cases, a granulomatous reaction occurs, leading to tumor-like lesions (amebomas) or to segmental narrowing of the bowel lumen. The area of intestine maximally involved is usually the cecum and ascending colon followed by rectum, sigmoid colon, and, finally, descending colon.[35]

A great deal of attention has been drawn to the significance of the intestinal carrier state of *E. histolytica*. Many state that the protozoan is an obligate pathogen and that excretion of the agent is invariably associated with active infection. This view is supported by the finding that most carriers will have intermittent symptoms of intestinal disease.[15] Others have maintained that *E. histolytica* can live intraluminally without invasion or production of a mucosal lesion.[36] Faust[37] performed an autopsy study of persons dying from accidental causes to look at the relationship between intestinal carriage and intestinal pathology. He noted ulceration in certain cases of clinically inactive "carriers," while in 6 of 13 patients, he found amebae in the intestinal lumen without demonstrable tissue pathology. In 4 of the patients without evidence of tissue injury, large numbers of amebae were present in the luman. When dysentery symptoms (bloody, mucoid stools) develop, trophozoites and red blood cells are usually present in stools, and cysts are noticeably absent. In the

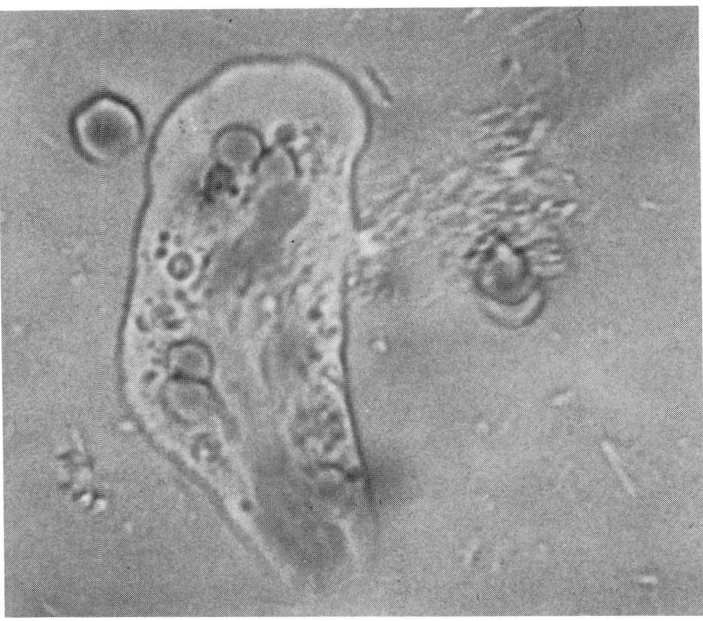

Figure 2.1. Live *Entamoeba histolytica* trophozoite with ingested red blood cells. Unidirectional movement along with cytoplasmic streaming was noted (saline preparation, ×1000). This photomicrograph was taken directly from stool specimen from a patient with diarrhea. Prepared by Mr. Bernard J. Marino of the Houston City Health Department.

dysenteric form of illness, the trophozoites are large and usually contain ingested red cells (Figure 2.1). In the intermittent, milder form of diarrhea seen in chronic carriers, the trophozoites which emerge during the period of symptomatology usually are smaller and often contain ingested red cells.[36]

Quadrinucleate cysts are formed from two successive divisions of cells with single nuclei. Each of the four nuclei undergoes division, forming eight daughter nuclei which then become eight uninucleate amebae. The life cycle of *E. histolytica* in humans begins with the ingestion of cysts. Encystation or hatching occurs in the lower ileum and colon. The trophozoites invade the colonic mucosa, multiply by binary fission which is completed in 10–15 min, and establish themselves in mucosal ulcers. Multiplication continues, with a percentage of amebae remaining in the lumen primarily as trophozoites in diarrheal stools or as cysts in milder diarrhea and in formed stools (see Figures 2.1 and 2.2). Trophozoites excreted in stool rapidly perish and are unimportant in the propagation of human illness. The precyst stage is smaller than the trophozoite, and a cyst wall forms about the amebae in 1–2 hr (encystation). Cysts found may be either immature uninucleate or mature quadrinucleate cells. The immature cyst matures in the external environment and is then ready to be ingested and complete the life cycle. Cysts are protected by a wall

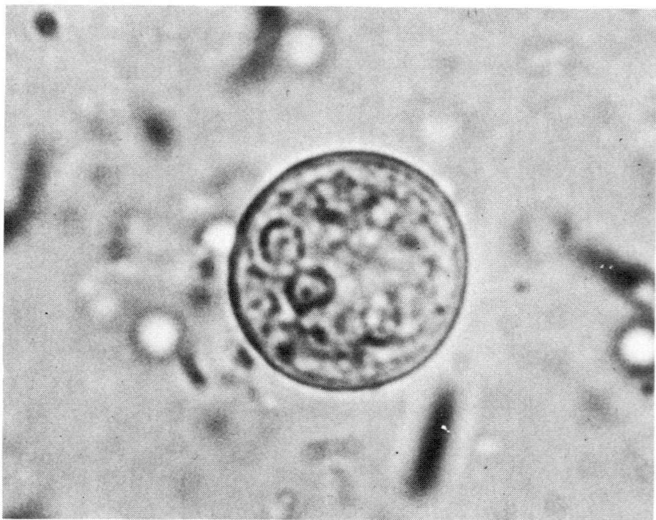

Figure 2.2. Cyst of *Entamoeba histolytica* seen in a merthiolate–iodine–formalin (MIF)-stained preparation from a clinical specimen showing two visible nuclei (×1000). Material kindly furnished by Mr. Bernard J. Marino of the Houston City Health Department.

which imparts an ability to withstand pH, a considerable degree of desiccation, and temperature changes. At room temperature, the cysts remain viable for 9–28 days, while at lower temperature they remain viable for a period of 4 months.[38,39] Cysts die rapidly in heavily polluted water but remain viable for 1–5 weeks if the bacterial contamination is low. Chlorine does not efficiently kill the cysts, and filtration methods are necessary to assure water safety.[39] The minimum period of time between ingestion of cysts and development of symptoms is 8 days. In volunteer experiments, the incubation period ranged from 20 to 95 days.[4]

The importance of the bacterial flora of the intestine to disease pathogenesis was apparent soon after identification of the causative agent.[2,4,6] Since these early observations, enteric bacteria were shown to enhance the virulence of *E. histolytica* in studies of experimental animals.[40] In gnotobiotic guineas pigs, bacteria were necessary to allow intestinal invasion to occur.[40] Undoubtedly, the beneficial effects of tetracycline drugs in amebiasis (and perhaps metronidazole to some degree) represent effects on intestinal flora.

E. histolytica may spread via the portal bloodstream to the liver. The typical hepatic lesion is necrosis leading to abscess formation. The abscess consists of a central zone of hepatic necrosis with an enlarging periphery of trophozoites. The abscess material generally is bacteriologically sterile. By direct extension and rupture, the hepatic lesion may spread to involve pleura, lung, peritoneum, pericardium, and any other body region, particularly if rupture into an hepatic vein occurs. The skin may become involved by direct spread from the bowel, from the anus, or from a colonic–cutaneous fistula which may follow a surgical procedure. Grossly, these indolent cutaneous ulcers show marked induration and overhanging edges. Parasites are readily found.

Evidence that amebae reach the liver via the portal vein is based on the finding of parasites in the capillaries of the gut and in thrombi in branches of the portal vein in the liver.[41] Amebae carried to the liver by the portal circulation are filtered into the portal capillaries, producing occlusion of the capillary lumen and subsequent focal liver necrosis. Most of the amebae which reach the liver fail to become established and are destroyed. Amebae which reach the liver and survive multiply, producing hepatic necrosis rather than inflammation. In the liver, the cytolytic *E. histolytica* trophozoites apparently are able to survive and multiply in the absence of bacteria. *E. histolytica* cysts are not found in tissues. The abscess extends concentrically, and the trophozoites are found at the leading edge of extending necrosis. The abscess contains necrotic liver tissue and few leukocytes. If untreated and progressive, the abscess will extend to the liver surface, where direct extension to other organs or rupture into hollow viscera or serous cavities may occur. Healing after specific therapy results in little damage to the liver, since there is minimal inflammation or tendency toward fibrosis. Liver tissue adjacent to hepatic abscesses is uninvolved except for minimal congestion and edema. Whether amebic hepatitis without abscess formation is a valid entity has not been resolved. It must be an unusual form of hepatic amebiasis if it does occur at all.[42,43] It is well recognized that patients with intestinal amebiasis may have tender hepatomegaly (5%), whereas liver abscess formation is slightly less common, occurring in between 1 and 3% of patients with intestinal amebiasis.[25,26,44] In all probability, small liver abscesses commonly occur as a result of intestinal amebiasis, but spontaneous resolution prevents evolution into frank liver abscesses.[45,46]

Factors which predispose patients to development of an abscess of the liver remain unresolved. Tissue sensitization from recurrent portal injection of amebae may be one factor, and, in addition, bacteria may play an early role. Cultures of amebae injected into portal vein produced liver abscess in guinea pigs only if the animals previously had been sensitized by injections of amebae fragmented by freezing and thawing.[47] Kondo (cited in Reference 32) noted that if amebae were injected into the portal venous system of kittens, bacteria had to be added to the inoculum in order to develop an abscess. If bacteria are necessary, they generally are not able to establish themselves in the liver, since 60–86% of hepatic abscess cultures are bacteriologically sterile.[15,48] The explanation for the involvement of the right lobe of the liver in 56–96% of studied cases has been elucidated. Sérégé[49,50] first demonstrated two blood currents in the portal vein by injections of ink into the portal system. Blood from the cecal area of the intestine (the site most frequently involved in intestinal amebiasis) was shown by this technique to drain through the superior mesenteric vein to the right lobe, while blood traversing through the inferior mesenteric and splenic veins from other intestinal regions flowed through the portal vein to the left lobe. Copher and Dick[51] later confirmed that two separate laminar streams of flow were maintained in the portal vein, one predominantly from the superior mesenteric vein to the right lobe of the liver and the other primarily from the inferior mesenteric and splenic veins to the left lobe.

The pathogenicity of *E. histolytica* may be enhanced among certain patients, such as those receiving immunosuppressive therapy or corticosteroids.[52-56] In addition, pregnant women show an increased frequency and severity of amebiasis.[57-59] Whether this is related to levels of hydrocortisone, estrogen, or other hormones in pregnancy or because of other nutritional, immunologic, or circulatory changes remains unknown.[58] It appears that hormonal alterations also play a role in the pathogenesis of amebic liver abscess. This is further suggested by the finding that while during the reproductive years the ratio of hepatic amebiasis in males to females is 10:1, in prepubertal children there is an equal incidence of liver abscess among males and females.[60]

CLINICAL ASPECTS

Amebic Colitis

The incubation period is usually one to four weeks[22] but may be as long as one year.[61] The onset of symptoms is usually gradual, with diarrhea, abdominal discomfort, and flatulence occurring before the dysentery. Abdominal pain and tenesmus are common complaints. The most common clinical condition is acute diarrhea, although the more striking dysentery form has been better characterized.[44,62] In areas where amebic and bacillary dysenteries have occurred and were studied, the differences in clinical symptoms were striking (Table 2.2). Patients with amebiasis have an appearance of well-being with complaints of abdominal pain and tenesmus, while patients with shigellosis are acutely ill and toxic, and many are dehydrated. Patients with colonic amebiasis usually have low-grade fever (oral temperature, $\leq 101°F$) or are afebrile. Abdominal tenderness and hepatomegaly may be other findings. Stools retain a fecal form in many cases of amebiasis but contain an admixture of blood and blood-stained mucus. Anemia is not a feature except in chronic, long-standing disease. Leukocytosis is common, reaching as high as 25,000 cells/mm³. Leukocytes are not prevalent in stools of patients with amebiasis, in sharp contrast to the finding in bacillary dysentery.[44,62]

TABLE 2.2
Comparison between Amebic and Bacillary Dysenteries

	Amebic	Bacillary
Onset	Gradual	Sudden
Clinical appearance	Usually nontoxic	Often toxic
Dehydration	Unusual	Common
Tenesmus	Severe	Moderate to mild
Hepatomegaly	Common	Uncommon
Stool appearance	Blood and mucus; stools may be semiformed	Blood and mucus; stools less commonly formed
Fecal leukocytes	Uncommon	Common
Colonic ulcerations	Segmental	Diffuse

A chronic intestinal infection may develop after the initial diarrheal illness. In such cases, recurrent diarrhea and dysentery may be interrupted by periods of constipation and vague abdominal discomfort. Weight loss is common, and complications of the infection may occur in patients with chronic or recurrent symptoms. Intestinal amebiasis has become an important problem in male homosexuals.[20,63]

Liver Abscess

The frequency of liver abscess development in amebic dysentery is between 1 and 3%; approximately 5% of cases will have hepatomegaly. The ratio of liver abscess among males to females is 7–10:1. Liver abscess may occur in the presence or absence of intestinal symptoms. About 40% of patients with amebic liver abscess will complain simultaneously of diarrhea. Half of patients with hepatic abscess will give a history of a previous episode of dysentery, and 10% will have dysentery at the time of presentation.[64] Approximately 15% of patients with a liver abscess without a prior or present history of diarrhea will have *E. histolytica* cysts in stool. The right lobe is more frequently involved than the left in a ratio of 9:1. Multiple hepatic abscesses are found in less than 1 in 5 cases. The pus from an hepatic abscess is classically described as "anchovy paste," probably from the admixture of disintegrated hepatocytes and blood. Just as often, it will be creamy white in color, and on occasion material will be yellow, green, or chocolate in color. Characteristically, the abscess material is not foul-smelling and is bacteriologically sterile. The consistency varies widely.

Patients presenting with liver abscess may have an acute illness lasting a week, while others will have been chronically ill for many months. Pain is present in most patients over the right hypochondrium and lower right anterior chest. Pain may be pleuritic or may be referred to the right shoulder. A common complaint is nonproductive cough, and a sustained fever is often seen. Hepatomegaly is found in a majority of cases. The most useful physical sign is tenderness to palpation in the liver area. A localized area of tenderness may be located between the ribs, and edema overlying the ribs may be found. In large abscesses, a mass may actually be visible in the right subcostal or epigastric area. In half the cases, changes in the right lung base will be found due to elevation and immobility of the diaphragm with compression of the lower lobe of the right lung. Decreased diaphragmatic excursion, dullness to percussion, rales, atelectasis, and occasionally a right-sided pleural effusion can be found. Jaundice is unusual, and most often indicates an intrahepatic obstructive lesion. Abnormal laboratory findings consist of elevated sedimentation rate, leukocytosis (12,000–28,000 cells/mm^3), and a normocytic–normochromic anemia.

Extension of the abscess from the liver to adjacent organs occurs. Involvement of lung and pleura follows extension through the diaphragm, and patients may develop pleural effusion or frank empyema. Rupture of the abscess into the peritoneal cavity is associated with a high mortality rate. Extension from the liver may also involve pericardium, stomach, duodenum, small and large intestine, spleen, inferior vena cava, hepatic veins, and renal pelvis, or a fistulous communication to the skin surface may occur. When the abscess ruptures into a hepatic vein, it may disseminate to any organ, including lung and brain. In these cases, multiple abscesses may develop.

COMPLICATIONS OF INTESTINAL AMEBIASIS

Perforation

Perforation of the bowel with development of peritonitis is an unusual complication, particularly since effective forms of therapy have become available. In cases of fatal amebiasis, perforation is the most common complication and undoubtedly plays a major role in the outcome.[65] Perforation may occur in any area of the colon, although the most common site is the cecum. Further sequelae include abscess formation and generalized peritonitis. Abscesses may rupture into adjacent viscera or may form fistulas draining to the skin surface. Perforation in amebiasis is usually an insidious event and characteristically is seen in the severely ill patient, resulting in a gradual deterioration. The best means of verifying this complication is to see free air in the peritoneal cavity on radiographic examination of the abdomen.

Treatment of intestinal perforation is usually conservative.[66,69] When laparotomy is undertaken, the bowel wall will be friable, and attempts to suture may lead to larger areas of perforation. In other cases, surgery will fail to localize the area of perforation, and the patient is exposed to unneeded surgery. Rarely, a patient with amebiasis under therapy may develop a classical "acute abdomen" where a colonic ulceration has eroded through the gut wall. Once the amebic infection is well controlled by drugs, the gut wall will be sufficiently healthy to allow surgical repair and suture.[64] The treatment of a localized intraabdominal abscess secondary to intestinal perforation includes antiamebicides and antibacterial agents to control infection, followed by surgical drainage.

Ameboma

An ameboma is a nonabscess mass of the intestine associated with amebiasis. Amebomas may arise in two settings: secondary to an intense local inflammatory reaction from mucosal ulceration or a fibrolipomatous tumor involving the entire thickness of the bowel. Amebomas may occur anywhere in the colon but are most common in the cecum and sigmoid colon. The clinical findings usually include localized pain and a hard, tender mass often fixed in the cecal area or freely movable in the transverse or descending colon. Biopsy shows granulation tissue, and *E. histolytica* often are found in histologic examination. Occasionally *E. histolytica* may be found in the presence of a colonic carcinoma or other intestinal lesion, including actinomycosis, regional enteritis, or diverticulosis.[64]

Stricture

Annular narrowing of the colonic lumen occurs in the presence or absence of ameboma. While stricture is classically a complication of chronic disease, it may be seen in acute amebiasis. Pain, constipation, and intestinal obstruction are the usual findings. Involvement of the rectum or sigmoid colon may be diagnosed by digital examination or sigmoidoscopy. It may be difficult to differentiate the lesion from carcinoma or from lymphogranuloma venereum.

Miscellaneous Complications

Hemorrhage secondary to erosion into a blood vessel by an amebic ulceration can cause a brisk hemorrhage which may be fatal. Intussusception is a rare but well-recognized complication which may result when an ameboma or segmental bowel thickening forms the apex of the intussusception. Ischiorectal abscess, fistulas, and rectal prolapse are recognized complications of intestinal amebiasis.

DIAGNOSIS

Establishing the diagnosis of intestinal amebiasis is usually difficult in view of the common intestinal carriage of *E. histolytica* cysts and the difficulty many laboratories have in identifying the causative agent. In patients with dysentery where large, unidirectionally motile trophozoites contain red cells, the diagnosis is not difficult (see Figure 2.1). In less obvious cases, three freshly passed stools collected over a three-day period will usually reveal the agent.[70,71] Stool examination should include direct, flotation, and staining methods. Even better than fresh stool is material obtained from ulcers at endoscopy, scrape or biopsy material from mucosal ulceration, or a blind rectal scraping with a glass spatula. In amebiasis, sigmoidoscopy may be normal, either because the parasite may not have invaded the bowel wall or because involvement may be confined to other areas of the colon. In general, endoscopic findings can vary so widely that they rarely are helpful in making a diagnosis.[72] There is general agreement that the diagnosis of intestinal amebiasis cannot be confirmed definitively unless hematopagy of trophozoites is documented. Unfortunately, this finding is reported in less than half of the cases of amebiasis.

Few technicians in diagnostic laboratories are properly trained to identify intestinal protozoans, and there often exists a lack of interest among laboratory personnel to pursue a difficult diagnosis when so many negative results are obtained. There is no doubt that the condition is misdiagnosed.[24] It may be difficult to differentiate *E. histolytica* from other intestinal protozoans,[73] and the untrained technician or clinician often mistakes fecal white cells for *E. histolytica* cysts or trophozoites, and vice versa. Because of misdiagnosis, patients may receive potentially toxic drugs for no purpose, while curative therapy may be withheld in other situations. The finding of *E. histolytica* cysts in stool specimens may be the focal point of attention by laboratory personnel and the attending physician, and patients with shigellosis or ideopathic ulcerative colitis may not receive proper therapy.[74] On the other hand, many cases of amebiasis fail to be properly diagnosed, and fatalities still occur in the United States. Failure to establish a proper diagnosis usually centers about errors in clinical judgment or laboratory inexperience. Clinicians must be aware that patients with amebiasis may present with bloody diarrhea, intestinal perforation, toxic dilatation of the colon, or ulcerative colitis. It must be learned that freshly passed stool or rectal scrapings are needed for optimal identification of the invasive trophozoites. In selected cases, sigmoidoscopy should be performed, and direct sampling of ulcerations or rectal biopsy material should be obtained and examined.[75] Cathartics and enemas should not be used to prepare the patient prior to endoscopy, since they may interfere with identification of the agent. Because of problems with identification of *E. histolytica* trophozoites in stool and the frequent finding of cysts in those without symptoms, serologic procedures may prove to be the optimal means of establishing a diagnosis of amebiasis.

Stool Examination

The examiner must be able to differentiate various intestinal protozoa from fecal leukocytes. Patients should not have received antibiotics, antiprotozoal drugs, or antidiarrheal compounds containing kaolin, pectin, bismuth, or magnesium hydroxide for one to two weeks prior to the examination, since they interfere with parasite identification.[12] Material obtained through a proctoscope or by mucosal scraping is preferred. A rectal swab should not be employed, as the protozoan will adhere to cotton. Stool specimens should be passed directly onto dry paper or into an empty stool container; trophozoites are lysed on contact with water. If more than 2 hr will elapse before direct microscopic examination, the specimen should be refrigerated at 4°C. A portion of the specimen should be placed as soon as possible in polyvinyl alcohol (PVA) fixative to preserve the trophozoites. This is primarily useful later to confirm the diagnosis of amebiasis. Direct screening examinations are carried out using a wet-mount preparation in physiologic saline, methylene blue, and, in suspicious cases, iodine. The methylene blue and iodine preparations are useful in differentiating *E. histolytica* cysts from leukocytes, and the iodine solution offers further help in identifying the double membranes of the cyst and multiple nuclei. The trophozoites of *E. histolytica* often contain ingested red blood cells. Definitive diagnosis of amebiasis should include examination of material preserved in PVA. This also serves as a permanent record for later review. Specimens negative on direct examination for cysts should be reexamined after concentration by the zinc sulfate flotation method[73] and the formalin–ether technique.[76] No fewer than three freshly passed stools need be examined before ruling out intestinal amebiasis. The merthiolate–iodine–formalin (MIF) procedure[77] is useful to preserve any organisms present, and, like the formalin–ether technique, the examination can be carried out at leisure. When *E. histolytica* is identified by any of the direct staining techniques, it is advisable to return to the PVA fixative and make a permanently stained slide employing either the trichrome[78] or an iron–hematoxylin stain.[79] The smaller nonpathogenic ameba *Entamoeba hartmanni* is differentiated from the pathogen *E. histolytica* by measurement using an ocular micrometer.[80] Rectal biopsy to look for intramucosal trophozoites may be useful in cases with equivocal findings on stool examination. When material is obtained from an extraintestinal site, as, for example, liver abscess fluid, the last few milliliters of aspirate may be more revealing, since the trophozoite can usually be found only at the periphery of the abscess.[81] Laboratories identifying *E. histolytica* should refer on a regular basis material preserved in formalin or PVA to their state health department for confirmation, and local laboratories should be encouraged to participate in proficiency testing programs under the direction of the regional labora-

TABLE 2.3
Structural Differences among the Amebae Found in the Large Intestine of Humans

Amebae	Peripheral chromatin and chromatid bars	Karyosomal chromatin	Nuclei in cyst	Other bodies
Entamoeba histolytica	+	Small, centric	1–4	Red blood cells (trophozoite)
Entamoeba coli	+	Large, centric	1–8	0
Endolimax nana	0	Large, blot-like	1–4	0
Iodamoeba bütschlii	0	Large	1	Large glycogen vacuoles (cyst)
Dientamoeba fragilis	0	Broken and clumped	No cyst	0

tory.[14] Table 2.3 highlights morphologic differences among the various amebae found in the intestine of humans.

Other Laboratory Procedures

Serology testing as performed by state departments of health (usually an indirect hemagglutination technique) is a valuable adjunct to establishing the diagnosis of amebiasis. This is particularly true in the case of liver abscess (see "Serology," below).

Hepatic amebiasis (liver absess) is suggested in patients with elevation of the right hemidiaphragm and tenderness or a mass in the right upper quadrant. The most helpful new laboratory developments in diagnosing a liver abscess are technetium-99m sulfur colloid and gallium-67 citrate scans and computerized axial tomography (CAT). Figure 2.3 indicates how a liver scan may be useful in detecting the presence and determining the extent of an amebic abscess. The CAT scan may be capable of defining smaller lesions than the currently available scanning procedures. The radionuclide image demonstrates a space-occupying lesion (abscess, hematoma, or malignancy). The technetium scan is particularly helpful in identifying lesions in the left lobe. Gallium scanning may show increased activity near the periphery of the lesion which is also characteristic of large neoplastic processes with central necrosis.[82] The gallium scan has been shown to be useful in following the progress of therapy. Ultrasonic scanning may not be as accurate as scintiscanning in detecting an abscess, but it offers the advantage of determining whether the lesion is fluid-filled or solid.[83] B-mode ultrasonography added to a radionuclide-image procedure may prove to be the optimal means of detecting liver abscess.

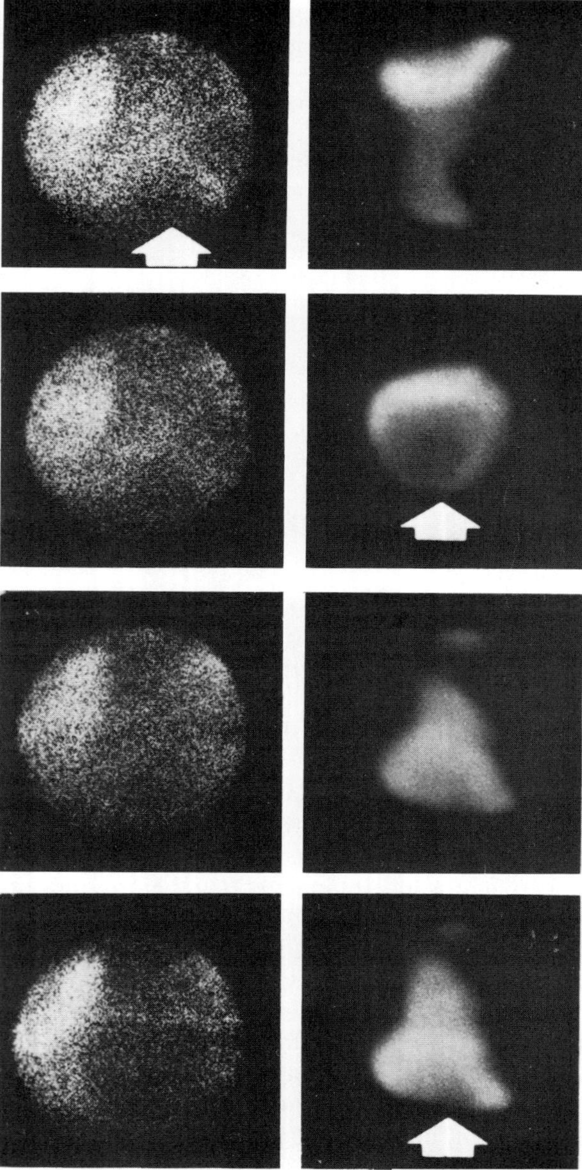

Figure 2.3. Liver scan of a 29-year-old male with a large solitary, avascular mass (arrows) due to *Entamoeba histolytica* in the posterior right lobe of the liver. Hepatic perfusion was performed using 5 mCi ^{99m}Tc. Provided by Robert N. McConnell, University of Texas Medical School at Houston. Top row: Pictures represent 4-sec intervals. Bottom row: 20-min delayed static linear images of anterior, left anterior oblique, right lateral, and posterior views, respectively.

is fluid-filled or solid.[83] B-mode ultrasonography added to a radionuclide-image procedure may prove to be the optimal means of detecting liver abscess.

Cultivation of *E. histolytica* may be used in establishing a diagnosis, but lack of availability of the technique generally limits the usefulness of such an approach. Axenic methods are used in most centers to obtain pure cultures of amebae, while monaxenic techniques, allowing one bacterial strain to grow with the amebae, may be used in the research laboratory.[84,85] The LER medium of Boeck and Drbohlav which was described in 1925[8] is still employed. A number of other media are available, including liver extract,[86] egg yolk infusion,[87] alcohol–egg extract,[88] and charcoal media.[89] Cultivation of *E. histolytica* from stool has been used successfully in diagnosing amebiasis in field studies.[90,91] Amebic antigen detection by counterimmunoelectrophoresis is a useful means of rapid and specific diagnosis of amebiasis, particularly in invasive disease such as liver abscess.[92]

SEROLOGY

Craig[93,94] demonstrated that patients with amebiasis had complement-fixing serum antibody to the causative agent. The antigen was an alcohol extract of an *E. histolytica* culture. Other procedures include amebae immobilization reaction,[95] indirect hemagglutination (IHA) and complement-fixation tests,[96,97] latex slide agglutination procedure,[98] fluorescent antibody technique,[99] countercurrent immunoelectrophoresis,[100] and gel diffusion preciptin (GDP).[101] Currently, most state health department laboratories employ the indirect hemagglutination test. Approximately 85% of the persons with symptomatic intestinal disease and nearly 100% of those with extraintestinal amebiasis have significant humoral antibody titers.[73,102,103] The serologic test is particularly useful in the United States due to the low level of antibody which exists in the general population.[104] The test is of great usefulness in diagnosing amebic liver abscess, since stool specimens are usually negative for the agent and the serologic procedure is nearly always positive (in 92–98% of cases). Also, serologic evaluation is of value in determining the importance of *E. histolytica* in patients with inflammatory bowel disease when the protozoan is visualized in stool specimens.[105] This is particularly important, since corticosteroids used in inflammatory bowel disease are contraindicated in amebiasis. A limitation of serologic procedures to establish a diagnosis of amebiasis relates to the failure of a humoral immune response to asymptomatic intestinal infection.[106] Also, an elevated titer does not distinguish between current or previous infection,[102] although a titer $\geq$ 1:512 generally indicates a recent or active infection.[103] GDP has been suggested as the best test for invasive amebiasis in view of its simplicity, reproducibility, and low cost.[101] IHA is the most useful as an epidemiologic tool, because prolonged persistence of antibodies after illness allows the study of disease prevalence.

TREATMENT

In the 19th century, ipecacuarrha (ipecac) was used for the treatment of dysentery. In 1912, Vedeer (cited in Reference 107) demonstrated that its derivative emetine could kill amebae *in vitro,* and Rogers [107] successfully treated two patients with amebic dysentery and one with liver abscess by parenteral emetine. Due to cardiovascular toxicity, this drug is rarely used today.

The objectives of therapy are to control symptoms, to destroy amebae in the bowel lumen, to prevent spread of amebae to other tissues, and to irradicate invasive amebae. Metronidazole (Flagyl) is the most effective single drug for all forms of symptomatic amebiasis and is given to children and adults regardless of the disease expression, including liver abscess (Table 2.4).[108–110] Failure to respond to metronidazole occasionally occurs with hepatic amebiasis, and other drugs may then be effective.[110–114] Liver abscess may on rare occasion develop after a full course of appropriate therapy for intestinal amebiasis.[114,115] Although most patients will respond to metronidazole alone, the occurrence of relapses and development of a liver abscess after therapy have encouraged many to suggest the use of an additional drug in combination with metronidazole, such as diiodohydroxyquin or chloroquine.[114,116] When the course of metronidazole is completed for the treatment of intestinal amebiasis, a drug active against cysts, such as diiodohydroxyquin, probably should be given to adults. Diiodohydroxyquin has important yet unusual side effects, including optic atrophy and blindness.[117,118] Patients who are critically ill or who are unable to take medication by mouth should initially be treated with emetine or, preferably, with dehydroemetine.[108–111] There is little doubt that a carrier state exists for *E. histolytica* whereby the organism is excreted in the cyst form in the absence of overt clinical symptoms. Liver abscess occurs in such patients, which indicates the potential hazards of long-term intestinal carriage. Also, it appears that decreased host resistance will stimulate the agent to produce intestinal invasion and symptoms. It is for these reasons many advocate treating asymptomatic intestinal carriers, particularly if the individuals live in areas where disease is not hyperendemic.

There is a lack of agreement on the optimal course of therapy of intestinal amebiasis due to unavailability or toxicity of drugs or because

TABLE 2.4
Antimicrobial Therapy of Amebiasis

	First choice	Alternative[a]
Asymptomatic cyst excretor	Diloxanide furoate (Furamide)[b] 500 mg (p.o.) t.i.d. for 10 days (adults), 20 mg/kg/day for 10 days (children)	Diiodohydroxyquin (Diodoquin) 650 mg (p.o.) t.i.d. for 5–10 days (adults), 40 mg/kg/day for 10 days (children) or Metronidazole (Flagyl) 750 mg (p.o.) t.i.d. for 5 days (adults), 50 mg/kg/day for 5 days (children)
Intestinal amebiasis	Metronidazole (Flagyl) 750 mg (p.o.) t.i.d. for 5–10 days (adults), 50 mg/kg/day for 10 days (children) plus Diiodohydroxyquin (Diodoquin) 650 mg (p.o.) t.i.d. for 21 days (adults), 40 mg/kg/day for 21 days (children)	Dehydroemetine[b] 90mg/day (i.m. or deep s.c.) (adults), 1 mg/kg/day (children) for 10 days plus either Diiodohydroxyquin (same dosage and duration as under "First choice") or Diloxanide furoate[b] (same dosage and duration as above)
Liver abscess (or other extraintestinal diseases)	Metronidazole (Flagyl) 750 mg (p.o.) t.i.d. for 5–10 days (adults), 50 mg/kg/day for 10 days (children) (Many would also administer chloroquine for 21 days; see dosage under "Alternative")	Dehydroemetine[b] (same dosage and duration as above) plus Chloroquine 150 mg base (p.o.) b.i.d. for 21 days–10 weeks (adults), 10 mg/kg/day for 21 days (children) plus Diiodohydroxyquin (same dosage and duration as under "Intestinal amebiasis")

[a]Some combinations are untested.
[b]Drugs not currently licensed; available from Parasitic Disease Drug Service, Center for Disease Control (404-329-3311 or 404-329-3644).

of high relapse rates after therapy. Diiodohydroxyquin is no longer marketed (it can be obtained on request from Searle Laboratories), diloxanide furoate[119] is not yet licensed, and metronidazole is suspected of being mutagenic for bacteria and carcinogenic in rats and mice,[120] indicating the therapeutic dilemma which exists in management of patients with amebiasis. Table 2.4 offers our suggestions for the therapy of the various forms of amebiasis. The best form of therapy for the asymptomatic cyst excretor (if treated) is diloxanide furoate[119] (which is available through the Center for Disease Control, 404-329-3311) or diiodohydroxyquin.[121]

Metronidazole represents the cornerstone of therapy for other symptomatic forms. Emetine or the synthetic dehydroemetine is useful for very ill patients or those unable to take oral drugs. Dehydroemetine is more rapidly excreted and has a more favorable liver–heart concentration and therefore is less toxic than the natural compound emetine.[122] It is available from the Center for Disease Control. Ideally, stool specimens are examined by concentration techniques for *E. histolytica* one month and two months after the course of therapy to establish a therapeutic response.

Corticosteroids should not be given to patients with amebiasis unless absolutely necessary because of underlying disease such as inflammatory bowel disease. Corticosteroids have been shown to increase the likelihood of developing liver abscess in experimental infection,[52] and case reports indicate a worsening of clinical amebic infection in those receiving steroid therapy for other reasons.[24,53,55]

In most cases, chemotherapy is curative of liver abscess without surgical intervention. In large abscesses, closed-needle aspiration is useful during drug therapy, although bacteria may be introduced by the procedure,[25,123] and in other cases, particularly when multiple abscesses occur (usually in children), surgical drainage may be necessary.[64,124]

Historically, when surgery has been performed in patients with intestinal amebiasis, it occurred when the diagnosis was not established and complications of surgery were common. The following are appropriate indications for surgery[125,126]:

1. Liver abscesses failing to respond to chemotherapy and closed-needle aspiration. Here, laparotomy and open drainage are performed.
2. Perforation of the bowel with localized abscess development. Open drainage is undertaken.
3. Perforation of the bowel with peritonitis. The perforated segment is either resected or exteriorized and a proximal colostomy performed. Reanastomosis can be carried out after recovery.
4. Fulminating amebic colitis with extreme toxemia, hyperpyrexia, tachycardia, abdominal distension, etc., which fails to respond to amebic chemotherapy and intensive medical measures, including nasogastric suction, intravenous therapy, and correction of acid–base balance and electrolyte abnormalities. Surgery also may be indicated in the patient who has persistent ulcerative colitis after completing a course of therapy providing the infection is eradicated.[126] If laparotomy reveals multiple areas of gangrene, sloughing, or perforation, subtotal colectomy and colostomy should be carried out. Ileorectal anastomosis can be carried out after recovery if the rectum returns to normal.

Percutaneous aspirations of a liver abscess may be safely performed by using a large-bore needle inserted through the ninth or tenth interspace in the right midaxillary line under guidance by physical examination and radiographic findings (for an abscess of the right lobe). Aspiration is reserved for those with a large abscess not showing clinical response after two to four days of therapy or if rupture appears to be imminent because of abscess size and location; it may also be important to aspirate left lobe abscesses to prevent rupture into the pericardium, which is highly fatal. The sole indications for open drainage of an amebic liver abscess are secondary bacterial infection which fails to respond to combined anti-amebic–antibacterial therapy or rupture of a liver abscess with development of intraabdominal abscess and peritonitis. Rupture into the lung with abscess formation is usually managed medically where spontaneous drainage occurs by erosion through a bronchus with establishment of a bronchohepatic fistula. Empyema may best be treated by chest tube and continuous pleural drainage. Rupture into the pericardium requires repeated needle aspiration. Brain abscess, which is frequently lethal, should be treated by early drainage, since medical therapy is incomplete in effecting a cure.[127]

REFERENCES

1. Lösch, F. Massenhafte Entwickelung von Amöben im Dickdarm. *Virchows Arch. Pathol. Anat* **65:**196–211, 1875.
2. Councilman, W. T., Lafleur, H. A. I. Amoebic dysentery. *Johns Hopkins Hosp. Rep. Rep. Pathol.* **7:**(7–9) 395–548, 1891.
3. Walker, E. L. A comparative study of the amoebae in the Manila water supply, in the intestinal tract of healthy persons, and in amoebic dysentery. *Philipp. J. Sci.* **6:**259–279, 1911.
4. Walker, E. L., Sellards, A. W. Experimental entamoebic dysentery. *Philipp. J. Sci. Sect. B* **8:**253–331, 1913.
5. Dobell, C. *The Amoebae Living in Man.* John Bale, Sons & Danielsson Ltd., London, 1919, 155 pp.
6. Westphal, A. Betrachtungen und experimentelle Unterschungen zur Virulenz der *Entamoeba histolytica* beim Menschen. *Arch. Schiffs Trop. Hyg.* **41:**262–280, 1937.
7. Baetjer, W. A., Sellards, A. W. Continuous propagation of amoebic dysentery in animals. *Johns Hopkins Hosp. Bull.* **25:**165–173, 1914.
8. Boeck, W. C., Drbohlav, J. The cultivation of *Endamoeba histolytica. Am. J. Hyg.* **5:**371–407, 1925.
9. Spector, B. K. A comparative study of cultural and immunological methods of diagnosing infections with *Endamoeba histolytica. J. Prev. Med.* **6:**117–128, 1932.
10. Deschiens, R. Le rôle de la flore bactérienne, associée a l'amibe dysentérique, dans l'amibiase. *Ann. Int. Pasteur* **61:**5–32, 1938.
11. Padilla y Padilla, C. A., Padilla, G. M. *Amebiasis in Man: Epidemiology, Therapeutics, Clinical Correlations and Prophylaxis.* Charles C. Thomas, Springfield, Ill., 1974.

12. Juniper, K., Jr. Amebiasis in the United States. *Bull. N.Y. Acad. Med.* **47:**448–461, 1971.
13. Brooke, M. M. Epidemiology of amebiasis in the U.S. *J. Am. Med. Assoc.* **188:**519–521, 1964.
14. Burrows, R. B. Prevalence of amebiasis in the United States and Canada. *Am. J. Trop. Med.* **10:**172–184, 1961.
15. Craig, C. F. *The Etiology, Diagnosis and Treatment of Amebiasis.* Williams & Wilkins, Baltimore, 1944.
16. Andrews, J. Incidence of intestinal protozoa with special reference to epidemiology of amoebiasis in population of Fresnillo, Zacatecas, Mexico. *Am. J. Hyg.* **19:**713–733, 1934.
17. Hinman, E. H., Kampmeier, R. H. Clinical intestinal amebiasis; study of 400 cases from Charity Hospital at New Orleans. *Am. J. Trop. Med.* **17:**263–278, 1937.
18. Ivanhoe, G. L. Studies on the transmission of amebiasis in a children's home in New Orleans. *Am. J. Trop. Med.* **23:**401–419, 1943.
19. Frye, W. W., Meleney, H. E. Investigations of *Endamoeba histolytica* and other intestinal protozoa in Tennessee: IV. A study of flies, rats, mice and some domestic animals as possible carriers of the intestinal protozoa of man in a rural community. *Am. J. Hyg.* **16:**729–749, 1932.
20. Kean, B. H. Venereal amebiasis. *N.Y. State J. Med.* **76:**930–931, 1976.
21. Hardy, A. V., Spector, B. K. Occurrence of infestations with *E. histolytica* associated with water-borne epidemic diseases. *Public Health Rep.* **50:**323–334, 1935.
22. McCoy, G. W., Hardy, A. V., Gorman, A. E., *et al.* Epidemic amebic dysentery: The Chicago outbreak of 1933. *Natl. Inst. Health Bull.* No. 166, 1936.
23. LeMaistre, C. A., Sappenfield, R., Culbertson, C., *et al.* Studies of a water-borne outbreak of amebiasis, South Bend, Indiana: I. Epidemiological aspects. *Am. J. Hyg.* **64:**30–45, 1956.
24. Krogstad, D. J., Spencer, H. C., Jr., Healy, G. R., *et al.* Amebiasis: Epidemiologic studies in the United States, 1972–1974. *Ann. Intern. Med.* **88:**89–97, 1978.
25. Abbruzzese, A. A. Hepatic amebiasis. *Am. J. Gastroenterol.* **54:**464–469, 1970.
26. Sheehy, T. W. Amebic liver abscess. *GP* **38:**94–104, 1968.
27. Elsdon-Dew, R. Amebiasis as a world problem. *Bull. N.Y. Acad. Med.* **47:**438–447, 1971.
28. Jarumilinta, R., Kradolfer, F. The toxic effect of *Entamoeba histolytica* on leucocytes. *Ann. Trop. Med. Parasitol.* **58:**375–381, 1964.
29. Eaton, R. D. P., Meerovitch, E., Costerton, J. W. The functional morphology of pathogenicity in *Entamoeba histolytica*. *Ann. Trop. Med. Parasitol.* **64:**299–304, 1970.
30. Knight, R., Bird, R. G., McCaul, T. F., Fine structural changes at *Entamoeba histolytica* rabbit kidney cell (RK13) interface. *Ann. Trop. Med. Parasitol.* **69:**197–202, 1975.
31. Mattern, C. F. T., Keister, D. B., Caspar, P. A. Experimental amebiasdis: III. A rapid *in vitro* essay for virulence of *Entamoeba histolytica*. *Am. J. Trop. Med. Hyg.* **27:**882–887, 1978.
32. Anderson, H. H., Bostick, W. L., Johnstone, H. G. *Amebiasis: Pathology, Diagnosis and Chemotherapy.* Charles C. Thomas, Springfield, Ill., 1953.
33. Woolley, P. G., Musgrave, W. E. The pathology of intestinal amebiasis. *J. Am. Med. Assoc.* **45:**1371–1378, 1905.
34. Harris, H. F. Amoebic dysentery. *Am. J. Med. Sci.* **115:**384–413, 1898.
35. Clark, H. C. The distribution and complications of amebic lesions found in 186 postmortem examinations. *Am. J. Trop. Med.* **5:**157–171, 1925.
36. Hoare, C. A. Parasitological reviews: The commensal phase of *Entamoeba histolytica*. *Exp. Parasitol.* **1:**411–427. 1962.

37. Faust, E. C. Amebiasis in the New Orleans population as revealed by autopsy examination of accident cases. *Am. J. Trop. Med.* ,**21**:35–48, 1941.
38. Stone, W. S. A method of producing encystment in cultures of *Endomoeba histolytica. Am. J. Trop. Med.* **15**:681–684, 1935.
39. Brady, F. J., Jones, M. F., Newton, W. L. Effect of chlorination of water on viability of cysts of *Endamoeba histolytica. War Med.* **3**:409–419, 1943.
40. Phillips, B. P., Wolfe, P. A., Rees, C. W., *et al.* Studies on ameba–bacteria relationship in amebiasis; comparative results of intracecal inoculation of germ-free, monocontaminated, and conventional guinea pigs with *Entamoeba histolytica. Am. J. Trop. Med.* **4**:675–692, 1955.
41. Palmer, R. B. Changes in the liver in amebic dysenterry; with special reference to the origin of amebic abscess. *Arch. Pathol. (Chicago)* **25**:327–335, 1938.
42. Kean, B. H. The nature of diffuse amebic hepatitis. *Am. J. Dig. Dis.* **2**:342–347, 1957.
43. Powell, S. J. The serum protein pattern, liver function tests and hematological findings in the differential diagnosis of amebic liver abscess. *Am. J. Trop. Med. Hyg.* **8**:337–341, 1959.
44. Payne, A. M. M. Amoebic dysentery in Eastern India. *Lancet* **1**:206–209, 1945.
45. James, K. L. Surgical complications of amoebic dysentery. *Proc. R. Soc. Med.* **39**:766–768, 1946.
46. Nandi, A. K. Amoebic hepatitis and hepatic abscess: Diagnosis and management. *J. Indian Med. Assoc.* **25**:87, 1955.
47. Maegraith, B. G., Harinasuta, C. Experimental amoebic infection of liver in guinea pigs: I. Infection via the mesenteric vein and via the portal vein. *Ann. Trop. Med.* **48**:421–433, 1954.
48. Rogers, L. Amoebic liver abscess: Its pathology, prevention and cure. *Lancet* **1**:463–469, 569–575, 677–684, 1922.
49. Sérégé, H. Contribution a l'étude de la circulation du sang porte dans le foie et des localizations lobaires hépatiques. *J. Med. Bordeaux* **32**:271–275, 291–295, 312–314, 1901.
50. Sérégé, H. Etude sur l'indépendence anatomique et physiologique des lobes du foie. *J. Méd Bordeaux* **32**:327–357, 1902.
51. Copher, G. H., Dick, B. M. "Stream line" phenomena in the portal vein and the selective distribution of portal blood in the liver. *Arch. Surg.* **127**:408–419, 1928.
52. Biagi, F., Robledo, E., Servin, H., et al. Influence of some steroids in the experimental production of amebic hepatic abscess. *Am. J. Trop. Med. Hyg.* **12**:318–320, 1963.
53. Eisert, J., Hannibal, J. E., Sanders, S. L. Fatal amebiasis complicating corticosteroid management of pemphigus vulgaris. *N. Engl. J. Med.* **25**:843–845, 1959.
54. McAllister, T. A. Diagnosis of amoebic colitis on routine biopsies from rectum and sigmoid colon. *Br. Med. J.* **1**:362–364, 1962.
55. Kanani, S. R., Knight, R. Relapsing amoebic colitis of 12 years' standing exacerbated by corticosteroids. *Br. Med. J.* **2**:613–614, 1969.
56. Mody, V. R. Corticosteroids in latent amoebiasis. *Br. Med. J.* **2**:1399, 1959.
57. Wagner, V. P., Smale, L. E., Lischke, J. H. Amebic abscess of the liver and spleen in pregnancy and the puerperium. *Obstet. Gynecol.* **45**:562–565, 1975.
58. Abioye, A. A. Fatal amoebic colitis in pregnancy and puerperium: A new clinicopathological entity. *J. Trop. Med. Hyg.* **76**:97–100, 1973.
59. Lewis, E. A., Antia, A. U. Amoebic colitis: Review of 295 cases. *Trans. R. Soc. Trop. Med. Hyg.* **63**:633–638, 1969.
60. Brandt, H., Tamayo, R. P. Pathology of human amebiasis. *Hum. Pathol.* **1**:351–385, 1970.
61. Craig, C. F. The occurrence of endamebic dysentery in the troops serving in the El Paso district from July, 1916 to December, 1916. *Mil. Surg.* **40**:286–302, 423–434, 1917.

62. Martin, G. A., Garfinkel, B. T., Brooke, M. M. *et al.* Comparative efficacy of amebicides and antibiotics in acute amebic dysentery used alone and in combination in five-hundred thirty-eight cases. *J. Am. Med. Assoc.* **151:**1055–1059, 1953.
63. Schmerin, M. J., Gelston, A., Jones, T.A C. Amebiasis: An increasing problem among homosexuals in New York City, *J. Am. Med. Assoc.* **238:**1386–1387, 1977.
64. Wilmot, A. J. *Clinical Amoebiasis.* F. A. Davis Co., Philadelphia, 1962.
65. Kean, B. H., Gilmore, H. R., Jr., Van Stone, W. W. Fatal amebiasis: Report of 148 fatal cases from the Armed Forces Institutes of Pathology. *Ann. Intern. Med.* **44:**831–843, 1956.
66. Evans, T. C. The surgical aspect of amoebiasis. *Trans. R. Soc. Trop. Med. Hyg.* **19:**282–311, 1925.
67. Ochsner, A., DeBakey, M. Surgical amebiasis. *New Int. Clin.* **1:**68–99, 1942.
68. Hawe, P. The surgical aspect of intestinal amebiasis. *Surg. Gynecol. Obstet.* **81:**387–404, 1945.
69. Barker, E. M. Colonic perforations in amoebiasis. *S. Afr. Med. J.* **32:**634–638, 1958.
70. Sawitz, W. G., Faust, E. C. The probability of detecting intestinal protozoa by successive stool examinations. *Am. J. Trop. Med.* **22:**131–136, 1942.
71. Stamm, W. P., II. The laboratory diagnosis of clinical amoebiasis. *Trans. R. Soc. Trop. Med. Hyg.* **51:**306–312, 1957.
72. Rail, G. A. The use of the sigmoidoscope in the diagnosis and prognosis of amoebic dysentery. *J. Trop. Med. Hyg.* **49:**68–69, 1946.
73. Healy, G. R. Laboratory diagnosis of amebiasis. *Bull. N.Y. Acad. Med.* **47:**478–493, 1971.
74. Reller, L. B. Rivas, E. N., Masferrer, R., *et al.* Epidemic Shiga-bacillus dysentery in Central America: Evolution of the outbreak in El Salvador, 1969–70. *Am. J. Trop. Med. Hyg.* **20:**934–940, 1971.
75. Cifarelli, P. S. Acute amebic colitis: Prospective analysis. *N.Y. State J. Med.* **69:**815–818, 1969.
76. Healy, G. R., Kagan, I. G., Melvin, D. M. Parasitic infections. In H. L. Bodily (ed.), *Diagnostic Procedures for Bacterial, Mycotic and Parasitic Infections.* American Public Health Association, New York, 1970, pp. 724–790.
77. Sapero, J. J., Lawless, D. K. The "MIF" stain-preservation technic for the identification of intestinal protozoa. *Am. J. Trop. Med.* **2:**613–619, 1953.
78. Alger, N. A simple, rapid, precise stain for intestinal protozoa. *Am. J. Clin. Pathol.* **45:**361–362, 1966.
79. Tompkins, V. N., Miller, J. K. Staining intestinal protozoa with iron–hematoxylin–phosphotungstic acid. *Am. J. Clin. Pathol.* **17:**755–758, 1947.
80. Gleason, N. N., Goldman, M., Carver, R. K. Size and nuclear morphology of *Entamoeba histolytica* and *Entamoeba hartmanni* trophozoites in culture and in man. *Am. J. Hyg.* **77:**1–14, 1963.
81. Brooke, M. M. Laboratory diagnosis of amebiasis. *Proc. VI Congr. Trop. Med.* **3:**369–384, 1958.
82. Miyamoto, A. T., Thadepalli, H., Mishkin, F. S. [67]Gallium images of amebic liver abscess. *N. Engl. J. Med.* **291:**1363, 1974.
83. Matthews, A. W., Gough, K. R., Rhys Davies, E., *et al.* The use of combined ultrasonic and isotope scanning in the diagnosis of amoebic liver disease. *Gut* **14:**50–53, 1973.
84. Taylor, A. E. R., Baker, J. R. *The Cultivation of Parasites In Vitro.* Blackwell, Scientific Publishers, Oxford, 1968, pp. 377.
85. Diamond, L. S. Axenic cultivation of *Entamoeba histolytica. Science* **134:**336–337, 1961.
86. Cleveland, L. R., Collier, J. The various improvements in the cultivation of *Entamoeba histolytica. Am. J. Hyg.* **12:**606–613, 1930.

87. Balamuth, W. Improved egg yolk infusion for cultivation of *Entamoeba histolytica* and other intestinal protozoa. *Am. J. Clin. Pathol.* **16**:380–384, 1946.
88. Nelson, E. C. Alcoholic extract medium for the diagnosis and cultivation of *Endamoeba histolytica. Am. J. Trop. Med.* **27**:545–552, 1947.
89. McQuay, R. M. Charcoal medium for growth and maintenance of large and small races of *Entamoeba histolytica. Am. J. Clin. Pathol.* **26**:1137–1141, 1956.
90. McQuay, R. M. Parasitologic studies in a group of furloughed missionaries: 1. Intestinal protozoa. *Am. J. Trop. Med. Hyg.* **16**:154–160, 1967.
91. Robinson, G. L. The laboratory diagnosis of human parasitic amoebae. *Trans. R. Soc. Trop. Med. Hyg.* **62**:285–294, 1968.
92. Mahajan, R. C., Ganguly, N. K., Datta, D. V. Diagnosis of hepatic amoebiasis. *Lancet* **1**:651, 1976.
93. Craig, C. F. Observations upon the hemolytic, cytolytic and complement-binding properties of extracts of *Endamoeba histolytica. Am. J. Trop. Med.* **7**:225–240, 1927.
94. Craig, C. F. Complement fixation in the diagnosis of infections with *Endamoeba histolytica. Am. J. Trop. Med.* **8**:29–37, 1928.
95. Biagi, F. F., Buentello, L. Immobilization reaction for the diagnosis of amebiasis. *Exp. Parasitol* **11**:188–190, 1961.
96. Keesel, J. F., Lewis, W. P., Pasquel, C. M., *et al.* Indirect hemagglutination and complement fixation tests in amebiasis. *Am. J. Trop. Med. Hyg.* **14**:540–550, 1965.
97. Maddison, S. E., Powell, S. J., Elsdon-Dew, R. Application of serology to the epidemiology of amebiasis. *Am. J. Trop. Med. Hyg.* **14**:554–557, 1965.
98. Morris, M. N., Powell, S. J., Eldson-Dew, R. Latex agglutination test for invasive amoebiasis. *Lancet* **1**:1362–1363, 1970.
99. Goldman, M. Evaluation of a fluorescent antibody test for amebiasis, using two widely differing ameba strains as antigen. *Am. J. Trop. Med. Hyg.* **15**:694–700, 1966.
100. Krupp, I. M. Comparison of counterimmunoelectrophoresis with other serologic tests in the diagnosis of amebiasis. *Am. J. Trop. Med. Hyg.* **23**:27–30, 1974.
101. Patterson, M., Healy, G. R., Shabot, J. M. Serologic testing for amoebiasis. *Gastroenterology* **78**:136–141, 1980.
102. Juniper, K., Jr., Worrell, C. L., Minshew, M. C., *et al.* Serologic diagnosis of amebiasis. *Am. J. Trop. Med. Hyg.* **21**:157–168, 1972.
103. Krupp, I., Antibody response in intestinal and extraintestinal amebiasis. *Am. J. Trop. Med. Hyg.* **19**:57–62, 1970.
104. Milgram, E. A., Healy, G. R., Kagan, I. G. Studies on the use of the indirect hemagglutination test in the diagnosis of amebiasis. *Gastroenterology* **50**:645–649, 1966.
105. Healy, G. R., Kraft, S. C. The indirect hemagglutination test for amebiasis in patients with inflammatory bowel disease. *Am. J. Dig. Dis.* **17**:97–104, 1972.
106. Healy, G. R., Kagan, I. G., Gleason, N. N. Use of the indirect hemagglutination test in some studies of seroepidemiology of amebiasis in the Western Hemisphere. *Health Lab. Sci.* **7**:109–116, 1970.
107. Rogers, L. The rapid cure of amoebic dysentery and hepatitis by hypodermic injections of soluble salts of emetine. *Br. Med. J.* **1**:1424–1425, 1912.
108. Scott, F., Miller, M. J. Trials with metronidazole in amebic dysentery. *J. Am. Med. Assoc.* **211**:118–120, 1970.
109. Powell, S. J. Therapy of amebiasis. *Bull. N. Y. Acad. Med.* **47**:469–477, 1971.
110. Powell, S. J., Elsdon-Dew, R. Evaluation of metronidazole and MK-910 in invasive amebiasis. *Am. J. Trop. Med. Hyg.* **20**:839–841, 1971.
111. Griffin, F. M., Jr. Failure of metronidazole to cure hepatic amebic abscess. *N. Engl. J. Med.* **288**:1397, 1973.
112. Henn, R. M., Collin, D. B. Amebic abscess of the liver: Treatment failure with metronidazole. *J. Am. Med. Assoc.* **224**:1394–1395, 1973.

113. Stillman, A. E., Alvarez, V., Grube, D. Hepatic amebic abscess: Unresponsiveness to combination of metronidazole and surgical drainage. *J. Am. Med. Assoc.* **229**:71–72, 1974.
114. Weber, D. M. Amebic abscess of liver following metronidazole therapy. *J. Am. Med. Assoc.* **216**:1339–1340, 1971.
115. Pittman, F. E., Pittman, J. C. Amebic liver abscess following metronidazole therapy for amebic colitis. *Am. J. Trop. Med. Hyg.* **23**:146–150, 1974.
116. Powell, S. J., Elsdon-Dew, R. Chloroquine in amoebic dysentery. *Trans. R. Soc. Trop. Med. Hyg.* **65**:540, 1971.
117. Pittman, F. E., Westphal, M. C. Optic atrophy following treatment with diiodohydroxyquin. *Pediatrics* **54**:81–83, 1974.
118. Warning on diiodohydroxyquin. *Med. Lett. Drugs Ther.* **16**:71–72, 1974.
119. Wolfe, M. S. Nondysenteric intestinal amebiasis: Treatment with diloxanide furoate. *J. Am. Med. Assoc.* **224**:1601–1604, 1973.
120. Is Flagyl dangerous? *Med. Lett. Drugs Ther.* **17**:53–54, 1975.
121. Most, H. Treatment of common parasitic infections of man encountered in the United States: 2. *N. Engl. J. Med.* **287**:698–702, 1972.
122. Schwartz, D. E., Herrero, J. Comparative pharmacokinetic studies of dehydroemetine and emetine in guinea pigs using spectrofluorometric and radiometric methods. *Am. J. Trop. Med.* **14**:78–83, 1965.
123. MacLeod, I. N., Powell, S. J., Wilmot, A. J. Hepatic amoebiasis. *Br. Med. J.* **2**:827, 1966.
124. Powell, S. J. Drug therapy of amoebiasis. *Bull. W.H.O.* **40**:953–956, 1969.
125. Theron, P. Surgical aspects of amoebiasis. *Br. Med. J.* **2**:123–126, 1947.
126. Stein, D., Bank, S. Surgery in amoebic colitis. *Gut* **11**:941–946, 1970.
127. Hughes, F. B., Faehnle, S. T., Simon, J. L. Multiple cerebral abscesses complicating hepathopulmonary amebiasis. *J. Pediatr.* **86**:95–96, 1975.

3

Giardiasis

INTRODUCTION

Giardia lamblia, a flagellated protozoan, was described in detail by Lambl in 1859.[1] Although Lambl is credited with the discovery, Leeuwenhoek actually may have been the first to describe the agent in his own diarrheal stool in 1681.[1] Initially, the agent was felt to be a normal inhabitant of the upper intestinal tract of humans,[2] and it was considered to be nonpathogenic. Major support for its low-grade pathogenicity was offered by the finding of asymptomatic cyst excretion in nearly 10% of persons throughout the world. In the 1950s, a series of volunteer experiments[3,4] established the infectivity of the protozoan. During the last two decades, *G. lamblia* has been shown to be an important cause of acute diarrhea in certain high-risk populations (particularly, American travelers to the Soviet Union, those traveling to developing parts of the world, and persons visiting ski resorts or camping areas of the Rocky Mountains) as well as the causative agent of recurrent and/or chronic diarrhea and malabsorption in all parts of the world.

PATHOGENESIS

Drinking of contaminated water is the most common way in which the infective cysts reach the target organ. In other situations, hand-to-food-to-mouth or hand-to-mouth transmission may occur from a cyst excretor to a susceptible individual. The inoculum size necessary to induce infection is low. Rendtorff[3] reported that 8 of 22 adult volunteers (36%) became infected after ingestion of 10–25 *G. lamblia* cysts. In another experiment, *G. lamblia* was shown to remain viable and infective

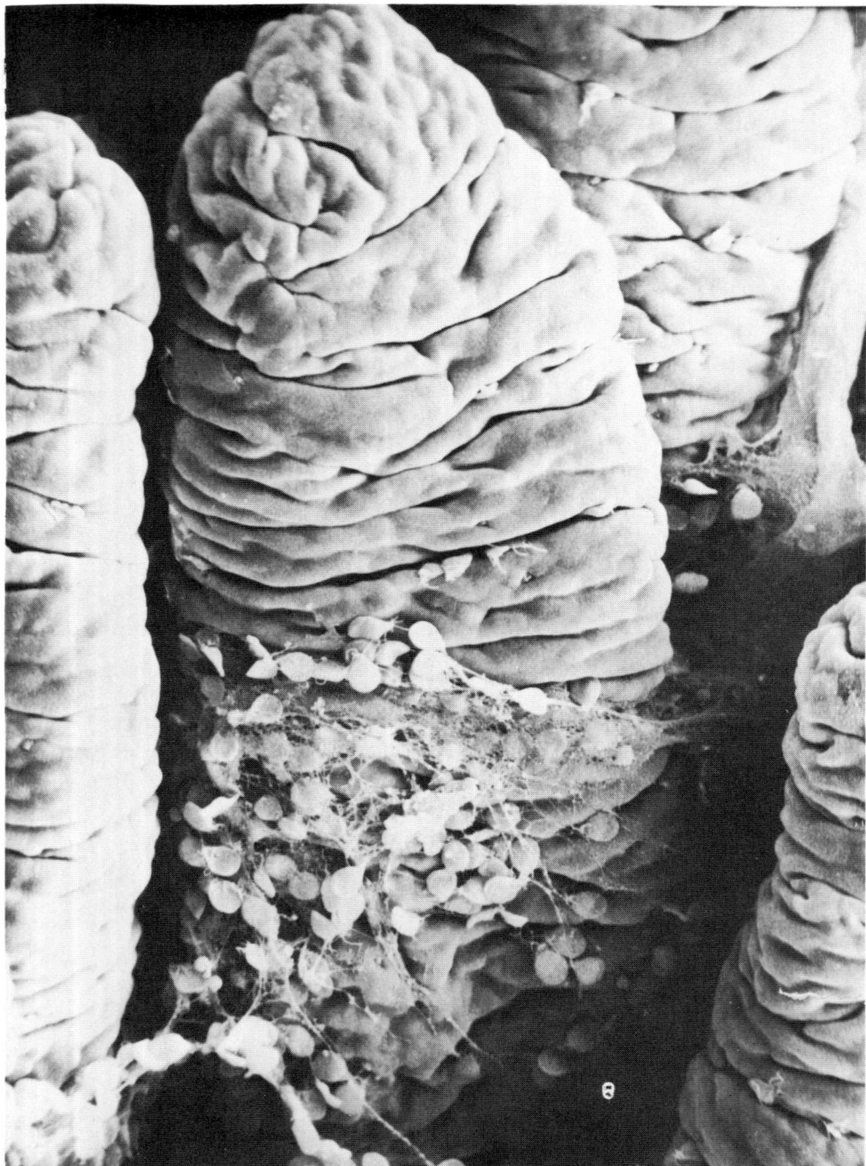

Figure 3.1. During acute infection in the mouse, *Giardia* hover in the mucus coat, wedge into furrows, or cling to the surfaces of jejunal villi with their adhesive disks (×708). Reprinted from Owen *et al.*[89]

for at least 16 days in tap water stored at 8°C,[4] indicating the stability of the infective cysts.

After ingestion, the organisms encyst in the upper small intestine, and each divides into two trophozoites which subsequently mature. In the infected person, the trophozoites line the small-intestinal mucosa and may interfere with absorption through mechanical means (Figure 3.1). Neither the density of the protozoans nor the degree of mucosal injury as found on biopsy completely correlates with the degree of symptomatology. There appears to be a correlation between intraepithelial lymphocyte counts and occurrence of malabsorption.[5] The sucking disk of the trophozoite has been shown by electron microscopy to produce damage to the small-bowel microvilli.[6,7] Histologically, focal areas of acute inflammation in the lamina propria and epithelium of the jejunal crypts and villi are found.[7,8] Polymorphonuclear leukocytes and eosinophils can be found between epithelial cells. Invasion of the trophozoites through the epithelium to the lamina propria may occur[6,9,10] and should be suspected in any person with steatorrhea or chronic diarrhea.[10] Occasionally, severe atrophy of jejunal mucosa with dense plasma cell infiltrate, with or without an underlying immunologic disorder, may occur.[11–13] The mucosal atrophy generally is reversible with therapy.[13] Patients with immunoglobulin deficiency may develop total villous atrophy in association with a *Giardia* infection.[14,15] Patients with giardiasis may have segmental involvement, so that multiple biopsies will be needed to show the intestinal lesion.[15]

Children appear to be more susceptible to *Giardia* than adults.[16–18] Conditions other than age which predispose to giardiasis are hypogammaglobulinemia, particularly where there is a deficiency in secretory IgA,[11,19,20] peptic ulcer, biliary tract disease, and pancreatitis.[21] Reduced gastric hydrochloric acid secretion as is seen in hypochlorhydria, achlorhydria, or following gastric resection has been shown to predispose patients to giardiasis.[16,20,22,23]

Disaccharidase deficiency, depression of other intestinal enzymes, and defects in vitamin B_{12} absorption have been described in patients with giardiasis.[24] Usually these intestinal changes are transient and disappear after treatment, although persistent carbohydrate intolerance may occur after successful treatment of the parasite.[14] As in other forms of acute infectious diarrhea involving the small bowel, an overgrowth of bacteria may occur in the upper gut of patients with giardiasis.[8,25] This overgrowth syndrome may contribute to the diarrhea and malabsorption.[25] In developing parts of the world, malnutrition contributes to the pathogenesis of giardiasis, and improvement in nutritional status may correct the associated malabsorption.[26] Intestinal plasma cells produce IgM early in infection,[27,28] followed by IgA and IgG production later in the evolution of the disease.[28] A role for locally produced immunoglobulin in giardial immunity has not been established.

EPIDEMIOLOGY

The causative agent is a ubiquitous protozoan which has worldwide distribution. Areas where the disease is hyperendemic are the Soviet Union (particularly in Leningrad),[29-32] the Rocky Mountain area of the United States,[33,34] Europe,[35,36] the Caribbean, and Latin America. *Giardia* infection is undoubtedly a more important cause of acute endemic diarrhea in the United States than appreciated.[34] The major reservoir of giardiasis appears to be water,[29,30,32,37-43] undoubtedly contaminated with human waste or possibly that from lower mammals.[38] One large community outbreak of giardiasis occurred in Rome, New York, and was traced to the municipal water supply which was contaminated with *Giardia*.[41] Because of the sparsity of humans in many remote regions of the Rocky Mountain area, it has been felt that contamination of surface water by lower mammals may explain the reservoir in these areas. Beavers appear to be particularly important carriers of *G. lamblia*.[38] Transmission may less commonly occur after ingestion of contaminated uncooked foods[44] or by direct person-to-person spread.[45,46]

The percentage of carriers of *G. lamblia* in the United States has been estimated at 3–7%[18,33,47] and as high as 20% for the southern part of the country.[18] The extent of person-to-person spread has not been established. Common-source outbreaks are most frequent, and while person-to-person spread has been uncommon in some studies,[40] secondary and tertiary contact spread were documented in others.[48]

Epidemics of giardiasis among infants and children in hospital nurseries,[49] custodial and residential institutions,[50,51] and day-care centers[52] have been reported. Person-to-person spread appears to be the most likely mode of transmission in these settings.[50,52] Transmission to ward helpers and family contacts was documented during these outbreaks.[49,52]

CLINICAL ASPECTS

The average incubation period in giardiasis is 8 days, with a range of 3–42 days.[31] Clinical manifestations are unpredictable[43] and vary from a total lack of symptomatology to an acute short-lasting diarrheal syndrome to a chronic or recurrent malabsorption syndrome. Patients usually have a short-lasting acute diarrheal disease with or without low-grade fever, nausea, and anorexia, while a small percentage develop an intermittent or more protracted course characterized by diarrhea, cramping, abdominal pain, bloating, and flatulence. In a series of 324 patients with giardiasis,[29] the frequency of occurrence of clinical symptoms was: diarrhea, 96%; weight loss, 62%; abdominal cramps, 61%; greasy stools, 57%; flatulence,

35%; vomiting, 29%; belching, 26%; and fever, 17%. Similar percentages have been reported in another study.[54]

Malabsorption is common in giardiasis and may be due to mucosal injury,[78] to a physical barrier to adsorption created by the shear numbers of *G. lamblia* trophozoites lining the intestinal surface,[6,55] to altered motility[56] with an intestinal stasis syndrome,[8] or to a competition between the protozoans and the host for nutrients and vitamins.[24,57] Diarrhea with or without overt malabsorption commonly lasts months or even years.[58] In addition to fat malabsorption, patients with giardiasis may have intolerance to meat.[59] The *Giardia* cysts usually disappear from stools after several weeks but may persist for more than several months.[3]

Giardiasis should be considered in any patient with protracted or intermittent symptoms, particularly, associated malabsorption, foul-smelling stools, flatulence, or weight loss. Although eosinophilia is not part of the syndrome, we have seen one patient with biopsy-proven giardiasis who gave an eight-year history of episodic explosive diarrhea associated with urticarial reactions and fever who experienced eosinophila (10 –20% of peripheral leukocytes) during his bouts of diarrhea. He responded to a standard course of metronidazole. Along with other enteropathogens, *G. lamblia* may have a venereal mode of transmission among male homosexuals.[60–62] Both giardial proctitis and acute watery diarrhea may be the forms of disease encountered. Fecal–oral[61] and fecal–rectal[60] modes of spread have been implicated.

DIAGNOSIS

There exists a differing opinion with regard to the efficiency of direct stool examination in diagnosing giardiasis (see Figures 3.2–3.4 for the appearance of the cysts and trophozoites of *G. lamblia*). Some say that the great majority of cases (76%) can be properly diagnosed by a single examination of a stool specimen, with the probability of proper diagnosis increased (90%) by a second examination,[63] while others have indicated the difficulty of making the diagnosis even after repeated examination of stool specimens.[15,64] One study indicated that stools are commonly negative for the causative agent early in the infection.[31] In certain cases with negative results on stool examination, it may be necessary to wait up to three weeks after exposure to *G. lamblia* to repeat the stool examination before assuming that the diagnosis is not giardiasis. Stool examination was compared to small-bowel aspiration in patients with diarrhea, and the protozoan was found in only 50% of stools where a small-bowel locus of infection was documented.[65] Also, in many cases, persons excrete the cysts intermittently, with cycles of negativity lasting as long as 2–30

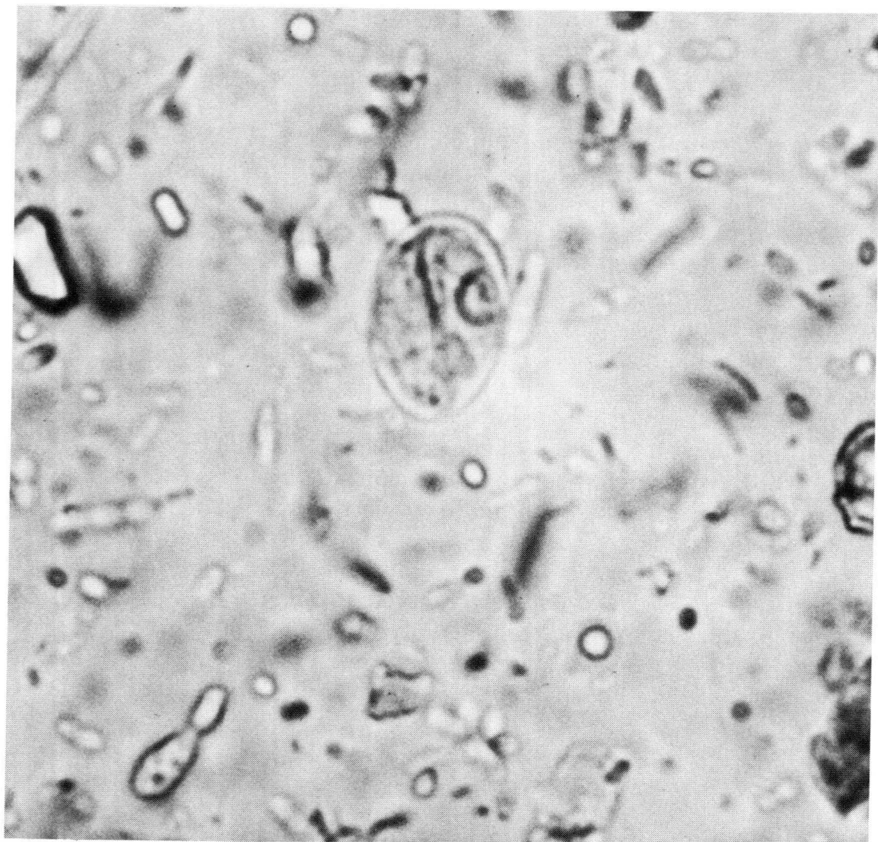

Figure 3.2. Cyst of *Giardia lamblia* in an MIF-stained preparation from clinical material. Note the characteristic oval shape of the organism and the retraction of cytoplasm from some parts of the cyst wall (×1000). Material kindly furnished by Mr. Bernard J. Marino of the Houston City Health Department.

days.[66,67] Antibiotics, antacids, and antidiarrheal compounds may cause a temporary disappearance of parasites from stool or interfere with recognition of the parasites. Purgatives have not improved the rate of *Giardia* identification in a collected stool specimens.[67]

The sensitivity of stool examination can be improved by using a zinc sulfate concentration technique.[47] In cases where the diagnosis is suggested and stools are negative, aspiration and/or biopsy of the duodenum or upper jejunum should be performed. Since the organism lives in the upper intestine, this procedure is more reliable than examination of stool specimens.[15,65] The importance of duodenal aspiration in making the di-

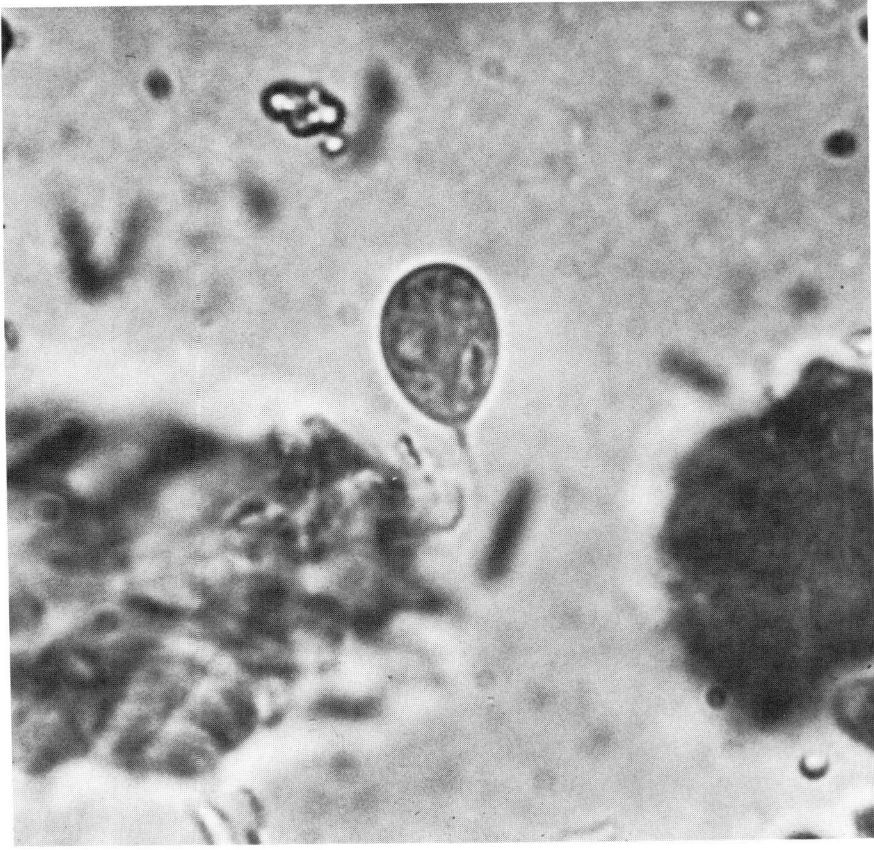

Figure 3.3. Precystic trophozoite form of *Giardia lamblia* in an iodine-stained preparation from a clinical specimen showing a single external flagellum ($\times$1000). Material kindly furnished by Mr. Bernard J. Marino of the Houston City Health Department.

agnosis of giardiasis is not a new observation.[2] Duodenal biopsy probably represents the optimal means of diagnosing giardiasis, where a touch preparation from mucus adhering to the biopsy section[65] is stained with Giemsa's or Masson's trichrome stain after fixation in Bouin's solution.[9] Electron microscopic examination of intestinal material may be useful in nondiagnostic cases.[68] An alternative method is the commercially available Entero-test (produced by Hedeco, Mountain View, California 94043), where a nylon string is affixed to a weighted gelatin capsule and swallowed. Four hours later, the string is withdrawn, and duodenal contents (bile-stained mucus adherent to the string) are examined microscopically for *G. lamblia.*[69–71] In selected cases, it may be advisable to

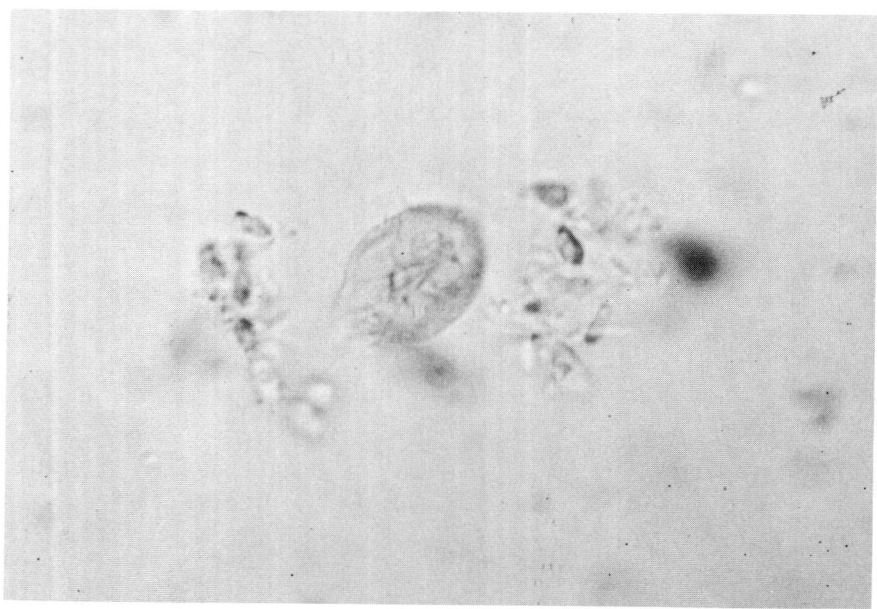

Figure 3.4. *Giardia lamblia* trophozoite in an MIF-stained preparation from a small-bowel aspirate of a patient with acute diarrhea (×1000). Note the pear-shaped body with two large subspherical nuclei within the bilaterally symmetrical organism.

administer secretin intravenously (Secretin-Boots, Warren-Teed Pharmaceuticals, Inc., distributor, Columbus, Ohio 43215) before studying duodenal juice for *G. lamblia*.[72] The optimal pH for survival of *G. lamblia* trophozoites is 6–7,[73] and the agent is actively destroyed when the pH of duodenal contents is lowered.[45] Secretin stimulates the pancreas to produce a watery alkaline juice, raising the pH of duodenal contents, and it also reduces gut motility. An altered small-bowel pattern is seen on X ray in giardiasis.[47,56,74]

TREATMENT

The key to treatment is proper laboratory diagnosis. Because of the occasional difficulty in establishing the diagnosis, some have advised empiric therapy despite the absence of laboratory confirmation in settings where diagnosis is likely.[53] Quinacrine (Atabrine), given in a dosage of 100 mg t.i.d. for seven days, is the optimal form of therapy in adults with laboratory-confirmed giardiasis and will result in a cure rate of 95–100%.[63,74–76] The pediatric dosage is 7 mg/kg daily (maximum 300 mg/

day) in three divided doses for seven days. Quinacrine is significantly less expensive than metronidazole. Important side effects of quinacrine are toxic psychosis, yellow staining of skin and sclera, and exfoliative dermatitis. Metronidazole (Flagyl) is a suitable alternative agent, although it is not currently licensed for use in treatment of giardiasis. It is given in a dosage of 250 mg t.i.d. for ten days for adults and 20 mg/kg daily (maximum 750 mg/day) in divided doses for ten days for children. While the cure rate in giardiasis may be slightly lower for metronidazole compared to quinacrine (95% vs. 100%),[76] metronidazole probably is better tolerated and may have other, non-*Giardia* antimicrobial activity which may prove beneficial. Some have suggested that metronidazole be considered the treatment of choice.[77,78] It has been used successfully in a dosage of 2 g daily for three days.[79] It is our current practice to employ quinacrine in clear-cut cases of giardiasis but to prescribe metronidazole for patients treated empirically without a definitive diagnosis. Both quinacrine and metronidazole are available only in pill form, requiring special formulation into a liquid or powder preparation for use with small children. The bitter taste of these preparations may make therapy of children difficult, if not impossible, due to lack of compliance.

The third available drug is furazolidone, which may or may not be less effective than the other two.[76,80] However, it is available in a liquid preparation which children can tolerate. The significantly lower cost of furazolidone is an advantage, particularly in developing countries. Patients, particularly those with more protracted symptoms, may, on occasion, fail to respond to a course of these recommended therapies. Such individuals may not have *Giardia* in stool, but duodenal aspirates will remain positive. Other patients may become asymptomatic after quinacrine, only to have a recurrence at some later time. Multiple courses of therapy, perhaps using alternative drugs, would be indicated. Tinidazole may prove to be the most efficacious drug and may be useful even in a single oral dose, although it is not yet licensed for use.[81–83] It does not produce gastric side effects. Other newer agents with antigiardial activity, such as nimorazole and ornidazole, will be tested in future studies.

One of the difficulties in clinical drug trials is the fact that the illness is usually self-limiting and that *Giardia* tend to disappear spontaneously without treatment[3,66] and may recur later after an interval of 20–30 days.[66] There is a dispute over whether persons without symptoms should receive therapy. Most say that asymptomatic cyst excretors should be treated since they are the usual reservoir of infection.[63] A less prevalent opinion is that the organism is ubiquitous, that asymptomatic infection is common and short-lived, and that treatment is unnecessary.[66] Table 3.1 presents a summary of antimicrobial agents used for the treatment of giardiasis.

TABLE 3.1
Antimicrobial Therapy of Giardiasis

Drug	Dosage and duration		Comment
	Children	Adults	
Quinacrine (Atabrine)	7 mg/kg/day (p.o.) in equally divided doses t.i.d. for 7 days (maximum 300 mg/day)	100 mg (p.o.) t.i.d. for 7 days	Most effective drug for laboratory-confirmed giardiasis; low cost
Metronidazole (Flagyl)	20 mg/kg/day (p.o.) in equally divided doses q.i.d. for 10 days (maximum 750 mg/day)	250 mg (p.o.) t.i.d. for 10 days	Perhaps the best choice for empirical therapy of unconfirmed cases; not approved by FDA
Furazolidone (Furoxone)	5 mg/kg/day (p.o.) in divided doses q.i.d. for 7 days	100 mg (p.o.) q.i.d. for 7 days	Slightly less effective; low cost; available as a liquid for use in pediatrics

IMMUNITY

Despite the ubiquity of the agent in nature and the undoubtedly common occurrence of exposure, humans are extremely susceptible to infection, which indicates that immunity is, at best, relative. In volunteer studies, all 13 adults males ingesting 10^2–10^6 cysts became ill,[3] verifying the susceptibility of humans to *G. lamblia.* Acquired immunity of a relative degree appears to occur, since short-term residents in Colorado have a higher rate of infection than long-term residents.[84]

An antigen for serologic evaluation of infection was prepared from *G. lamblia* obtained from duodenal juice, from jejunal biopsies, and from *G. lamblia* cysts of patients giardiasis.[27] Employing an indirect immunofluorescent antibody procedure, Ridley and Ridley were able to document a humoral immune response to infection, particularly in those patients with malabsorption (89% were positive), which could be correlated roughly with the degree of histologic involvement of the intestine.[27] The test may be impractical in view of the difficulty in obtaining a satisfactory cyst antigen. Improved techniques are being established.[85] Now that techniques for artificial cultivation of *Giardia* are being developed,[86] a ready supply of antigen may be produced, and serologic studies may be forthcoming. A model of murine giardiasis (due to *Giardia muris*) has been developed[87] in which animals were shown to develop prolonged resistance after a primary infection.

PREVENTION

Infection is best prevented by avoiding the ingestion of tap water in high-risk areas such as the Soviet Union or of surface water in Rocky Mountain states. Water can be rendered noninfective if it is boiled for 10 min or if treated with iodine solutions.[40,63] Chlorinating per se may not inactivate the cysts,[37,41] but properly functioning water treatment systems employing sedimentation, flocculation, and filtration should successfully remove *Giardia* cysts from water.[88] Uncooked or unpeeled fruits and vegetables may be sources of infection in areas of endemicity.

REFERENCES

1. Dobell, C. A. The discovery of intestinal protozoa in man. *Proc. R. Soc. Med.* **13:**1–5, 1920.
2. Paulson, M., Andrews, J. The incidence of human intestinal protozoa in duodenal aspirates. *J. Am. Med. Assoc.* **94:**2063–2065, 1930.
3. Rendtorff, R. C. The experimental transmission of human intestinal protozoan parasites: II. *Giardia lamblia* cysts given in capsules. *Am. J. Hyg.* **59:**209–220, 1954.
4. Rendtorff, R. C., Holt, C. J. The experimental transmission of human intestinal protozoan parasites: IV. Attempts to transmit *Endamoeba coli* and *Giardia lamblia* cysts by water. *Am. J. Hyg.* **60:**327–338, 1954.
5. Wright, S. G., Tomkins, A. M. Quantification of the lymphocytic infiltrate in jejunal epithelium in giardiasis. *Clin. Exp. Immunol.* **29:**408–412, 1977.
6. Morecki, R., Parker, J. G. Ultrastructural studies of the human *Giardia lamblia* and subjacent jejunal mucosa in a subject with steatorrhea. *Gastroenterology* **52:**151–164, 1967.
7. Takano, J., Yardley, J. H. Jejunal lesions in patients with giardiasis and malabsorption: An electron microscopic study. *Bul. Johns Hopkins Hosp.* **116:**413–429, 1965.
8. Yardley, J. H., Takano, J., Hendrix, T. R. Epithelial and other mucosal lesions of the jejunum in giardiasis: Jejunal biopsy studies. *Bull. Johns Hopkins Hosp.* **115:**389–406, 1964.
9. Brandborg, L. L., Tankersley, C. B., Gottlieb, S., *et al.* Histological demonstration of mucosal invasion by *Giardia lamblia* in man. *Gastroenterology* **52:**143–150, 1967.
10. Saha, T. K., Ghosh, T. K. Invasion of small intestinal mucosa by *Giardia lamblia* in man. *Gastroenterology* **72:**402–405, 1977.
11. Hermans, P. E., Huizenga, K. A., Hoffman, H. N., *et al.* Dysgammaglobulinemia associated with nodular lymphoid hyperplasia of the small intestine. *Am. J. Med.* **40:**78–89, 1966.
12. Levinson, J. D., Nastro, L. J. Giardiasis with total villous atrophy. *Gastroenterology* **74:**271–275, 1978.
13. Blenkinsopp, W. K., Gibson, J. A., Haffenden, G. P. Giardiasis and severe jejunal abnormality. *Lancet* **1:**994, 1978.
14. Hoskins, L. C., Winawer, S. J., Broitman, S. A., *et al.* Clinical giardiasis and intestinal malabsorption. *Gastroenterology* **53:**265–279, 1967.
15. Ament, M. E., Rubin, C. E. Relation of giardiasis to abnormal intestinal structure and

function in gastrointestinal immunodeficiency syndromes. *Gastroenterology* **62**:216–226, 1972.

16. Yardley, J. H., Bayless, T. M. Giardiasis. *Gastroenterology* **52**:301–304, 1967.
17. Veghelyi, P. Giardiasis in children. *Am. J. Dis. Child.* **56**:1231–1241, 1938.
18. Cortner, J. A. Giardiasis, a cause of celiac syndrome. *Am. J. Dis. Child.* **98**:311–316, 1959.
19. Zinneman, H. H., Kaplan, A. P. The association of giardiasis with reduced intestinal secretory immunoglobulin A. *Am. J. Dig. Dis.* **17**:793–797, 1972.
20. Wolfe, M. S. Giardiasis. *J. Am. Med. Assoc.* **233**:1362–1365, 1975.
21. Sheehy, T. W., Holley, H. P., Jr. *Giardia*-induced malabsorption in pancreatitis. *J. Am. Med. Assoc.* **233**:1373–1375, 1975.
22. Vachon, A., Paliard, P., Moulinier, B., *et al.* Diagnostic par biopsie jéjunale d'une diarrhée chronique à lamblia avec syndrome de dénutrition (2 observations). [Diagnosis by jejunal biopsy of chronic lamblia diarrhea with a denutrition syndrome. 2 cases.] *Arch. Mal. Appar. Dig.* **52**:355–359, 1963.
23. Slonim, J. M., Ireton, H. J., Smallwood, R. A. Giardiasis following gastric surgery. *Aust. N.Z. J. Med.* **6**:479–480, 1976.
24. Cowen, A. E., Campbell, C. B. Giardiasis—A cause of vitamin B_{12} malabsorption. *Am. J. Dig. Dis.* **18**:384–390, 1973.
25. Tandon, B. N., Tandon, R. K., Satpathy, B. K., *et al.* Mechanism of malabsorption in giardiasis: A study of bacterial flora and bile salt deconjunction in upper jejunum. *Gut* **18**:176–181, 1977.
26. Mayoral, L. G., Tripathy, K., Garcia, F. T., *et al.* Intestinal malabsorption and parasitic disease: The role of protein malnutrition (abstract). *Gastroenterology* **50**:856–857, 1966.
27. Ridley, M. J., Ridley, D. S. Serum antibodies and jejunal histology in giardiasis associated with malabsorption. *J. Clin. Pathol.* **29**:30–34, 1976.
28. Thompson, A., Rowland, R., Hecker, R., *et al.* Immunoglobulin-bearing cells in giardiasis (letter). *J. Clin. Pathol.* **30**:292–294, 1977.
29. Brodsky, R. E., Spencer, H. C., Jr., Schultz, M. G. Giardiasis in American travelers to the Soviet Union. *J. Infect. Dis.* **130**:319–323, 1974.
30. Jokipii, L., Jokipii, A. M. Giardiasis in travelers: A prospective study. *J. Infect. Dis.* **130**:295–299, 1974.
31. Jokipii, A. M., Jokipii, L. Prepatency of giardiasis. *Lancet* **1**:1095–1097, 1977.
32. United States Department of Health, Education and Welfare, Center for Disease Control. *Giardia lamblia* infection in travelers to the Soviet Union. *Morbid. Mortal. Week. Rep.* **23**:78–79, 1974.
33. Schultz, M. G. Giardiasis (editorial). *J. Am. Med. Assoc.* **233**:1383–1384, 1975.
34. Wanner, R. G., Atchley, F. O., Wasley, M. A. Association of diarrhea with *Giardia lamblia* in families observed weekly for occurrence of enteric infections. *Am. J. Trop. Med. Hyg.* **12**:851–853, 1963.
35. Thompson, R. G., Karandikar, D. S., Leek, J. Giardiasis, an unusual cause of epidemic diarrhoea. *Lancet* **1**:615–616, 1974.
36. Andersson, T., Forssell, J., Sterner, G. Outbreak of giardiasis: Effect of a new antiflagellate drug, tinidazole. *Br. Med. J.* **2**:449–451, 1972.
37. Moore, G. T., Cross, W. M., McGuire, D., *et al.* Epidemic giardiasis at a ski resort. *N. Engl. J. Med.* **281**:402–407, 1969.
38. United States Department of Health, Education and Welfare, Center for Disease Control. Waterborne giardiasis outbreaks—Washington, New Hampshire. *Morbid. Mortal. Week. Rep.* **26**:169–170, 175, 1977.
39. Brady, P. G., Wolfe, J. C. Waterborne giardiasis. *Ann. Intern. Med.* **81**:498–499, 1974.

40. Wright, R. A., Spencer, H. C., Brodsky, R. E., *et al.* Giardiasis in Colorado: An epidemiologic study. *Am. J. Epidemiol.* **105**:330–336, 1977.

41. Shaw, P. K., Brodsky, R. E., Lyman, D. O., *et al.* A communitywide outbreak of giardiasis with evidence of transmission by a municipal water supply. *Ann. Intern. Med.* **87**:426–432, 1977.

42. Wright, R. A Giardial infection from water (letter). *Ann. Intern. Med.* **82**:589–590, 1975.

43. Horowitz, M. A., Hughes, J. M., Craun, G. F. Outbreaks of waterborn disease in the United States. 1974. *J. Infect. Dis.* **133**:588–593, 1976.

44. Bryan, F. L. Diseases transmitted by foods. *USDHEW Publ.* No. (CDC) 75-8237, 1975, p. 21.

45. Petersen, H. Giardiasis (lambliasis). *Scand. J. Gastroenterol.* **7**(Suppl. 14):1–44, 1972.

46. Belding, D. L. *Textbook of Parasitology*, 3rd ed. Appleton-Century-Crofts, New York, 1965, p. 126.

47. Mahmoud, A. A., Warren, K. S. Algorithms in the diagnosis and management of exotic diseases: II. Giardiasis. *J. Infect. Dis* **131**:621–624, 1975.

48. Kettis, A. A., Thoren, G. Inter- and intrafamilial distribution of *Giardia lamblia* infection. *Scand. J. Infect. Dis.* **6**:349–353, 1974.

49. Ormiston, G., Taylor, J., Wilson, G. S. Enteritis in a nursery home associated with *Giardia lamblia*. *Br. Med. J.* **2**:151–154, 1942.

50. Brown, E. H *Giardia lamblia*. The incidence and results of infestation of children in residential nurseries. *Arch. Dis. Child.* **23**:119–128, 1948.

51. Yoeli, M., Most, H., Hammond, J., *et al.* Parasitic infections in a closed community: Results of a 10-year survey in Willowbrook State School. *Trans. R. Soc. Trop. Med. Hyg.* **66**:764–776, 1972.

52. Black, R. E., Dykes, A. C., Sinclair, S. P., *et al.* Giardiasis in day-care centers: Evidence of person-to-person transmission. *Pediatrics* **60**:486–491, 1977.

53. Simpson, G. E. Epidemic giardiasis (letter). *Med. J. Aust.* **1**:601–602, 1975.

54. Walzer, P. D., Wolfe, M. S., Schultz, M. G. Giardiasis in travelers. *J. Infect. Dis.* **124**:235–237, 1971.

55. Veghelyi, P. Celiac disease imitated by giardiasis. *Am. J. Dis. Child.* **57**:894–899, 1939.

56. Peterson, G. M. Intestinal changes in *Giardia lamblia* infestation. *Am. J. Roentgenol.* **77**:670–677, 1957.

57. Zamcheck, N., Hoskins, L. C., Winawer, S. J., *et al.* Histology and ultrastructure of the parasite and the intestinal mucosa in human giardiasis: Effects of atabrine therapy (abstract). *Gastroenterology* **44**:860, 1963.

58. Cain, G. D., Moore, P., Jr., Paterson, M. Malabsorption associated with *Giardia lamblia* infestation. *South. Med. J.* **61**:532–534, 1968.

59. Halstead, S. B., Sadun, E. H. Alimentary hypersensitivity induced by *Giardia lamblia*: Report of a case of acute meat intolerance. *Ann. Intern. Med.* **62**:564–569, 1965.

60. Kacker, P. P. A case of *Giardia lamblia* proctitis presenting in a VD clinic. *Br. J. Vener. Dis.* **49**:318–319, 1973.

61. Meyers, J. D., Kuharic, H. A., Holmes, K. K. *Giardia lamblia* infection in homosexual men. *Br. J. Vener. Dis* **53**:54–55, 1977.

62. Mildvan, D., Gelb, A. M., William, D. Venereal transmission of enteric pathogens in male homosexuals: Two case reports. *J. Am. Med. Assoc.* **238**:1387–1389, 1977.

63. Wolfe, M. S. Giardiasis. *N. Engl. J. Med.* **298**:319–321, 1978.

64. Paine, T. F., Jr., Gluck, F. W. A puzzling case of giardiasis. *J. Am. Med. Assoc.* **236**:2425–2426, 1976.

65. Kamath, K. R., Murugasu, R. A comparative study of four methods for detecting

Giardia lamblia in children with diarrheal disease and malabsorption. *Gastroenterology* **66**:16–21, 1974.

66. Rendtorff, R. C. Giardia in water (letter). *Ann. Intern. Med.* **82**:280–281, 1975.

67. Danciger, M., Lopez, M. Number of *Giardia* in the feces of infected children. *Am. J. Trop. Med. Hyg.* **24**:237–242, 1975.

68. Klima, M., Gyorkey, P., Min, K. W., *et al.* Electron microscopy in the diagnosis of giardiasis. *Arch. Pathol. Lab. Med.* **101**:133–135, 1977.

69. Beal, C. B., Viens, P., Grant, R. G., *et al.* A new technique for sampling duodenal contents: Demonstration of upper small-bowel pathogens. *Am. J. Trop. Med. Hyg.* **19**:349–352, 1970.

70. Bezjak, B. Evaluation of a new technic for sampling duodenal contents in parasitologic diagnosis. *Am. J. Dig. Dis.* **17**:848–850, 1972.

71. Thomas, G. E., Goldsmid, J. M., Wicks, A. C. Use of the Enterotest duodenal capsule in the diagnosis of giardiasis: A preliminary study. *S. Afr. Med. J.* **48**:2219–2220, 1974.

72. Sagaró, E., Blanco, E., Fragoso, T., *et al.* Duodenal intubation with secretin stimulus for diagnosis of giardiasis. *Arch. Dis. Child.* **52**:505–507, 1977.

73. Haiba, M. H. The pH of the alimentary tract in normal and *Giardia*-infected culture mice. *Parasitology* **44**:387–391, 1954.

74. Babb, R. R., Peck, O. C., Vescia, F. G. Giardiasis. A cause of traveler's diarrhea. *J. Am. Med. Assoc.* **217**:1359–1361, 1971.

75. Hartman, H. R., Kyser, F. A. Giardiasis and its treatment: A clinical study. *J. Am. Med. Assoc.* **116**:2835–2839, 1941.

76. Bassily, S., Farid, Z., Mikhail, J. W., *et al.* The treatment of *Giardia lamblia* infection with mepacrine, metronidazole and furazolidone. *J. Trop. Med. Hyg.* **73**:15–18, 1970.

77. Ament, M. E. Diagnosis and treatment of giardiasis. *J. Pediatr.* **80**:633–637, 1972.

78. Marsden, P. D., Schulz, M. G. Intestinal parasites. *Gastroenterology* **57**:724–750, 1969.

79. Green, E., Lynch, D. M., McFadzean, J. A., *et al.* Treatment of giardiasis. *Br. Med. J.* **3**:411–412, 1974.

80. Craft, J. C., Murphy, T., Nelson, J. D., Furazolidone and quinarcine for treatment of giardiasis in children (abstract). In *Proceedings of 19th Interscience Conference on Antimicrobial Agents in Chemotheraphy*, Boston, Mass., October 3, 1979.

81. Salih, S. Y., Abdalla, R. E. Symptomatic giardiasis in Sudanese adults and its treatment with tinidazole. *J. Trop. Med. Hyg.* **80**:11–13, 1977.

82. El Masry, N. A., Farid, Z., Miner, W. F. Treatment of giardiasis with tinidazole. *Am. J. Trop. Med. Hyg.* **27**:201–202, 1978.

83. Levi, G. C., de Avila, C. A., Amato Neto, V. A. Efficacy of various drugs for treatment of giardiasis: A comparative study. *Am. J. Trop. Med. Hyg.* **26**:564–565, 1977.

84. Wright, R. A., Vernon, T. M. Epidemic giardiasis at a resort lodge. *Rocky Mount. Med. J.* **73**:208–211, 1976.

85. Moody, A. H. Improved method for the pure preparation of faecal cysts for use as antigen. *Trans. R. Soc. Trop. Med. Hyg.* **70**:338, 1976.

86. Fortess, E., Meyer, E. A. Isolation and axenic cultivation of *Giardia trophozoites from the guinea pig. J. Parasitol.* **62**:689, 1976.

87. Roberts-Thomson, I. C., Stevens, D. P., Mahmoud, A. A., *et al.* Acquired resistance to infection in an animal model of giardiasis. *J. Immunol.* **117**:2036–2037, 1976.

88. Fair, G. M., Geyer, J. C. *Water Supply and Waste-Water Disposal.* John Wiley & Sons, New York, 1954.

89. Owen, R. L., Nemanic, P. C., Stevens, D. P. Ultrastructural observations on giardiasis in a murine model. *Gastroenterology* **76**:757–769, 1979.

4

Bacillary Dysentery

INTRODUCTION

Bacillary dysentery is a common diarrheal syndrome generally caused by one of 32 serotypes of *Shigella* and less commonly by invasive strains of *E. coli.* Many cases of dysentery remain undiagnosed after laboratory examination. *Campylobacter* recently has been shown to produce a dysentery syndrome, and other causes will be identified in future studies. The term "dysentery" was used by Hippocrates to indicate a condition characterized by the frequent passage of stools containing blood and mucus and accompanied by straining and painful defecation. At the end of the 19th century, the causative agents were identified, and the two forms of dysentery, bacillary and amebic, were distinguished. Much of the dysentery described in older writings is felt to be bacillary (shigellosis) in origin due to rarity of liver involvement. Outbreaks of bacillary dysentery through the first World War were as important in deciding the outcome of most military campaigns as war-related injuries. The most characteristic clinical picture of shigellosis is dysentery (bloody, mucoid stools) in which the passage of numerous small-volume stools is associated with variable degrees of fever, systemic toxicity, fecal urgency, and tenesmus. The causative agent may produce less striking diarrhea without fever.

BACTERIOLOGY

In the identification of *Shigella* and *Salmonella,* most laboratories use an enrichment broth (primarily for *Salmonella* isolation) and two or more plating media, followed by biochemical identification of lactose-negative colonies showing a characteristic fermentation reaction on triple sugar–

iron (TSI) and lysine–iron agar (LIA) slants. Commonly employed media for initial plating of stool specimens include *Shigella–Salmonella* (SS), MacConkey, eosin–methylene blue (EMB), xylose–lysine–deoxycholate (XLD), Hektoen enteric agar, and Tergitol 7 agars.

The media inhibit the growth of bile-sensitive bacteria, thereby producing a selective environment for the growth of the relatively bile-resistant *Salmonella* and *Shigella* organisms. Multiple plates are employed,[1] since these media also inhibit the growth of all other bacteria and are thus primarily useful in detecting the agents when they are present in large numbers (more than 10^3/g of stool). It is customary to streak lightly on a minimally inhibitory medium such as MacConkey, XLD, Tergitol 7, or EMB and plate heavily on a more inhibitory medium such as SS agar.

During active infection where the patient is clinically ill, the infecting strain generally is present in stool in concentrations between 10^3 and 10^9 viable bacteria/g. During convalescence, *Shigella* proliferation decreases to 10^2–10^3 cells/g of feces, which influences laboratory identification. The sooner after passage that the stool specimen is processed and the more culture plates processed, the greater the likelihood of identifying the causative agent. In certain research centers, fluorescent antibody techniques have been employed to detect *Shigella* strains in diarrheal stools when present in lower numbers.[2] In areas where *Shigella dysenteriae* 1 (the Shiga bacillus) is endemic, the use of nonselective media such as MacConkey or Tergitol 7 is essential due to strict growth requirements of the organism.[3,4] When a bacterial isolate gives a characteristic reaction, it is confirmed as *Shigella* by biochemical reactions and then it is serogrouped and typed by slide agglutination. There are four serogroups of *Shigella:* group A, *S. dysenteriae* (10 serotypes); group B, *S. flexneri* (6 serotypes); group C, *S. boydii* (15 serotypes); and group D, *S. sonnei* (1 serotype). Antiserum for determining group- and type-specific antigenicity is commercially available.

In most parts of the world, the vast majority of cases of bacillary dysentery are caused by a *Shigella* strain. A small percentage of cases are secondary to infection by an invasive *E. coli*. These bacteria are classified biochemically as *E. coli*, yet biologically they closely resemble *Shigella*. Their similarity to *Shigella* strains is further suggested by the finding that most invasive *E. coli* antigenically resemble *Shigella* strains,[5] and most will agglutinate with *Shigella* antisera. Invasiveness by these bacteria is a chromosomally mediated virulence property. There is a clear relationship between serotype based on O and H antigens and invasiveness. Important O groups include 28, 112, 115, 124, 136, 143, 144, 147, and 152. It may be that serotyping of *E. coli* will prove to be of value in screening for enteroinvasive *E. coli. Campylobacter, Yersinia,* and *Vibrio parahemolyticus* strains may produce dysentery and will be discussed in Chapter 8.

PATHOGENESIS

The primary virulence property of strains of *Shigella* and *Shigella*-like *E. coli* is invasiveness, whereby the infecting strain is capable of penetrating the epithelial lining of the gut.[6] The property of invasiveness appears to be chromosomally mediated, and the segment of genome involved is located near the purine E and lactose–galactose regions.[7] Primates, including humans, are the only animal order naturally susceptible to infection by *Shigella*. A great deal of knowledge about pathogenesis of bacillary dysentery has come from experimental animal studies employing animal models (either monkeys with natural susceptibility or guinea pigs made susceptible by starvation and pretreatment with opiates). Shigellosis in starved, opium-treated guinea pigs is a rapidly fatal disease, with death occurring within 48–72 hr due to extensive small-bowel involvement.[8] The experimental infection in this model resembles the rare fulminating human infection, the ekiri syndrome,[9] in which a similar small-bowel lesion occurs and mortality is common. Dysentery bacilli penetrate intact epithelial lining and reach the lamina propria within a few hours. Epithelial changes range over a wide spectrum from severe degenerative alterations to increased cellular activity.[8]

Naturally occurring shigellosis in monkeys resembles the disease in humans in that oral administration of virulent dysentery bacilli leads to an acute colitis within 48 hr.[10] *Shigella* organisms are found in decreasing numbers from the luminal epithelial cells to deep crypt cells to the lamina propria. The superficial nature of infection explains the rarity of obtaining positive blood cultures from patients with shigellosis. The small bowel is normally spared in the monkey model. Dysentery bacilli invade the colonic mucosa from the intestinal lumen, and organisms have a preference for the cytoplasm of colonic epithelial cells. Prior to invasion, the bacteria attach to the surface epithelium, as shown by phase-contrast time-lapse cinemicrography.[11] Bacterial invasion unevenly affects epithelial cells, with disappearance of goblet cells and extrusion of epithelial cells, leading to formation of microulcers at the luminal surface. Crypt abscesses develop secondary to a focal accumulation of inflammatory cells. Bacillary dysentery has been produced in cynomolgus monkeys when a virulent *Shigella* strain was given either by direct injection into the cecal lumen[12] or by oral challenge. In cecal challenge, a lower inoculum size produced illness, and there was a greater percentage of stools containing blood and mucus.

Volunteer experiments have helped to establish the occurrence of a biphasic illness which depends upon the site of intestinal localization of the infecting *Shigella* strain. Twelve hours after ingestion of a virulent *Shigella* strain, the bacteria were shown to transiently multiply in the small intestine to concentrations of 10^7–10^9 cells/ml of luminal content. Occasionally, the infecting strain could be found in the stomach for periods of 20 hr despite low pH. Abdominal cramps and fever usually were found during this early phase of infection. After one to three days, the *Shigella* strain could no longer be cultivated from small-bowel fluids, the temperature became lower, and pain and abdominal tenderness were confined to lower abdominal quadrants. Urgency, tenesmus, and dysentery commonly were seen at this time when the organisms were confined to the colon (see "Clinical Features").

Table 4.1 reveals the stool findings in 59 adult students with diarrhea acquired while in Mexico. Twenty-nine of the students had a *Shigella* strain isolated from diarrheal stools and were considered to have shigellosis. Thirty students were diagnosed as having diarrhea due to enterotoxigenic *E. coli* (ETEC) as determined by documenting a fourfold or greater rise in serum antibodies to heat-labile toxin (LT) during illness by the passive immune hemolysis technique [13] (15 students) or by identifying an LT-producing *E. coli* in diarrheal stools (15 students). It was our intention to determine whether an early, watery diarrhea could be detected in naturally occurring shigellosis and to compare the weight and water content of diarrheal stools with those seen in a known small-bowel secretory diarrheal syndrome due to ETEC. During the first 24 hr of stool collection, a significantly greater weight of stool was passed by students with shigellosis when compared to the group with seroconversion to LT ($p < 0.01$) or the combined ETEC group ($p < 0.001$). The percentage of water in stool

TABLE 4.1
Stool Weight and Water Content in Shigellosis and Enterotoxigenic *Escherichia coli* Diarrhea among Students in Mexico

| | | Stool findings (mean values) | | | |
| | | Day 1 | | Day 2 | |
Infection	Number of students	Total wt. (g)	Percentage water[a]	Total wt. (g)	Percentage water[a]
Shigellosis	29	285	86	191	81
Enterotoxigenic *E. coli*					
Antitoxin seroconversion	15	121	75	115	73
All cases[b]	30	113	80	153	75

[a]Percentage of water was determined by weighing a wet aliquot of stool, drying it in a constant-temperature heating block for 1 hr, and then calculating (dry weight/wet weight × 100).
[b]Cases in which LT-producing *E. coli* was isolated from diarrheal stools were added to those showing seroconversion.

during day 1 of observation was significantly (*p* <0.01) greater for the *Shigella* group than for those with LT-producing *E. coli* as determined by antitoxin seroconversion. The water content of stool was significantly (*p* <0.01) higher on day 1 compared to day 2 of stool collection for those with shigellosis. No significant differences in stool weight or water content were found between the 29 students with shigellosis when compared to the 30 students with diarrhea due to ETEC on the second day of observation. This study supports the volunteer studies showing an early, watery diarrhea in patients with shigellosis followed by decreasing volumes of stool with lower water content as disease progresses.

A series of studies using rhesus monkeys also have helped to clarify the two forms of clinical shigellosis. Rout *et al.*[14] showed that following oral inoculation with virulent *Shigella,* watery diarrhea and/or colitis developed in various animals. While net secretion of sodium and water occurred in the colon of both groups, only those with diarrhea (without dysentery) had active jejunal secretion of sodium and water. Kinsey and associates[15] found that when the small bowel was bypassed by challenging rhesus monkeys intracecally, the dysentery form alone developed, and water and sodium secretion was demonstrated only for the colon. It is likely that increased stool volume and higher water content in early shigellosis reflect active secretion of electrolytes and fluid from jejunal and colonic surfaces. Small-bowel participation in illness and watery diarrhea may represent an early and self-limiting phase, as demonstrated by a decreasing stool weight and water content and disappearance of the organism from small-bowel secretions as disease progresses.

Although there is general agreement that invasiveness is the primary virulence characteristic of *Shigella* strains, the importance of toxin production in the pathogenesis of the diarrheal syndrome has not been resolved entirely. In the early part of this century, the Shiga bacillus was shown to elaborate a neurotoxin which produced paralysis and death in mice and rabbits. More recently, the toxin of the Shiga bacillus was shown to have enterotoxic and cytotoxic properties,[16] a factor which may relate to the unusual severity of illness by this agent. *S. flexneri* and *S. sonnei* may also produce *in vitro* a cell-free cytotoxin which resembles Shiga toxin.[17,18] Patients with infection due to *S. flexneri* and *S. sonnei* have been shown to develop antibody which neutralizes Shiga toxin, suggesting a role for the toxin in human illness. How these exotoxins contribute to clinical illness has been explained by several mechanisms. Release of the toxin in the small bowel, leading to outpouring of fluid and electrolytes, may explain the watery diarrhea phase of early infection,[19] or toxins may be active after mucosal penetration by virulent organisms which contribute to the tissue damage and inflammatory reaction. The released exotoxins also may explain the resistance of virulent *Shigella* strains to phagocytosis. Virulent and avirulent *Shigella* strains are equally susceptible to phagocytosis, but virulent strains are highly lethal to macrophages.[20]

EPIDEMIOLOGY

A majority of bacillary dysentery cases which occur in the United States are spread from person to person by the fecal–oral route. Fecal excretion of the infecting strain of *Shigella* usually lasts for one to four weeks if not treated. Long-term excretion (greater than a year) rarely occurs but has been documented in patients residing in custodial institutions and in others, often with coexistent intestinal parasite infestation.[21,22] A study carried out in a residential institution for the mentally retarded demonstrated a role for hand transmission in shigellosis. Ten percent of persons with positive stool cultures for *Shigella* had positive finger cultures for the same strain, while other patients had *Shigella* organisms recovered from cultures of fingers and hands at a time when the stool findings were negative.[23] Clustering of cases, suggesting a common source vehicle, is more characteristic of disease in confined populations and in those traveling from the United States to developing areas of the world. Occasionally, food- and waterborne outbreaks occur in the United States, in which large numbers of persons may become affected. A continuing common source (contaminated food) may explain a significant percentage of the diarrhea including shigellosis of travelers from the United States to Latin America.[24] The finding of *Shigella* in stools of 27 to 223 (12%) asymptomatic students in Mexico suggests that healthy transient carriers may be a reservoir of *Shigella* organisms and a potential source of infection in this setting.[25]

Clinical illness is most common in children between the ages of six months and ten years. Women are more likely to become affected than men, presumably because of closer contact with infected children. Children under the age of six months rarely become infected. In parts of the world where breast-feeding is discouraged, a severe form of diarrhea may occur in newborns,[26] but it is unusual among breast-fed newborns.[27]

Soon after *E. histolytica* and dysentery bacilli were identified in the early part of the 20th century, it was found that both agents produced sporadic illness, while institutional ("asylum") dysentery was invariably bacillary dysentery.[28] Shigellosis has been shown in more recent investigations to be a particularly important problem in any area where persons are housed closely together, such as residential institutions for the retarded, day-care centers, nursery schools, kindergartens, elementary schools, Indian reservations, and cruise ships. Preschool children in day-care centers may play an important role in the epidemiology of shigellosis.[29,30] In these reported studies, the preschool children were the most susceptible to secondary infection and often were responsible for introduction of illness into families. Secondary transmission of *Shigella* infection is common, from a high of 60% for those under one year of age in a family where an index case is introduced to approximately 20% for persons of all ages.[23] Transmission rates of shigellosis are increased by crowding and by reduced income and personal hygiene. The unusual communicability of shigellosis is partially explained by the finding of a low inoculum of bacteria (fewer than 200 viable cells) necessary to produce illness in humans.[31] Such a low dose is unique to shigellosis among bacterial pathogens and also helps to explain why shigellosis is the most common form of bacterial diarrhea acquired by microbiology laboratory workers. Flies may play a role in disease transmission, especially in tropical climates.[32–34] Dysentery in tropical parts of the world is most prevalent during peak fly seasons and bacteriologic studies of flies indicate that they may harbor the pathogenic organisms.[23]

In certain areas of the world, water serves as a vehicle of disease transmission. Wells contaminated with feces are a problem in rural areas of the developing world. Institution of running water and toilet facilities is associated with a decrease in rates of diarrhea from all causes in these areas. *Shigella* strains remain viable in water at room temperature for periods up to six months.[33] Wells may be located in areas adjacent to cesspools and privies in developing regions, or septic-tank discharge may drain into lakes or other surface waters and contaminate water supplies and bathing or swimming[35] areas. Water chlorination, if properly maintained, will remove the threat of disease transmission. Water transmission is, however, relatively more important to the epidemiology of typhoid fever and cholera than to that of shigellosis. Historically, when water sanitation facilities were instituted in an area where enteric infection was hyperendemic, the incidence of typhoid fever fell, but the prevalence of bacillary dysentery remained unchanged.[33]

There is indirect evidence that household-type toilets may be efficient transmitters of *Shigella* organisms. Hutchinson[36] was able to trace the spread of an infecting *Shigella* strain to children in a nursery school to contaminated toilets. The epidemic strain was recovered readily from the bathroom floor and toilet seats for a period as long as 17 days. Bacteria remain in the toilet bowl through adsorption to the porcelain surface of the bowl, and droplets produced by flushing toilets may efficiently spread infecting bacteria.[37] Considering the low number of organisms necessary to produce dysentery, the toilet must play a role in transmission of shigellosis and perhaps other enteric infections. Studies need to be carried out to evaluate the importance of the toilet to endemic diarrhea.

Shigella strains are responsible for between 10 and 20% of acute diarrhea worldwide. Since bacillary dysentery is often a serious infection producing a striking illness, it is diagnosed in approximately 20% of patients with diarrhea who are admitted to the hospital. Although the frequency of bacillary dysentery cases reflects the level of sanitation and nutritional development, the relative importance of the disease remains remarkably constant from one country to another. Cycling epidemics of dysentery every 20 years have been commented upon since the beginning of the 17th century.[38] Since the early 1900s, when *Shigella* serotypes became identifiable, the cyclic pattern of shigellosis has been confirmed.[39] Early in the 20th century, *S. dysenteriae* 1 was the most important serotype, followed by serotypes of *S. flexneri* and, more recently, by *S. sonnei,* with a cyclic interval of 20–30 years. This epidemiologic observation has suggested that it takes a certain number of years for herd immunity to reach a critical level before one strain is replaced by another. Currently, *S. sonnei* accounts for between 60 and 80% of cases reported in the United States, and *S. flexneri* serotypes account for most of the remaining cases. *S. dysenteriae* 1 is an unusual cause of bacillary dysentery in the United States.

During the fall of 1971, there were a series of diarrhea outbreaks in the United States which were caused by an invasive *E. coli* that had contaminated Camembert and Brie cheese imported from France.[40] Except for this one epidemic, invasive strains of *E. coli* rarely have been implicated in diarrhea cases in the United States.

CLINICAL FEATURES

In its classic form, bacillary dysentery is a biphasic illness characterized by the onset of fever followed by abdominal pain and watery diarrhea (Figure 4.1). During the first 24–48 hr of clinical illness, a small number of voluminous liquid stools are passed, while later in the illness there is a change to a greater number of stools with smaller volume (fractional stools). Soon thereafter, blood and mucus may be seen in stools (dysentery), and patients characteristically complain of fecal urgency, tenesmus, and painful defecation. The disease appears to be an expression of a descending infection of the intestinal tract, with the early symptoms corresponding to small-bowel infection and later ones, to a colitis. The sequence of events is sufficiently characteristic in many patients so that an accurate diagnosis can be made by history. Children often present with the early form of the disease, and an enteric infection may not be suspected because of the absence of diarrhea. Systemic toxicity and hyperpyrexia in such patients may be associated with a seizure.

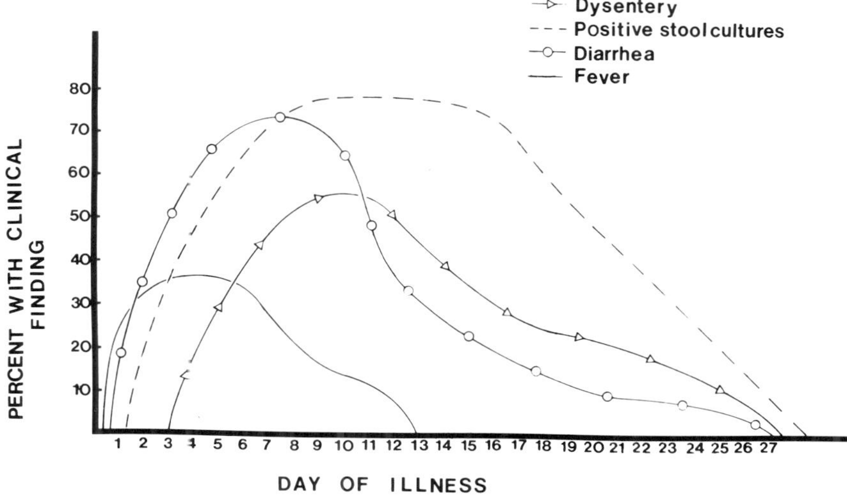

Figure 4.1. Frequency and duration of clinical findings in induced bacillary dysentery. Adapted from data of DuPont *et al.*[19]

The proper diagnosis is made when diarrhea begins. In older children and in most adults, a physician is consulted later in the course of the infection, and dysentery is often the complaint. Figure 4.1 shows the frequency and duration of clinical features and results of stool microbiology during bacillary dysentery. Fever is often the first manifestation, followed by watery diarrhea. As the colitis phase develops, fever becomes less impressive or absent. Abdominal pain and diarrhea occur in nearly all patients with shigellosis; fever is documented in about one-third, stool mucus in one-half, and gross blood in 40% of patients. Stool cultures are positive for the infecting strain during the early infection in slightly more than two-thirds of patients, and stool cultures may remain positive for a month or longer in a small percentage of patients who are untreated. Long-term intestinal carriers of *Shigella* organisms are unusual but may be found among children housed in custodial institutions or persons with coexistent parasitic intestinal infestation.[21,22]

Respiratory symptoms including coryza, cough, and chest pain are common in patients with shigellosis, and pneumonia may occur rarely. A small percentage of patients will present with a picture of sepsis, and a *Shigella* strain or coliform organism may be isolated from blood.[41,42] A shocklike syndrome, which probably reflects extensive mucosal inflammation, may be seen without apparent bacteremia. A hemolytic–uremic syndrome rarely complicates bacillary dysentery.[43] Infants and young children can present with a seizure which generally is felt to be related to the temperature elevation and not to the presence of a circulating neurotoxin. During later stages of infection in malnourished children, profound intestinal protein loss may occur. *S. dysenteriae* 1 (the Shiga bacillus) characteristically produces a more severe clinical illness compared to Sonne or Flexner disease, and mortality rates among untreated patients with Shiga dysentery approximate 20% during epidemics in developing countries. The unusual virulence of this organism probably relates to the nature and quantity of toxin elaborated which has enterotoxic and cytotoxic properties.[16]

Shigellosis is one of the diagnoses to consider when a male homosexual develops diarrhea. Other conditions, including salmonellosis, amebiasis, giardiasis, gonococcal proctitis, and lymphogranuloma venereum infection, also should be considered in a male homosexual with diarrhea. Studies in such populations have indicated a venereal mode of transmission. *Shigella* strains also may cause vulvovaginitis in children and adults, chronic urinary tract infection, bacteremia, arthritis, osteomyelitis, conjunctivitis, iritis and corneal ulceration, hepatitis, and wound infection.[44]
[−46] The relationship of shigellosis to Reiter's syndrome (arthritis, urethritis, and conjunctivitis) has been known since the early part of this century. Recently, a group of patients with post-*Shigella* Reiter's syndrome was found to be HLA-B27-positive, a finding which was particularly common in those with chronic symptomatology.[47] Although patients with sickle-cell anemia have a predilection for infection with *Salmonella*, infection with *Shigella* in this group of patients has been reported rarely.[48]

DIAGNOSIS

Bacillary dysentery should be considered in any patient with fever and diarrhea, particularly when the temperature is excessive and the diarrhea protracted or in persons with acute colitis. The colitis is generally characterized by fecal urgency, tenesmus, painful defecation, and passage of scanty stools with blood and mucus. Physical findings are nonspecific and may include systemic toxicity, fever, and abdominal tenderness, especially in the lower quadrants. Hemorrhoids can be present and painful. Rectal examination or proctoscopy will often cause extreme discomfort. Sigmoidoscopic examination will usually demonstrate distal colonic and rectal involvement with edematous, hyperemic, granular mucosa and excess mucoid secretions. As illness progresses, small ulcerations may be found. The peripheral leukocyte count is not characteristic, although often there is a leukocytosis or leukopenia, and frequently there is a shift to the left in the white count (increased number of immature neutrophils). Direct microscopic examination of stool or mucus in stool mixed care-

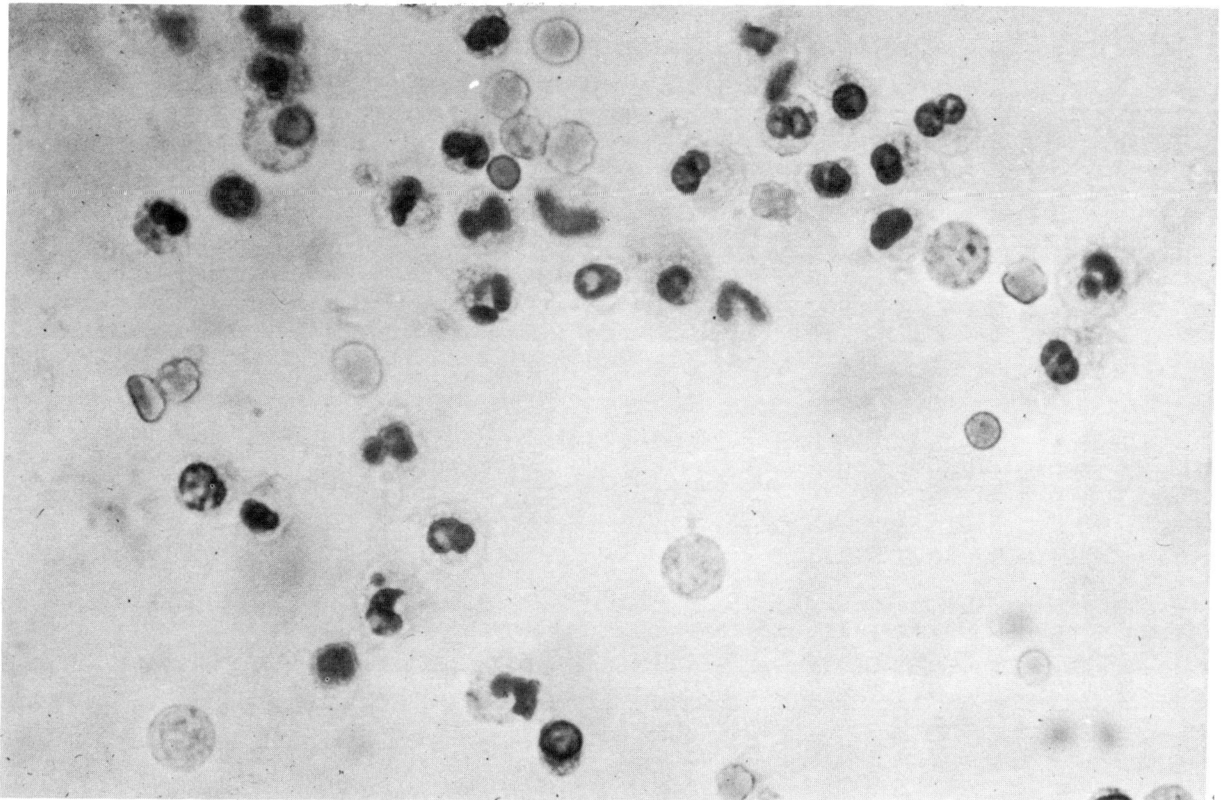

Figure 4.2. A methylene blue wet-mount preparation of stool from a patient with shigellosis. The numerous polymorphonuclear leukocytes indicate the presence of a diffuse colitis ($\times$ 400).

fully with methylene blue and place under a coverslip will be helpful in evaluating patients with possible shigellosis.[49] Numerous polymorphonuclear leukocytes (see Figure 4.2) generally are present, particularly in the later stages of disease, at which time a diffuse colitis can be found. Early in the small-bowel phase of infection, leukocytes may not be readily identified in stool smears. A fecal exudative reaction also is characteristic of gastroenteritis due to *Salmonella, Yersinia enterocolitica,* and *Campylobacter fetus;* the colitis associated with idiopathic inflammatory bowel disease and certain cases of antibiotic-associated pseudomembranous enterocolitis. A large number of leukocytes indicates a pathologic process, diffuse colitis, and not an etiologic diagnosis.[50]

Pathogenicity of a *Shigella* or *E. coli* strain isolated from a patient with diarrhea can be verified by testing in the guinea pig eye (Sereny) model.[51] A heavy suspension of bacteria is dropped into the conjunctival sac of a guinea pig, and one to seven days later, purulent keratoconjunctivitis is seen when the strain is capable of invading epithelial cells (Figure 4.3). This test is reliable if the strain is tested within one month of primary isolation. Strains stored for a longer period of time may lose the capacity for a positive reaction. Serologic evaluation of a patient with bacillary dysentery is not helpful in making an etiologic diagnosis, since the antibody levels generally rise after the patient has recovered. Serologic stud-

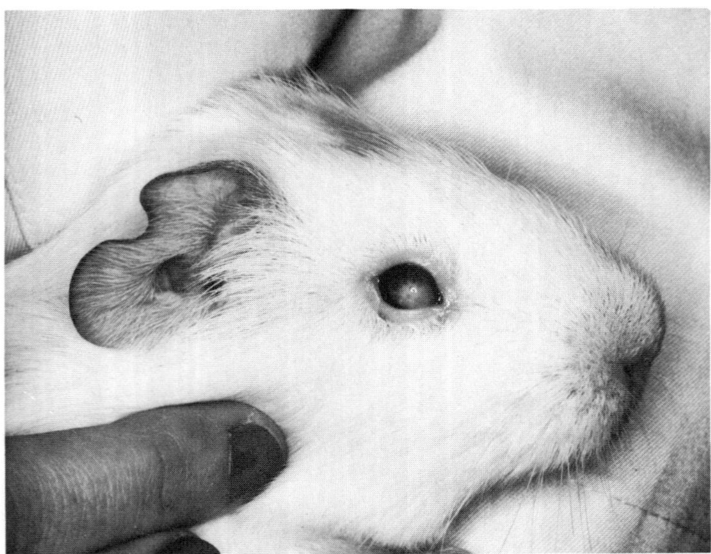

Figure 4.3. Serény test for invasiveness. An invasive *Escherchia coli* or *Shigella* isolate will produce purulent keratoconjunctivitis in a guinea pig within one to seven days.

ies are useful as an epidemiologic tool to define the level of endemicity of certain serotypes of *Shigella* and to document the occurrence of infection in an epidemic situation.[52]

IMMUNOLOGY OF SHIGELLOSIS

During shigellosis, a rise in humoral antibody and intestinal antibody (coproantibody) can often be demonstrated. Employing a macroscopic hemagglutination technique, specific *Shigella* antibodies were detected in sera of volunteers experimentally infected with a virulent *Shigella* strain.[19] Forty-nine percent of the volunteers developed a fourfold rise in humoral antibody, regardless of the occurrence of clinical symptoms. Among the volunteers with diarrhea, 62% experienced *Shigella* seroconversion, compared to 70% of those with *Shigella* isolated from stool, 75% of those with bloody, mucoid stools, and 83% of those with fever. This study demonstrated that humoral antibody increases were common in those experiencing intestinal replication of the virulent bacterial strain (positive stool isolation) and were most frequent when extensive mucosal invasion by the *Shigella* strain occurred, as indicated by the presence of bloody, mucoid stools or fever. In the latter cases, antibody-producing cells apparently were reached and effectively stimulated by the invasive bacteria. Baseline antibody titers varied widely between <1:15 and 1:7680. A correlation between baseline antibody level and susceptibility to illness could not be demonstrated. In fact, the volunteer with the highest baseline serum titer (1:7680) developed a severe diarrheal illness. Serum antibody increases generally occurred between 7 and 14 days after challenge and remained elevated for one to two months thereafter. Utilizing a passive hemagglutination technique, paired sera of 281 patients with Shiga dysentery were examined for humoral antibody development.[52] By the second day of symptomatology, antibodies could be detected. They reached maximum titers by the eighth or ninth day of disease, while the titer fell to insignificant levels (<1:40) by the fifth or sixth month. The antibody was sensitive to 2-mercaptoethanol, indicating that it was probably an IgM immunoglobulin.

Specific immunity following a bout of shigellosis can be shown by resistance to experimental infection in animals[53] and humans[54] and by decreased susceptibility to infection among persons living in areas of *Shigella* endemicity.[55-57] Primary infection probably produces resistance to infection by immunologic mechanisms operative after mucosal penetration by the bacteria, in contrast to the immunity from oral vaccination, which appears to influence subsequent adherence or penetration of bacteria.[54] Volunteers who had recovered from a previously induced infection were resistant to a second exposure to the same virulent strain when compared to a group of controls; however, the test organism proliferated in the gut to the same degree in both groups.[54] In these published studies, there was no correlation between baseline serum *Shigella* antibody levels and susceptibility.[19,53,54] The importance of *Shigella* toxin to the immunology of shigellosis is unknown.

Besredka[58] first indicated that the immunity conferred by an attack of dysentery or by vaccination was due to sensitization of the intestinal mucosa to dysentery bacilli. He was able to show in the early 1900s that serum antibody played little if any role in the immunity. The presence of *Shigella* agglutinins in feces during infection was first described by Davies in 1922[59] for patients with acute and chronic bacillary dysentery. These so-called coproantibodies have been further characterized by Burrows *et al.*,[60,61] Gordon *et al.*,[62] and Freter *et al.*[63] Intestinal antibodies develop earlier, disappear more quickly, and probably are more important to immunity than serum immunoglobulins.

Epidemiologic studies showing the development of resistance to shigellosis among individuals recurrently exposed to the prevalent serotypes of *Shigella*[55–57] have given support to the idea that a vaccine might be developed for the control of infection in high-risk areas. An effective immunizing agent would have usefulness in certain lower socioeconomic areas such as Indian reservations and in custodial institutions for the mentally retarded during an epidemic. Most illness in the United States is due to *S. sonnei* and *S. flexneri* 2, indicating the need for a bivalent preparation. It has been established that killed parenterally administered vaccines fail to protect animals against experimental infection[64,65] or to protect humans against naturally occurring shigellosis.[66,67] Living attenuated bacteria administered as an oral vaccine were, however, protective in animals subsequently challenged with virulent *Shigella* organisms. Formal *et al.*[68–70] employed spontaneously derived avirulent mutants of *Shigella* as well as *Shigella–E. coli* hybrids as oral vaccines. These attenuated strains were shown to impart protective immunity to volunteers which approximated that seen following recovery from disease.[54] In contrast to the immunity produced by prior illness, that seen following oral vaccination was operative at the gut level. Intestinal proliferation of the virulent strain, employed to test vaccine efficacy, was less in the vaccinated volunteers when compared to controls, as determined by recovery from stool specimens. This finding was in contrast to that of a similar study of the immune status of individuals following convalescence from disease, in which illness after challenge with a virulent organism was prevented without an effect on intestinal proliferation of the virulent test organism.[54]

The value of orally administered *Shigella* vaccines in controlling infection in areas of endemicity was demonstrated by Mel *et al.*[71,72] These workers used streptomycin-dependent mutant *Shigella* strains as oral immunizing agents. They found that immunity could be achieved if multiple (at least four) large doses of vaccine (greater than 10^{10} viable cells/dose) were administered after first altering gastric function with oral sodium bicarbonate. Serotype–specific protection followed vaccination and lasted between six months and one year. The vaccines that prevented development of clinical disease did not alter the rate of asymptomatic *Shigella* carriage. Strains combined as bivalent preparations were protective. In the future, immunologic control of shigellosis for very select populations may be possible. Improved vaccines which may be given in fewer doses containing lower numbers of bacteria are needed.

THERAPY OF BACILLARY DYSENTERY

Significant dehydration can occur in bacillary dysentery, particularly in infants and elderly patients. Fluid losses should be replaced by oral intake. If vomiting or extreme systemic toxicity is protracted, intravenous fluid replacement should be undertaken.

Since bacillary dysentery is generally a self-limiting disease, and because *Shigella* strains tend to develop resistance to antimicrobial agents in wide use,[73] some feel that chemotherapeutic agents are not indicated in the treatment of patients with mild shigellosis but should be reserved for the most severely ill patients.[74] However, we feel that a compelling case can be made for treating all persons infected by a *Shigella* strain with an antimicrobial agent. The major arguments are that humans represent the only important reservoir of human shigellosis; that the infection is uniquely communicable among bacterial enteropathogens, being easily transmitted from person to person by contact spread[23]; and that infecting strains are susceptible to a number of available antimicrobial agents. Asymptomatic carriers also may transmit an infectious inoculum to contacts. The other important reason for routine treatment of patients with shigellosis is that patients will have their clinical illness shortened.[75] These arguments are not applicable to the treatment of *Salmonella* gastroenteritis, in which humans are not the important reservoir, the dose of organisms necessary to produce illness in healthy persons is usually high, and antibiotics do not appear to shorten clinical illness but actually prolong the fecal shedding of the infecting strain.[76] Perhaps some of the misunderstandings centering about the need to treat shigellosis relate to the caution which has been put forth about treating the other common recognizable form of bacterial diarrhea, salmonellosis. The emergence of resistant *Shigella* isolates will require that periodic sensitivity testing be performed to determine changes in sensitivities.[77]

Nelson, Haltalin, and their associates demonstrated that orally absorbable antibiotics were more effective than those not readily absorbed.[78] They further established ampicillin as the treatment of choice of shigellosis and showed that it was more active when given parenterally.[79] This group also indicated that certain other drugs were relatively ineffective in the treatment of shigellosis, including furazolidone,[80] cephalexin,[81] and amoxicillin.[82]

In the treatment of shigellosis in children eight years of age or younger where the infecting strains are known to be sensitive, ampicillin is the antibiotic of choice. It is given in a dosage of 50–100 mg/kg/day in equally divided doses every 6 hr for 5 days. For infection due to strains of unknown sensitivity or in penicillin-allergic patients, trimethoprim (TMP) plus sulfamethoxazole (SMX) is the preferred treatment for shigellosis in young children[83] and should be given in a dosage of 10 mg TMP plus 50 mg SMX/kg/day in equally divided doses every 12 hr for 5 days. For adults with bacillary dysentery, a single oral dose (2.5 g) of tetracycline may be the most practical therapy.[31,84–86] Five to ten percent of adult patients will vomit the dose of drug, but it can be repeated.[86] It may even be effective in treatment of shigellosis due to resistant strains,[86] possibly because of the high intraluminal concentrations of drug. Single oral doses of doxycycline or ampicillin were not found to be effective.[31] Alternative forms of therapy for adults are TMP–SMX, given in a dosage of 160 mg TMP plus 800 mg SMX (p.o.) b.i.d. for 5 days, and oxolinic acid 750 mg (p.o.) b.i.d. for 5 days.[31] These drugs and dosages are summarized in Table 10.3, Chapter 10. Figure 4.4 shows the clinical and bacteriologic response to treatment of 68 volunteers experimentally infected with a virulent strain of *S. flexneri* 2a. The strain uniformly was sensitive to all antimicrobial agents, so that relative effectiveness of the drugs could be examined. In terms of temperature defervescence, decrease in number of diarrheal stools, and eradication of the infecting strain from stools during treatment, ampicillin given in a dosage of 500 mg q.i.d. for either 3 or 5 days, oxolinic acid given in a dosage of 750 mg b.i.d. for 5 days, and tetracycline given in a single oral dose of 2.5 g were each equally effective in the treatment of induced shigellosis when compared to the placebo-treated group.[87] There was no apparent clinical response among the six volunteers treated with cephalexin in a dosage of 500 mg q.i.d. In fact, two volunteers were still toxic with fever greater than 103°F 36 hr after therapy was initiated and had to be removed from the study. These results agree with those of a previously published study showing the ineffectiveness of cephalexin despite *in vitro* susceptibility of the infecting strains to cephalosporins.[81]

Although unlicensed for use in the treatment of shigellosis, oxolinic acid appears to be useful against strains resistant to ampicillin. A comparative study employing TMP–SMX versus oxolinic acid would be impor-

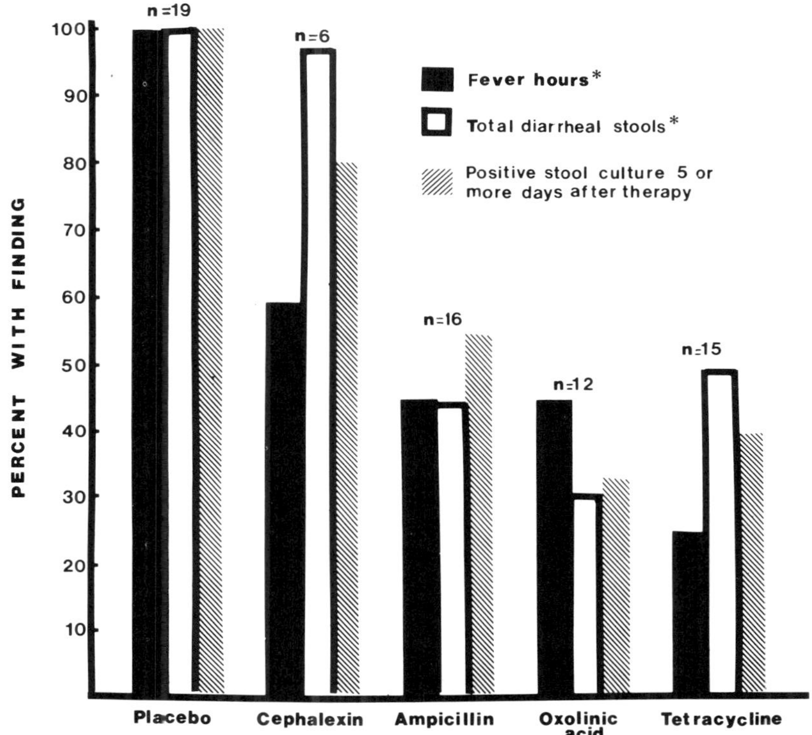

Figure 4.4. Clinical and bacteriologic response to treatment of induced bacillary dysentery due to an antibiotic-sensitive strain of *Shigella flexneri* 2a. *Expressed as percentage considering placebo value as 100%. From DuPont *et al.*[87]

tant to place them in proper perspective. Oxolinic acid is an antimicrobial agent with structure and antimicrobial activity similar to those of nalidixic acid. Oxolinic acid may be preferred to nalidixic acid in view of its more favorable pharmacology and decreased likelihood of developing resistant mutants.[88] Another advantage of this group of drugs is that resistance may not be mediated by a plasmid (R factor), limiting the potential for dissemination of resistance if the drug is widely employed. Also, the limited usefulness of this class of drugs in treating other infections (in contrast to the TMP–SMX combination) would make the development of general resistance among gram-negative bacilli less important.

Antidiarrheal compounds are commonly given to patients with acute diarrhea for the symptomatic relief of their illness. Such drugs probably have no role in the treatment of bacillary dysentery. In fact, there is evidence that drugs which inhibit motility of the gut, such as paregoric, loperamide, and diphenoxylate (Lomotil), should be avoided, since they can on occasion prolong the illness.[89] We have seen a small number of patients with salmonellosis or shigellosis treated with such motility-active drugs where progression to toxic dilatation of the colon developed, necessitating colectomy. The association of toxic megacolon with invasive bacterial diarrhea and ulcerative colitis when motility-active drugs were used to combat the symptoms of diarrhea has been noted by others.[91-92] These drugs should be avoided by any patient with high fever, systemic toxicity, or bloody, mucoid stools.

REFERENCES

1. Morris, G. K., Koehler, J. A., Gangarosa, E. J., *et al.* Comparison of media for direct isolation and transport of shigellae from fecal specimens. *Appl. Microbiol.* **19**:434–437, 1970.
2. Thomason, B. M., Cowart, G. S., Cherry, W. B., Current status of immunofluorescence techniques for rapid detection of shigellae in fecal specimens. *App. Microbiol.* **13**:605–613, 1965.
3. Mata, . J., Gangarosa, E. J., Cáceres, A., *et al.* Epidemic Shiga bacillus dysentery in Central America: I. Etiologic investigations in Guatemala, 1969. *J. Infect. Dis.* **122**:170–180, 1970.
4. Rahaman, M. M., Huq, I., Dey, C. R. Superiority of MacConkey's agar over *Salmonella-shigella* agar isolation of *Shigella dysenteriae* type 1. *J. Infect. Dis.* **131**:700–703, 1975.
5. Edwards, P. R., Ewing, W. H. *Identification of Enterobacteriaceae,* 3rd ed. Bergess, Minneapolis, 1972.
6. LaBrec, E. H., Schneider, H., Magnani, T. J., Jr. Epithelial cell penetration as an essential step in the pathogenesis of bacillary dysentery. *J. Bacteriol.* **88**:1503–1518, 1964.
7. Formal, S. B., Gemski, P., Jr., Baron, L. S., *et al.* A chromosomal locus which controls the ability of *Shigella flexneri* to evoke keratoconjunctivitis. *Infect. Immun.* **3**:73–79, 1971.
8. Takeuchi, A., Sprinz, H., LaBrec, E. H., *et al.* Experimental bacillary dysentery: An electron microscopic study of the response of the intestinal mucosa to bacterial invasion. *Am. J. Pathol.* **47**:1011–1044, 1965.
9. Shiga, K. The trend of prevention, therapy and epidemiology of dysentery since the discovery of its causative organism. *N. Eng. J. Med.* **215**:1205–1211, 1936.
10. Takeuchi, A., Formal, S. B., Sprinz, H. Experimental acute colitis in the rhesus monkey following peroral infection with *Shigella flexneri. Am. J. Pathol.* **52**:503–529, 1968.
11. Ogawa, H., Nakamura, A., Nakaya, R. Cinemicrographic study of tissue cell cultures infected with *Shigella flexneri. Jpn. J. Med. Sci. Biol.* **21**:259–273, 1968.
12. Takaska, M., Honjo, S., Fujiwara, T., *et al.* Shigellosis in cynomolgus monkeys (*Macaca irus*): VI. The inoculation with various doses of *Shigella flexneri* 2a into cecal lumen. *Jpn. J. Med. Sci. Biol.* **21**:275–281, 1968.
13. Evans, D. J., Jr., Evans, D. G. Direct serological assay for the heat-labile enterotoxin of *Escherichia coli,* using passive immune hemolysis. *Infect. Immun.* **16**:604–609, 1977.
14. Rout, W. R., Formal, S. B., Giannella, R. A., *et al.* Pathophysiology of *Shigella* diarrhea in the rhesus monkey: Intestinal transport, morphological, and bacteriological studies. *Gastroenterology* **68**:270–278, 1975.
15. Kinsey, M. D., Formal, S. B., Dammin, G. J., *et al.* Fluid and electrolyte transport in

rhesus monkeys challenged intracecally with *Shigella flexneri* 2a. *Infect. Immun.* **14**:368–371, 1976.

16. McIver, J., Grady, G. F., Keusch, G. T., Production and characterization of exotoxin(s) of *Shigella dysenteriae* type 1. *J. Infect. Dis.* **131**:559–566, 1975.

17. Keusch, G. T., Jacewicz, M. The pathogenesis of shigella diarrhea: VI. Toxin and antitoxin in *Shigella flexneri* and *Shigella sonnei* infections in humans. *J. Infect. Dis.* **135**:552–556, 1977.

18. O'Brien, A. D., Thompson, M. R., Gemski, P., *et al.* Biological properties of *Shigella flexneri* 2a toxin and its serological relationship to *Shigella dysenteriae* 1 toxin. *Infect. Immun.* **15**:796–798, 1977.

19. DuPont, H. L., Hornick, R. B., Dawkins, A. T., *et al.* The response of man to virulent *Shigella flexneri* 2a. *J. Infect. Dis.* **119**:296–299, 1969.

20. Yee, R. B., Buffenmyer, C. L. Infection of cultured mouse macrophages with *Shigella flexneri*, *Infect. Immun.* **1**:459–463, 1970.

21. DuPont, H. L., Gangarosa, E. J., Reller, L. B., *et al.* Shigellosis in custodial institutions. *Am. J. Epidemiol.* **92**:172–179, 1970.

22. Levine, M. M., DuPont, H. L., Khodabandelou, M., *et al.* Long-term *Shigella*-carrier state. *N. Engl. J. Med.* **288**:1169–1171, 1973.

23. Hardy, A.V., Watt, J. Studies of the acute diarrheal diseases: XVIII. Epidemiology. *Public Health Rep.* **63**:363–378, 1948.

24. Tjoa, W. S., DuPont, H. L., Sullivan, P., *et al.* Location of food consumption and travelers' diarrhea. *Am. J. Epidemiol.* **106**:61–66, 1977.

25. Pickering, L. K., DuPont, H. L., Evans, D. G., *et al.* Isolation of enteric pathogens from asymptomatic students from the United States and Latin America. *J. Infect. Dis* **135**:1003–1005, 1977.

26. Haltalin, K. C. Neonatal shigellosis: Reports of 16 cases and review of the literature. *Am. J. Dis. Child.* **114**:603–611, 1967.

27. Mata, L. J., Urrutia, J. J., Garcia, B., *et al.* Shigella infection in breast-fed Guatemalan Indian neonates. *Am. J. Dis. Child.* **117**:142–146, 1969.

28. Rogers, L. Bacillary dysentery. In *Dysenteries: Their Differentiation and Treatment.* Oxford University Press, Oxford, 1913, p. 268.

29. Weissman, J. B., Schmerler, A., Weiler, P., *et al.* The role of preschool children and day-care centers in the spread of shigellosis in urban communities. *J. Pediatr.* **84**:797–802, 1974.

30. Weissman, J. B., Gangarosa, E. J., Schmerler, A., *et al.* Shigellosis in day-care centers. Lancet **1**:88–90, 1975.

31. DuPont, H. L., Hornick, R. B. Clinical approach to infectious diarrheas. *Medicine (Baltimore)* **52**:265–270, 1973.

32. Davison, W. C. A bacteriological and clinical consideration of bacillary dysentery in adults and children. *Medicine* **1**:389–510, 1922.

33. Felsen, J. *Bacillary Dysentery, Colitis and Enteritis.* W. B. Saunders, Philadelphia, 1945.

34. Watt, J., Lindsay, D. R. Diarrheal disease control studies: I. Effect of fly control in a high morbidity area. *Public Health Rep.* **63**:1319–1334, 1948.

35. Rosenberg, M. L., Hazlet, K. K., Schaefer, J., *et al.* Shigellosis from swimming. *J. Am. Med. Assoc.* **236**:1849–1852, 1976.

36. Hutchinson, R. I. Some observations on the method of spread of sonne dysentery. *Month. Bull. Minist. Health* **15**:110–118, 1956.

37. Gerba, C. P., Wallis, C., Melnick, J. L. Microbiological hazards of household toilets: Droplet production at the fate of residual organisms. *Appl. Microbiol.* **30**:229–237, 1975.

38. Gettings, H. S. Bacillary dysentery. *Trans. Soc. Trop. Med. Hyg. (London)* **8**:111–136, 1914–1915.

39. Kostrzewski, J., Stypulkowska-Misiurewicz, H. Changes in the epidemiology of dysentery in Poland and the situation in Europe. *Arch. Immunol. Ther. Exp.* **16:**429–451, 1968.
40. Marier, R., Wells, J. G., Swanson, R. C., *et al.* An outbreak of enteropathogenic *Escherichia coli* foodborne disease traced to imported French cheese. *Lancet* **2:**1376–1378, 1973.
41. Haltalin, K. C., Nelson, J. D. Coliform septicemia complicating shigellosis in children. *J. Am. Med. Assoc.* **192:**441–443, 1965.
42. Henson, M. Bacillary dysentery with bacteremia. *Am. J. Med. Technol.* **22:**179–183, 1956.
43. Chesney, R., Kaplan, B. S. Hemolytic–uremic syndrome with shigellosis (letter). *J. Pediatr.* **84:**312–313, 1974.
44. Barrett-Connor, E., Conner, J. D. Extra-intestinal manifestations of shigellosis. *Am. J. Gastroenterol.* **52:**234–245, 1970.
45. Stern, M. S., Gitnick, G. L. *Shigella* hepatitis. *J. Am. Med. Assoc.* **235:**2628, 1976.
46. Gregory, J. E., Starr, S. P., Omdal, C. Wound infection with *Shigella flexneri* (letter). *J. Infect. Dis.* **129:**602–604, 1974.
47. Calin, A., Fries, J. F. An "experimental" epidemic of Reiter's syndrome revisited: Follow-up evidence on genetic and environmental factors. *Ann. Intern. Med.* **84:**564–566, 1976.
48. Evans, H. E., Sampath, A. C., Douglass, F., *et al.* Shigella bacteremia in a patient with sickle cell anemia. *Am. J. Dis. Child.* **123:**238–239,1972.
49. Harris, J. C., DuPont, H. L., Hornick, R. B. Fecal leukocytes in diarrheal illness. *Ann. Intern. Med.* **76:**697–703, 1972.
50. Pickering, L. K., DuPont, H. L., Olarte, J., *et al.* Fecal leukocytes in enteric infections. *Am. J. Clin. Pathol.* **68:**562–565, 1977.
51. Sereny, B. Experimental shigella keratoconjunctivitis: A preliminary report. *Acta Microbiol. Acad. Sci. Hung.* **2:**293–296, 1955.
52. Cáceres, A., Mata, L. J. Serologic response of patients with Shiga dysentery. *J. Infect. Dis.* **129:**439–443, 1974.
53. Honjo, S., Takasaka, M., Fukiwara, T., *et al.* Shigellosis in cynomolgus monkeys (*Macaca irus*): V. Resistance acquired by the repetition of experimental oral infection with *Shigella flexneri* 2a and fluctuation of serum agglutinin titer. *Jpn. J. Med. Sci. Biol.* **20:**341–348, 1967.
54. DuPont, H. L., Hornick, R., B., Snyder, M. J., *et al.* Immunity in shigellosis: II. Protection induced by oral live vaccine or primary infection. *J. Infect. Dis.***125:**12–16, 1972.
55. Cruickshank, R. Acquired immunity: Bacterial infections. *Mod. Trends Immunol.* **1:**107–109, 1963.
56. Hardy, A. V., Watt, J. The acute diarrheal diseases. *J. Am. Med. Assoc.* **124:**1173–1179, 1944.
57. DuPont, H. L., Gangarosa, E. J., Reller, L. B., *et al.* Shigellosis in custodial institutions. *Am. J. Epidemiol.* **92:**172–179, 1970.
58. Besredka, A. *Local Immunization.* Williams & Wilkins, Baltimore, 1927.
59. Davies, A. An investigation into the serological properties of dysentery stools. *Lancet* **2:**1009–1012, 1922.
60. Burrows, W., Elliott, M. E., Havens, I. Studies on immunity to Asiatic cholera: IV. The excretion of coproantibody in experimental enteric cholera in the guinea pig. *J. Infect. Dis.* **81:**261–281, 1947.
61. Burrows, W., Havens, I. Studies on immunity to Asiatic cholera: V. The absorption of immune globulin from the bowel and its excretion in the urine and feces of experimental animals and human volunteers. *J. Infect. Dis.* **82:**231–250, 1948.

62. Gordon, R. S., Bennet, I. L., Jr., Barnes, L. A. Field trial of *Shigella flexneri* III vaccine: III. Coproantibody studies. *J. Infect. Dis.* **86**:197–201, 1950.
63. Freter, R., De, S. P., Mondal, A., *et al.* Coproantibody and serum antibody in cholera patients. *J. Infect. Dis.* **115**:83–87, 1965.
64. Formal, S. B., Maenza, R. M., Austin, S., *et al.* Failure of parenteral vaccines to protect monkeys against experimental shigellosis. *Proc. Soc. Exp. Biol. Med.* **125**:347–349, 1967.
65. Honjo, S., Takasaka, M., Imaizumi, K., *et al.* Oral challenge with *Shigella flexneri* 2a in cynomolgus monkeys having extremely high titer of serum agglutinin. *Jpn. J. Med. Sci. Biol.* **21**:283–287, 1968.
66. Hardy, A. V., DeCapito, T., Halbert, S. P. Studies of acute diarrheal diseases: XIX. Immunization in shigellosis. *Public Health Rep.* **63**:685–688, 1948.
67. Higgins, A. R., Floyd, T. M., Kader, M. A. Studies in shigellosis: III. A controlled evaluation of a monovalent shigella vaccine in a highly endemic environment. *Am. J. Trop. Med. Hyg.* **4**:281–288, 1955.
68. Formal, S. B., LaBrec, E. H., Palmer, A., *et al.* Protection of monkeys against experimental shigellosis with attenuated vaccines. *J. Bacteriol.* **90**:63–68, 1965.
69. Formal, S. B., Kent, T. H., Austin, S., *et al.* Fluorescent-antibody and histological study of vaccinated and control monkeys challenged with *Shigella flexneri. J. Bacteriol.* **91**:2368–2376, 1966.
70. Formal, S. B., Kent, T. H., May, H. C., *et al.* Protection of monkeys against experimental shigellosis with a living attenuated oral polyvalent dysentery vaccine. *J. Bacteriol.* **92**:17–22, 1966.
71. Mel, D. M., Arsić, B. L., Nickolić, B. D., *et al.* Studies on vaccination against bacillary dysentery: 4. Oral immunization with live monotypic and combined vaccines, *Bull. W.H.O.* **39**:375–380, 1968.
72. Mel, D. M., Gangarosa, E. J., Radovanovic, M. L., *et al.* Studies on vaccination against bacillary dysentery: 6. Protection of children by oral immunization with streptomycin-dependent *Shigella* strains. *Bull. W.H.O.* **45**:457–464, 1971.
73. Farrar, W. E., Jr., Eidson, M. Antibiotic resistance in *Shigella* mediated by R factors. *J. Infect. Dis.* **123**:477–484, 1971.
74. Weissman, J. B., Gangarosa, E. J., DuPont, H. L., *et al.* Shigellosis: To treat or not to treat? *J. Am. Med. Assoc.* **229**:1215–1216, 1974.
75. Cheever, F. S. Treatment of shigellosis with antibiotics. *Ann. N.Y. Acad. Sci.* **55**:1063–1069, 1952.
76. Aserkoff, B., Bennett, J. V. Effect of antibiotic therapy in acute salmonellosis on the fecal excretion of salmonellae. *N. Engl. J. Med.* **281**:636–640, 1969.
77. Byers, P. A., DuPont, H. L., Goldschmidt, M. C. Antimicrobial susceptibilities of shigellae isolated in Houston, Texas, in 1974. *Antimicrob. Agents Chemother.* **9**:288–291, 1976.
78. Haltalin, K. C., Nelson, J. D., Hinton, L. V., *et al.* Comparison of orally absorbable and nonabsorbable antibiotics in shigellosis. *J. Pediatr.* **72**:708–720, 1968.
79. Haltalin, K. C., Nelson, J. D., Kusmiesz, H. T., *et al.* Comparison of intramuscular and oral ampicillin therapy for shigellosis. *J. Pediatr.* **73**:617–622, 1968.
80. Haltalin, K. C., Nelson, J. D. Failure of furazolidone therapy in shigellosis. *Am. J. Dis. Child.* **123**:40–44, 1972.
81. Nelson, J. D., Haltalin, K. C. Comparative efficacy of cephalexin and ampicillin for shigellosis and other types of acute diarrhea in infants and children. *Antimicrob. Agents Chemother.* **7**:415–420, 1975.
82. Nelson, J. D., Haltalin, K. C. Amoxicillin less effective than ampicillin against *Shigella in vitro* and *in vivo:* Relationship of efficacy to activity in serum. *J. Infect. Dis.* **129**:S222–S227, 1974.

83. Nelson, J. D., Kusmiesz, H., Jackson, L. H., *et al.* Trimethoprim–sulfamethoxazole therapy for shigellosis. *J. Am. Med. Assoc.* **235**:1239–1243, 1976.

84. Garfinkel, B. T., Martin, G. M., Watt, J., *et al.* Antibiotics in acute bacillary dysentery: Observations in 1408 cases with positive cultures. *J. Am. Med. Assoc.* **151**:1157–1159, 1953.

85. Lionel, N. D., Abeyasekera, F. J., Samarasinghe, H. G., *et al.* A comparison of a single dose and a five-day course of tetracylcine therapy in bacillary dysentery. *J. Trop. Med. Hyg.* **72**:170–172, 1969.

86. Pickering, L. K., DuPont, H. L., Olarte, J. Single-dose tetracycline therapy for shigellosis in adults. *J. Am. Med. Assoc.* **239**:853–854, 1978.

87. DuPont, H. L., Hornick, R. B., Snyder, M. J. Unpublished data.

88. Atlas, E., Clark, H., Silverblatt, F., *et al.* Nalidixic acid and oxolinic acid in the treatment of chronic bacteriuria. *Ann. Intern. Med.* **70**:713–721, 1969.

89. DuPont, H. L., Hornick, R. B. Adverse effect of Lomotil therapy in shigellosis. *J. Am. Med. Assoc.* **226**:1525–1528, 1973.

90. Pittman, F. E. Adverse effects of Lomotil (letter). *Gastroenterology* **67**:408–410, 1974.

91. Toxic megacolon—Medical Staff Conference, University of California, San Francisco. *West. J. Med.* **124**:122–127, 1976.

92. Brown, J. W. Toxic megacolon associated with loperamide therapy. *J. Am. Med. Assoc.* **241**:501–502, 1979.

5

Salmonellosis

INTRODUCTION

Salmonella gastroenteritis is a common problem in all areas of the world, regardless of economic development. It has become an even greater problem in developed countries where mass production and distribution of food products have occurred. In contrast, endemicity of typhoid or enteric fever, generally the most serious form of *Salmonella* infection, is invariably related to reduced economic development and sanitation. *Salmonella* as the causative agent of intestinal infection is readily recovered by routine diagnostic microbiologic procedures. In this chapter, we will focus on the important aspects of human salmonellosis and will examine the differences between typhoid and nontyphoid disease.

BACTERIOLOGY

Salmonella organisms have been identified from biologic material for the past 100 years. Along with *Shigella* strains, they are the agents sought when stools routinely are processed in the diagnostic bacteriology laboratory. When stool is cultured for *Salmonella*, it is customary to employ media containing variable concentrations of bile salts which selectively inhibit the growth of nonenteric bacteria. Blood, bone marrow aspirate, cerebrospinal fluid, and urine normally are bacteriologically sterile and therefore are best cultured for *Salmonella* on a nonselective medium such as blood agar.

The chance of recovering a *Salmonella* strain from stool is enhanced if the swab containing generous amounts of stool is incubated overnight in an enrichment broth such as selinite F or tetrathionate prior to plating on two or three different enteric media, for example, EMB, SS, MacConkey, Tergitol 7, XLD, brilliant green, or bismuth sulfite agar (the latter primarily for *S. typhi*). Lactose-negative colonies should be processed for *Salmonella* (and *Shigella*) by placing colonies on stab tubes containing TSI, LIA, urea, and motility medium. Strains giving alkaline (pink) slant and acid (yellow) butt in TSI (purple slant and yellow butt in LIA) with (or, rarely, without) black pigment, (hydrogen sulfide) are processed further by biochemical and serologic techniques. Other than *Salmonella cholerae-suis*, a few bioserotypes of *S. enteritidis*, and some strains of *S. typhi*, *Salmonella* strains produce hydrogen sulfide. *Salmonella* organisms yield positive methyl red and negative Voges–Proskauer test results. Table 5.1 lists the usual biochemical reactions of *Salmonella* isolates.

More than 1400 serotypes of *Salmonella* have been identified. The Kauffmann–White group and type classification depends upon somatic (O) antigens and flagellar (H) antigens by agglutination testing.[1] Groups are determined according to the presence of common O antigens. As *Salmonella* strains frequently possess multiple O and H antigens, some of which are different antigenic phases of the same anatomic structure, complete serotype identification has become a complex undertaking. To make matters worse, genotypic variations (mutations, sexual recombinations) and phenotypic variations may occur.

Most hospital diagnostic laboratories are capable of biochemically differentiating three species of *Salmonella: S. cholerae-suis, S. typhi*, and

TABLE 5.1
Important Biochemical Reactions of Salmonella

Reaction with test or substrate[a]	
Positive	Negative
Hydrogen sulfide	Urease
Methyl red	Voges–Proskauer
Motility	Potassium cyanide
Lysine decarboxylase	Phenylalanine deaminase
Ornithine decarboxylase	Lactose
Acid from glucose	Sucrose
Gas from glucose	Adonitol
Mannitol	Raffinose
Sorbitol	Malonate
Rhamnose	Oxidase
Maltose	Cetrimide
Xylose	
Trehalose	
Nitrate to nitrite	

[a]More than 90% of strains.

TABLE 5.2
Important Biochemical Reactions Commonly Used to Differentiate *Salmonella* Species

Species	Hydro-gen sulfide	Citrate (Sim-mons)	Ornithine decar-boxylase	Gas from glucose	Dulcitol	Trehalose	Arab-inose	Rham-nose
S.typhi	+	0	0	0	0	+	0	0
S. cholerae-suis	+	+[b] (delayed)	+	+	0	0	0	+
S. enteritidis	+	+	+	+	+	+	+	+

Reactions with test or substrate[a]

[a]Positive reaction (99% or more).
[b]Positive reaction after three or more days.

S. enteritidis.[1] Table 5.2 lists important biochemical tests which are useful in differentiating *Salmonella* species. Once *S. enteritidis* is identified by biochemical testing, it can be reported by the laboratory but should then be sent to a local or regional reference laboratory for serotyping.

VIRULENCE

The antigenic makeup of *Salmonella* strains undoubtedly relates to intrinsic virulence. The major antigens which are used to classify *Salmonella* are the Vi (envelope), O (somatic), and H (flagellar) antigens. The important role of the envelope antigen in pathogenicity of typhoid fever has been recognized for years. The term "Vi" was selected as the designation to denote its association with virulence.[2] The pathogenic potential of the Vi antigen may relate to its role in the protection of O antigen from antiserum and subsequent phagocytosis. Humans have been shown to be more susceptible to typhoid strains containing Vi, attesting to the importance of this virulence property.[3] During infection by *Salmonella* strains, serum agglutinins to the three antigens often develop and may on occasion be useful in diagnosing the infection. Although the human is the only natural host of the typhoid bacillus *(S typhi)*, other *Salmonella* strains commonly infect animals, especially poultry and reptiles. A standard animal assay for virulence of *Salmonella* strains (both typhoid and nontyphoid) is to determine the dose of bacteria required to produce mortality in 50% of mice when given by intraperitoneal inoculation (LD_{50}).

As with *Shigella* strains, a primary prerequisite of virulence for *Salmonella* is the ability to invade epithelial cells. The nature of the inflammatory response to invasion may determine the clinical expression of disease—bacteremia versus gastroenteritis (see "Pathogenesis"). Cell-wall lipopolysaccharides (LPSs) are important in virulence. LPS-deficient rough mutants found to be nonpathogenic have been employed as oral immunizing agents.[4] In addition to deficiency in cell-wall LPSs as a marker of avirulence, strains of *Salmonella* selected for resistance to chlorate were found to have reduced virulence in mice.[5] The knowledge that other bacterial enteropathogens such as *Shigella* and *E. coli* produce intestinal disease by at least two mechanisms, invasiveness and enterotoxigenicity,[6] has led to similar studies of *Salmonella* virulence. Living *Salmonella* organisms have been shown to cause fluid accumulation in rabbit ileal loop segments,[7,8] while crude culture filtrates failed to produce intestinal dilatation.[7] In separate studies, strains of *Salmonella* were shown to produce fluid accumulation in the suckling mouse model[9] and a skin permeability reaction in rabbits, similar to that produced by *V. cholerae* and enterotoxigenic *E. coli*.[10] The substances which produce intestinal secretion and increase capillary permeability may play a role in the mechanism of diarrhea produced by *Salmonella*.

In typhoid fever, a unique intracellular location of the bacteria renders them resistant to antimicrobial therapy and explains the occurrence of typhoid relapse which is seen in approximately 20% of patients who receive adequate treatment. A virulence property of *S. typhi* may be the ability to inhibit normal leukocyte metabolism, as manifested by the organisms' prevention of the initiation of an enhanced postphagocytic rate of oxygen consumption.[11]

PATHOGENESIS

The number of persons who develop disease after ingesting food containing *Salmonella* organisms, as with other enteric bacterial pathogens, directly relates to the number of bacteria ingested. In healthy adults, ID_{25} for typhoid bacilli is approximately 100,000 viable cells.[3] The dose in nature which is responsible for illness has not been easy to calculate in most instances. Since *Salmonella* infection is nearly always a food- or water-borne illness, it is reasonable to speculate that the normal infective dose is high in contrast to *Shigella* infection. However, among hospitalized patients and elderly persons living in nursing homes, person-to-person spread occurs, suggesting a lower inoculum size. It is likely that infection in the very young, the elderly, the debilitated, and particularly those with gastrointestinal disease (especially patients who have had gastrectomy) may be the result of a low dose of *Salmonella*.[12–14] Other than the dose of ingested bacteria, a major determinant of the development of clinical illness is the integrity of the gastric trap. Like other enteric bacterial pathogens, *Salmonella* organisms are quite susceptible to acid.[15] Patients with reduced gastric acid secretion, achlorhydria, and/or gastrectomy are not only more susceptible to salmonellosis[14,16,17] but more likely to develop a fulminating, cholera-like disease.[18,19]

The intestinal lesions and anatomic location of *Salmonella* in humans with illness have not been well characterized. Much of our information has been derived from experimental infection in various animal models. Rhesus monkeys fed *Salmonella* organisms developed symptoms similar to those seen in humans with *Salmonella* gastroenteritis, with diarrhea beginning after 24 hr.[20] The primary sites of monkey infection due to *Salmonella typhimurium* were found to be the colon and the ileal mucosa. Mild focal lesions also were noted in the stomach and jejunum. Histologically, the inflammatory lesion was nonspecific, while fluorescence studies showed that the *Salmonella* organisms were within colonic epithelial cells and lamina propria. Seven days after initiation of infection, only a few fluorescent bacilli were seen in the small bowel and colonic mucosa. *S. typhimurium* frequently was recovered from mesenteric lymph nodes, rarely in low density from liver and spleen, and never from the blood. Bacteria were invariably found to be deeper in the mucosa, less confined to the epithelium, but in lower densities when compared to experimental shigellosis employing the same animal model.[20] *Salmonella* found in the submucosa produced patchy inflammation, while *Shigella* organisms were more superficial, producing abscesses about the crypts extending into lymphoid patches of the monkey colon. The diarrhea induced by an infecting *Salmonella* strain in the rhesus monkey model is secondary to both an ileitis and a colitis. Alterations in intestinal transport of fluid and electrolytes could be shown in both large intestine and small bowel despite a lack of invasion into the upper gut mucosa.[21]

In typhoid fever of humans, a nonspecific enteritis was shown to develop in the upper gut soon after ingestion of *S. typhi*.[22] Random invasion by the organism produces degenerative and proliferative changes in the epithelial lining of villi, crypt cells, and lamina propria. Experimental typhoid has been well studied in the chimpanzee.[23-25] After the early invasion of the intestinal epithelium, there is rapid clearing of the invading strain, and extensive multiplication of the organisms occurs in regional lymph follicles and mesenteric lymph nodes.[23] From these sites, *S. typhi* spread to the thoracic lymph and then into the general circulation. Chimpanzees who recovered from infection with *S. typhi* were able to restrict the concentration and distribution of the virulent strain in the intestine after a subsequent challenge one and one-half years later. Also, the nonspecific reactive lymphoid hyperplasia and tissue reaction were less intense in animals recovering from previous typhoid infection. The typhoid fever which developed in chimpanzees after intravenous or intramesenteric lymph node challenge with *S. typhi* was identical to the illness produced in animals after oral inoculation.[24] These studies verify the systemic nature of the infection and suggest that an initial intestinal phase is not necessary for the establishment of typhoid fever.

A major factor which influences the nature of *Salmonella* infection appears to be the intestinal inflammatory response of the host.[26,27] Typhoid bacteria elicit a mononuclear response. Monocytes appear to facilitate the extraintestinal transit of the bacteria, and patients present with bacteremia or enteric fever. Most nontyphoid *Salmonella* strains stimulate a polymorphonuclear leukocytic exudate. The organisms are phagocytized and contained locally, and patients experience gastroenteritis. Stools examined microscopically will indirectly reflect the intestinal exudative response, mononuclear for typhoid and polymorphonuclear for nontyphoid salmonellosis.[27]

Since typhoid fever is a severe infection, with fatalities common among untreated cases, a great deal is known about the pathology of the disease. In uncomplicated disease early in the infection, mononuclear and polymorphonuclear leukocytes can be found in the upper-bowel mucosa. The mucosa is congested and edematous and often shows petechiae and ulcerations. The ulcers usually are oval-shaped, having a long axis parallel to the long axis of the intestine. The central portion of the ulcer is flat, and the edges are elevated and congested. There is adjacent mesenteric adenitis. The cut surface of lymph nodes shows focal necrosis and proliferation of mononuclear phagocytic cells in the sinusoids. Gram stains of the intestinal ulcer and the lymph node usually do not yield bacteria. The sites of ulceration are the terminal ileum, the cecum, and the proximal colon. Microscopically, the ulcers correlate with the location of ileal Peyer's patches and submucosal lymphoid nodules of the cecum. Within the ulcer base and adjacent lamina propria and submucosa are mononuclear phagocytic cells.

Nontyphoid *Salmonella* gastroenteritis is nearly always a self-limiting illness, and fatalities are uncommon. In a few fatal cases of nontyphoid salmonellosis studied, the intestinal lesions were of a diffuse nature.[28] The findings included dehydration, pleural petechiae, intestinal distention, hyperplasia of follicles, and Peyer's patches with diffuse hypermia of the entire small intestine. The colon showed even more striking changes, including swollen hyperemic mucosa, punctate hemorrhages, and superficial ulcerations. Mesenteric lymph nodes occasionally were involved in an inflammatory response. The colon has been confirmed by sigmoidoscopic examination and biopsy to be a major site of infection in *Salmonella* gastroenteritis.[29–31] These studies demonstrated histologic changes ranging from edema of the lamina propria and a focal or diffuse inflammatory infiltrate to a more intense colitis with disruption of surface epithelium and multifocal microabscesses. Extensive inflammatory changes were seen in some cases with severe edema, vascular congestion, infiltration of the lamina propria with round cells and polymorphonuclear leukocytes, interstitial hemorrhage, and abscesses in lamina propria and crypts, with erosions and ulcerations in crypt and surface epithelium.

Typhoid fever is the best-studied form of salmonellosis. After oral inoculation with virulent *S. typhi,* there is intestinal multiplication of bacteria. Stools are positive for *S. typhi* within 24 hr after ingestion and often remain so during the incubation period.[3] During the early stages of clinical illness, stools are no longer positive for the infecting strain, and the organism can be readily recovered from blood. The virulent organism usually reoccurs in the intestine during the second week, even though the patient may be recovering from clinical illness. This second intestinal phase of typhoid fever does not seem to be affected by chloramphenicol therapy. The sustained and stepwise febrile response in typhoid fever has been noted for more than two generations. The febrile component and systemic toxicity do not appear to be due to circulating endotoxin, since volunteers rendered tolerant to endotoxin experienced the same clinical illness following subsequent ingestion of virulent *S. typhi.*[32] Endotoxin may, however, play a role in the local inflammatory response, as there appears to be a disassociation of resistance to the systemic and local toxic effects of endotoxin during tolerance.[3] Endotoxin was shown in the latter report to influence the local inflammatory response by action on chemotactic, metabolic, and endogenous pyrogen-releasing activities of phagocytic cells.

EPIDEMIOLOGY

The epidemiology of typhoid and nontyphoid salmonellosis differs remarkably. Documented *Salmonella* isolates from humans other than the typhoid bacillus increased from 504 in 1942 to greater than 20,000 bacteriologically confirmed isolates annually since 1964. The ten most frequently reported serotypes from human and nonhuman sources in 1977 are listed in Table 5.3. The Center for Disease Control has estimated that the number of *Salmonella* infections each year in the United States may approach two million.[33] The annual cost in medical bills and loss of productivity in this single country because of *Salmonella* infection may be as high as one billion dollars.[34] The increase in the isolation of nontyphoid *Salmonella* can be explained by increased awareness of the agent, better reporting of cases, and a changing pattern of mass food processing and distribution.

The major reservoir of nontyphoid human salmonellosis is poultry

TABLE 5.3
The Ten Most Frequently Reported Serotypes of *Salmonella* from Human and
Nonhuman Sources in 1977 (U.S. Figures)[a]

Serotype	Frequency (%)	Ranking 1963–1967[b,c]
1. *S. typhimurium*	35	1 (30)
2. *S. newport*	8	3 (6)
3. *S. heidelberg*	6	6 (5)
4. *S. enteritidis*	5	2 (8)
5. *S. infantis*	5	4 (6)
6. *S. agona*	5	NL
7. *S. saint-paul*	2	7 (4)
8. *S. typhi*	2	8 (3)
9. *S. oranienburg*	2	NL
10. *S. montevideo*	2	NL

[a]*Annual Summary, 1977: Salmonella Surveillance,* United States Department of Health, Education and Welfare, Center for Disease Control, Atlanta, 1979.
[b]Numbers in parentheses represent percentage total.
[c]NL, Not listed.

and domestic livestock. Outbreaks have occurred from contaminated dried and whole milk, poultry, pork, shellfish, smoked whitefish, eggs, water, and carmine dye. Poultry and poultry products such as eggs are the most important source for human illness. There is generally a rise in reported cases of salmonellosis during late November due to the greater frequency of consumption of turkeys during the Thanksgiving holiday. Nearly all nontyphoid *Salmonella* organisms are pathogenic to poultry, particularly to young chicks. The chicks that survive to maturity become asymptomatic carriers.Market poultry as it is found in retail stores is contaminated with viable *Salmonella* in 50% of cases.[35] Egg surfaces are often contaminated by the hen's excreting a *Salmonella* strain. The organism can penetrate cracked eggs, and cross-spread to other eggs commonly occurs when eggs are cleaned in a common water bath. In the past, pet turtles have been associated with outbreaks of salmonellosis. With control of commercial production, this problem appears to be minimal at the present time.

As previously mentioned, most cases of *Salmonella* gastroenteritis develop following ingestion of a large inoculum of bacteria contaminating food. In the young, elderly, or debilitated, such as hospitalized patients, person-to-person spread of illness can occur, implying a lower inoculum size.[12,13] Human-to-human spread of salmonellosis, while far less common than in shigellosis, probably has been underestimated.[36] In certain situations where flies have access to human excreta containing *Salmonella*, the insects may serve as vectors of transmission. The common housefly has been shown to be particularly suited to harbor *Salmonella,* wherein the bacteria can be established and multiply efficiently.[37]

Humans are the only important reservoir of the typhoid bacillus, either a patient recovering from infection or an asymptomatic carrier. Rates of typhoid endemicity directly relate to two factors: lack of water sanitation and number of carriers of the infecting strain in the population. In the United States, small outbreaks of typhoid fever are seen when an undiagnosed carrier contaminates food, usually in a public restaurant. Sizable outbreaks result when fecal contamination of a drinking water supply occurs.[38]

CLINICAL FEATURES

There are four major clinical patterns of *Salmonella* infection of humans: (1) acute gastroenteritis, (2) typhoid (enteric) fever, (3) septicemia with or without localized infection, and (4) asymptomatic carrier state. The disease expression which results depends to a large extent upon the specific infecting strain, the general underlying health and immunologic status of the host, and the inoculum size. Patients infected with *S. typhi, S. paratyphi,* and *S. cholerae-suis* characteristically present with systemic features or enteric fever, while a majority of the approximately 1400 serotypes of *S. enteritidis* lead to an acute gastroenteritis without bloodstream invasion.

Acute Gastroenteritis

Acute gastroenteritis, the most common form of salmonellosis, can be caused by any of the subserotypes of *S. enteritidis* (see Table 5.3). Some of the more important subserotypes are *S. typhimurium, S. newport, S. javiana, S. agona, S. infantis, S. heidelberg, S. oranienburg, S. montevideo, S. muenchen, S. give, S. derby, S. anatum, S. saint-paul,* and *S. enteritidis.* Clinical symptoms develop 8–48 hr following the ingestion of contaminated food. It is common for symptoms to begin upon waking the day after eating the contaminated food. The most common complaints are headache, abdominal pain, fever, and diarrhea. Vomiting is seen, as are respiratory symptoms, particularly coughing. Stools are characteristically watery and often contain mucus and, rarely, blood. The diagnosis is suspected in the presence of a foodborne epidemic where the incubation period is greater than 6 hr and fever is a common finding.

Typhoid (Enteric) Fever

Classic typhoid fever is usually caused by *S. typhi*, although a similar illness may be seen in patients infected with nearly any *Salmonella* species or strain. Contaminated food or water is the usual source, and clinical symptoms develop after 3–60 days, with an average of 7–8 days. Bacteremia is the rule in these patients, and findings usually include fever, headache, and abdominal complaints, most commonly constipation, diarrhea, abdominal pain, and ileus. Other less common but important clinical features are symptoms of a respiratory infection such as cough, characteristic skin eruption (rose spots), and melena or hematochezia. The fever characteristically increases progressively during the first week of illness and decreases progressively during the second week of illness in patients with uncomplicated disease (see Figure 5.1). Rose spots representing cutaneous vasculitis are characteristically seen on the abdomen in clusters of delicate and small erythematous macules which blanch on light pressure (see Figure 5.2). Splenomegaly is common on physical examination, as is segmental ileus in which dilated loops of bowel give the sensation that air and fluid are being displaced when gentle but deep abdominal pressure is exerted by the hand.

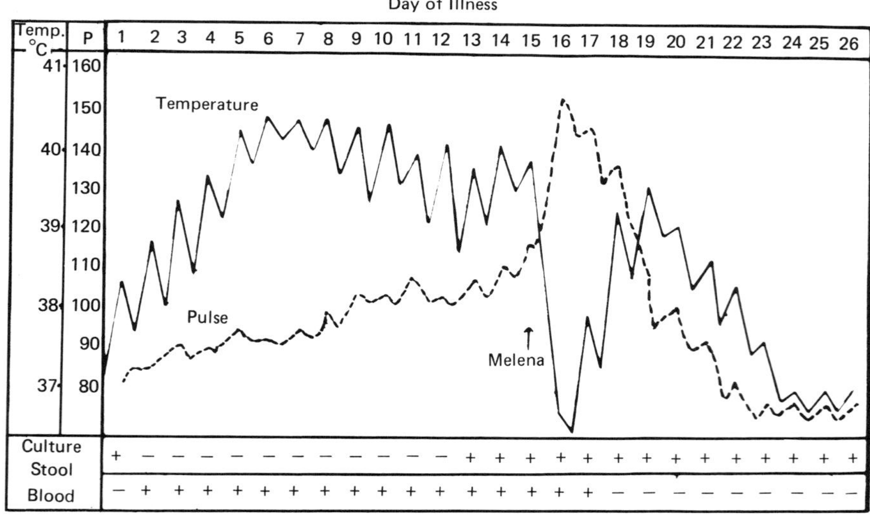

Figure 5.1. Simulated course in typhoid fever, showing early stepwise increase in temperature, relative bradycardia, biphasic stool excretion of *Salmonellla typhi*, positive blood cultures during the acute illness, and increase in pulse rate and decrease in temperature during intestinal hemorrhage.

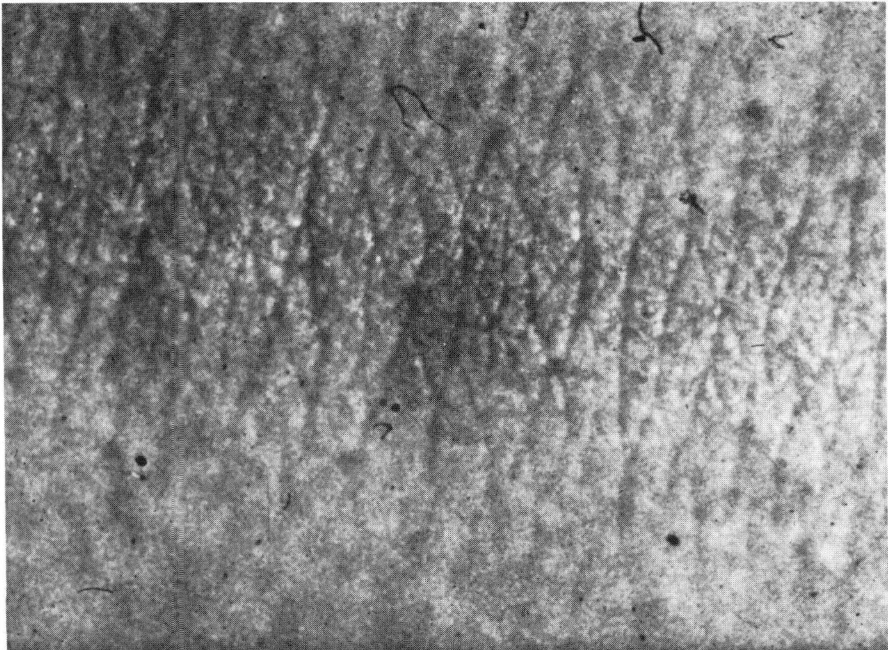

Figure 5.2. Rose spot in typhoid fever: delicate erythematous macules which blanch on pressure and occur in small numbers, often clustered on the surface of the abdomen.

Septicemia with or without Localized Infection

Salmonellosis occurs more frequently in patients with certain hematologic diseases such as sickle cell anemia, lymphoma and leukemia, and solid tumors (usually with metastases). Localized infections occur as cholecystitis, peritonitis, appendicitis, intraabdominal abscess, pneumonia, empyemia, pericarditis, arthritis, osteomyelitis, meningitis, endocarditis, mycotic aneurysms, urinary tract infection, or wound infection. *S. cholerae-suis* characteristically invades the bloodstream, which is apparent when one considers that most isolates reported are from blood and not stool cultures.[39]

Asymptomatic Carrier State

Following acute *Salmonella* gastroenteritis, *Salmonella* excretion may occur for one week to two months. Individuals also may ingest pathogenic organisms and excrete the strain for a short period in the absence of clinical manifestations. These persons contribute to the reservoir of infection. Chronic carriage of *Salmonella* is characteristic of typhoid carriers but rarely occurs with nontyphoid *Salmonella* in healthy persons.[40] Chronic carriage in the intestine or urinary tract may occur in persons with concomitant parasitic infection such as intestinal or urinary tract schistosomiasis. Oral antimicrobial therapy appears to prolong the intestinal carriage of nontyphoid *Salmonella*.[41] Approximately 3% of untreated patients with typhoid fever become intestinal carriers of *S. typhi* for longer than one year. The carrier rate for patients appropriately treated for typhoid fever is unknown, but it is probably lower than the 3% for those with untreated disease. The characteristic intestinal carrier is a

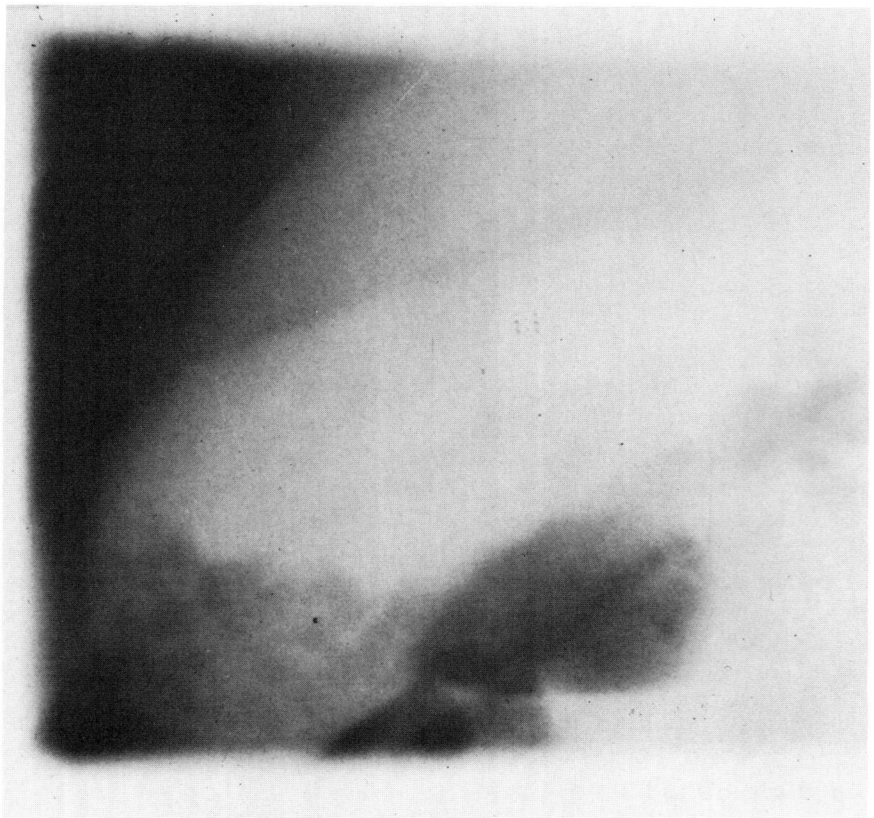

Figure 5.3. An adult intestinal carrier of *Salmonella typhi* undergoes oral cholecystography. Cholelithiasis is noted.

woman with gallbladder disease. Figure 5.3 shows cholelithiasis in a typhoid carrier as revealed by oral cholecystography. As many as 10^{11} virulent *S. typhi* may be excreted per gram of stool. The typhoid bacilli reside in gallbladder stones and in scarred foci of the intrahepatic biliary system and are excreted into the duodenum in high counts. Less commonly, persons may be chronic asymptomatic carriers of *Salmonella* from a presumed vascular source without biliary tract involvement.[42] In the management of typhoid carriers, antimicrobial therapy and occasionally cholecystectomy are the usual forms of therapy. In those persons in whom intestinal carriage cannot be interrupted, reassurance and education in the importance of personal hygiene are generally all that is required.

COMPLICATIONS

In *Salmonella* gastroenteritis, illness is usually mild, and mortality is seen in only 0.22% of patients, usually in infants or in debilitated or elderly adults. In most cases, complications relate directly to dehydration. In the very young and the elderly, fluid and electrolyte disturbances occur more commonly, and oral fluid therapy for those with mild to moderate disease and intravenous therapy for those with severe illness may be lifesaving (see Chapter 11 for rehydration solutions). Patients with achlorhydria or those having prior gastrectomy are more susceptible to developing a rapidly fatal dehydrating illness. In a small percentage of patients with nontyphoid salmonellosis, the intestine may be involved to an extensive degree with typhoid-like lesions, leading to perforation (see "Pathogenesis"). In typhoid fever, the major complications are intestinal perforation or hemorrhage, relapse of illness, and overwhelming sepsis with profound generalized metabolic and physiologic alterations.

Intestinal Perforation and Intestinal Hemorrhage

Perforation of the intestine is the most serious complication of typhoid fever. Perforation occurs in 1–3% of patients and was invariably associated with fatality in the years before the advent of antimicrobial therapy and modern surgery. The complication of intestinal hemorrhage occurs likewise in 1–3% of patients with typhoid fever, yet the prognosis is much better when compared to perforation. Each of these intestinal complications occurs most often in debilitated and malnourished persons treated late in their illness. Perforation and hemorrhage are characteristically seen during the second and third week of illness. Intestinal perforation occurs without relationship to severity of clinical symptoms. It is associated with increased abdominal pain, muscle rigidity, and abdominal distention with absent bowel sounds and general collapse. Peritonitis and intraabdominal abscess formation may complicate the perforation, while in other cases, clinical signs may be minimal, especially if a small tear in the paper-thin ileum develops. Free air generally is found under the diaphragm on a radiograph of the abdomen. Hemorrhage is a result of edema of Peyer's patches which undergo necrosis. Although intestinal bleeding may be profoundly acute, with massive blood loss, it more characteristically is slow and is not a life-threatening complication. Most studies have indicated that the occurrence of intestinal hemorrhage does not increase the mortality rate when compared to uncomplicated disease. A clinical finding suggesting intestinal hemorrhage is a drop in temperature at a time when the pulse rate increases unexpectedly. Hypotension or shock may be diagnosed. Melena is then noted (see Figure 5.1). Corticosteroids, which are often administered to the acutely ill patient, do not predispose patients to hemmorhage.

The optimal means of treating perforation of the intestine due to *S. typhi* initially was felt to be medical.[43,44] Such management included use of antibiotics, fluid replacement, and gastric suction to decompress bowel distention. The primary argument against surgical intervention was that the terminal ileum was paper thin in many places and was liable to perforate in more than one spot. Also, repair of the friable gut was shown to be impossible in many cases, and, in others, attempts to suture the leak merely resulted in further tears. Finally, it was shown that patients with intestinal perforation due to *S. typhi* infection were in poor general health, making a decision to perform surgery difficult. The clear exceptions to restricting therapy to medical measures were sudden perforation that occurred during the period of convalescence and recognized early (in the first 6 hr), perforation that progressed to intraabdominal abscess formation, or adhesions that caused obstruction. More recently, there has been a tendency in areas of typhoid endemicity to operate early when perforation is diagnosed.[45,46] These studies and the experience of other groups that have not published their data support the use of early surgery in the management of most patients with intestinal perforation. This approach appears to reduce morbidity and mortality. Multiple perforations are present in one-third of patients,[46] and it is unlikely that spontaneous closure would occur in a majority of these patients. Perforation of the cecum and proximal colon also may occur.[47] The aims of surgery are to drain purulent material and intestinal contents from the abdominal cavity and to prevent further intraabdominal contamination. Surgery consists of either simple closure of perforations in disease of minimal extent or, more commonly, wedge excision of the perforated ulcer. When multiple perforations are not present, ileal resection is the preferred treatment if there is bowel friability. In patients in whom the ileum is severely and extensively involved, ileostomy should be performed. In all patients with typhoid perforation, antimicrobial therapy should include chloramphenicol combined with an aminoglycoside (gentamicin, tobramycin, or amikacin) to treat typhoid organisms, colonic anaerobes, and other enteric gram-negative bacilli. The treatment of intestinal hemorrhage is blood replacement. The source of bleeding generally is an area of superficial ulceration of the ileum, and spontaneous closure is the rule.

Relapse

Relapse of typhoid fever is characterized by the return of symptomatology similar to that of the primary illness, including headache, chills, fever, malaise, and abdominal pain. The intensity of clinical illness is less severe than the initial disease, and fatalities rarely occur. Relapse occurs in about 20% of patients who have received therapy, compared to 9% in the preantibiotic era.[44] Blood and stool cultures are often positive during typhoid relapses, and rose spots occasionally are seen.

Miscellaneous Complications

As with other septicemic processes, a number of systemic and localized complications may arise. Patients with salmonellosis, even uncomplicated gastroenteritis, often present with respiratory symptoms, particularly a nonproductive cough. In certain patients, this represents the most significant early complaint. The chest radiograph is usually normal, although transient patchy infiltrates may be documented. Rarely, bacterial pneumonia can be documented, and the etiologic agent may be the infecting *Salmonella* strain, *S. pneumoniae,* or enteric gram-negative bacilli.

Hepatomegaly occurs in just under one-third of patients with enteric fever, and jaundice may be seen in about one-third of patients with hepatic enlargement.[48] Histologic changes in the liver include the appearance of "typhoid nodules," which consist of focal accumulations of mononuclear cells. Nephritis may complicate the hepatitis,[49] with an immune-complex glomerulitis being the most common form of kidney damage.[50] Kidney failure rarely may be associated with myoglobinuria.[51] Acute pancreatitis is a rare complication.

Hematologic changes occur, including thrombocytopenia[49] and disseminated intravascular coagulation.[52] Central nervous system involvement is more common than generally considered. A meningoencephalitis picture is not uncommon, and such patients frequently will have a cerebrospinal fluid pleocytosis, although recovery of a bacterial agent from cerebrospinal fluid is unusual. Patients may develop seizures or neuropsychiatric symptoms, myocarditis,[53,54] circulatory failure, or Reiter's syndrome[55] (as occurs in *Shigella* gastroenteritis). During enteric fever, there may be a transient suppression of tuberculin skin test reactivity.[56]

INSTITUTIONAL SALMONELLOSIS

Although there appears to be a greater susceptibility among institutionalized persons to virulent *Shigella* than *Salmonella* strains, there is an unexplained reversal in potential for spread within certain hospitalized or institutionalized populations. Shigellosis is more of a problem in custodial institutions for the mentally retarded, but salmonellosis is a far greater problem in hospitals and in homes for the elderly. Undoubtedly, the exposure of many patients to common foods, drugs, and materials which may become contaminated with a *Salmonella* strain is important in the latter settings.

Hospitalized patients appear to be unusually susceptible to *Salmonella* infection. Acute-care hospitals, pediatric wards (particularly newborn nurseries), psychiatric institutions, and homes for the elderly are the usual settings. The overall fatality:case ratio is approximately 2%.[57] There is usually a common vehicle such as contaminated food,[33,58] carmine dye,[59,60] platelet transfusions,[61] pharmaceutical products,[62] or contaminated human breast milk.[63] Common-vehicle outbreaks that occur most often among adult patients are often secondary to contaminated eggs, egg products, red meats, milk, or powdered food supplements.[33] Cross-infection is common through either person-to-person contact or by fomites. Outbreaks have been traced to contaminated hospital equipment,[64–67] furniture,[68] dust,[69,70] and air.[71] Hospital personnel may become infected asymptomatically and may serve as a reservoir for continuing spread.[72]

In institutional outbreaks of salmonellosis, a careful search should be made among patients and hospital personnel for both symptomatic and asymptomatic excretors of the epidemic strain. Personnel found to be harboring the organism should be transferred to low-risk areas of the hospital where there is minimal contact with patients or food preparation. "Enteric isolation" of patients with positive cultures should be instituted. Fomites can be cultured, especially when there is common contact with infected patients. Outbreaks may be averted by routinely isolating any patient admitted to the hospital with diarrhea, particularly infants and children. Strict stool isolation must be adhered to in any situation where stool cultures are positive for a *Salmonella* strain, and such patients should be discharged as early as possible from the hospital. Careful attention to infection control procedures should be instituted, including regular, effective hand-washing. Antimicrobial therapy has not been helpful in limiting the spread of infection and may actually contribute to increased transmissibility of the *Salmonella* strain.[73]

The problem of epidemic salmonellosis in newborn nurseries is one of great importance.[33,63–66,68,71,73–76] Rectal carriage of the infecting strain reaches 5% during extensive nursery outbreaks. In one epidemic, *Salmonella* was isolated from the hands of a nurse immediately after they had been washed.[68] Nursery outbreaks may be derived from a mother infected in the community transmitting the strain to the infant at the time of delivery.[66,75] It may be of significance that newborns appear to excrete *Salmonella* for a longer period of time during the convalescence period than adults. Asymptomatic carriage for more than six months is a finding in half of infected infants in well-studied epidemics.[74–76] These infants who excrete the strain during the postconvalescent stage probably serve as important sources of community-based infection. In two epidemics where families of infants involved in a hospital outbreak were studied, secondary rate of attack among household contacts ranged from 50 to 75%, although most of the secondary cases remained asymptomatic.[64,74,75]

CONDITIONS PREDISPOSING TO OR ASSOCIATED WITH SALMONELLOSIS

Approximately 10% of *Salmonella* isolates referred to local and national reference laboratories are from nonfecal sources. A majority of these represent positive blood cultures for *Salmonella* organisms. The frequency of bacteremia in nontyphoid *Salmonella* gastroenteritis is between 5 and 6%.[16,77] For the previously healthy individual, the prognosis is good despite the documentation of bacteremia.

Certain underlying diseases appear to predispose patients to progressive salmonellosis with bacteremia, including sickle-cell anemia and other conditions associated with hemolysis, alcoholism, lymphoma, leukemia, metastatic malignancy, schistosomiasis, liver disease,[78,79] postsurgery state,[78,80,81] chronic granulomatous disease (CGD) of children, and possibly glucose-6-phosphate dehydrogenase deficiency. Premature newborns and elderly persons are similarly predisposed. In the debilitated individual, profound metabolic and physiologic changes, including septic shock, may occur along with *Salmonella* bacteremia.

Salmonellosis and Hematologic Diseases

The coexistence of *Salmonella* sepsis and/or *Salmonella* osteomyelitis in patients with sickle-cell anemia has been a subject of general interest. The unusual susceptibility of patients with sickle-cell disease to progressive infection, including bacteremia and osteomyelitis, has been explained by anatomic alteration of the gut and bones and by an abnormality of immune responsiveness. It is reasonable to assume that vascular thromboses with infarction in the intestinal wall and cortical infarcts in bones are important in explaining the transit of *Salmonella* from the intestine to blood to bones. Separate but perhaps equally important factors are paralysis of the reticuloendothelial system (RES) by erythrophagocytosis of red cell fragments secondary to the invariable hemolysis in such patients or defective complement-mediated serum opsonizing activity for *Salmonella*. Kaye *et al.*[82] established an experimental model in mice which clearly showed the relationship between hemolysis and phagocytosis of red cell fragments, blockade of RES activity, and subsequent susceptibility to infection by *S. typhimurium*. Their studies support the notion that the RES and other phagocytic cells play a major role in control of intracellular parasites such as *Salmonella*. That hemolysis is a major predisposing event leading to salmonellosis is further suggested by the association of *Salmonella* infection with other hematologic disorders characterized by hemolysis, including malaria, bartonellosis, relapsing fever, and certain liver diseases.[83–85] Hand and King[86] demonstrated that half of a group of patients with sickle-cell anemia studied by them had abnormalities of the complement system, including defective functions of the alternative complement pathway and depressed C_3 levels. These patients showed a deficiency in serum opsonizing activity. That a generalized opsonic defect occurs in sickle-cell disease was further supported by the work of Field and Overturf.[87]

Patients with typhoid fever appear to have an increased frequency of glucose-6-phosphate dehydrogenase deficiency, suggesting a possible relationship. In this hematologic condition, the association with salmonellosis may relate to impaired RES function secondary to hemolysis; to defective bactericidal activity of the leukocytes[88]; or to increased serum iron levels.[89]

The frequency of bacterial infections, including systemic salmonellosis, is increased among patients with CGD of childhood. Persistent infection with a *Salmonella* strain may reflect survival of the bacteria in the macrophages of the RES protected from the effect of systemic antimicrobials. It has been shown in this condition that mononuclear cells have the same defects in killing bacteria as do polymorphonuclear leukocytes,[90-91] and since macrophages of the RES are derived from circulating monocytes, a similar defect exists in them.[92] Carriers for CGD may also have difficulty in intracellular killing of *Salmonella* in view of the recurrent *S. enteritidis* septicemia that was observed for over three and one-half years in one well-studied patient.[93]

Salmonellosis and Malignant Disorders

The relationship of malignancy to serious *Salmonella* infection was noted more than a half century ago.[94] While *Salmonella* bacteremia is seen in fewer than 10% of patients with gastroenteritis, in patients with malignant disorders, a positive blood culture can be obtained in 37% of cases.[16,77,95] Also, the incidence of focal infections such as pneumonia, meningitis, peritonitis, and urinary tract infection is greater in patients with underlying malignant diseases. There appear to be a number of factors which relate to the association of salmonellosis and malignancy: (1) malignancy may occasionally activate a latent infection (carrier); (2) antimicrobial agents which these patients receive serve to encourage the proliferation of *Salmonella* strains; (3) patients with malignant disorders may undergo a greater number of gastrointestinal surgical procedures or may have altered gastric physiology, including hypochlorhydria, either of which may predispose to salmonellosis[78,80,81]; and (4) specific immunologic defects may be present in some patients.

The immune deficiencies of patients with malignant disorders which play a role in predisposing them to *Salmonella* infections may be due to anergy, to a primary defect in cellular immunity, or to a compromise of the immune system secondary to the chemotherapy or radiotherapy for the primary disease. Enhanced susceptibility of mice to *Salmonella* infection occurs following a course of irradiation[96] or when the animals are treated with a low dose of hydrocortisone[97] or an alkylating agent such as nitrogen mustard.[98] Evidence was offered that humans receiving these antitumor therapies also show an increased susceptibility to *Salmonella* infection.[95]

Salmonella Bacteremia and Aneurysm of the Aorta

Large elastic arteries such as the aorta have a high degree of resistance to infection unless a vascular abnormality occurs, including atherosclerosis, cystic medionecrosis, and syphilitic arteritis.[99-102] An infected aortic aneurysm should be suspected in any patient with *Salmonella* bacteremia which recurs after a course of treatment or in one who expires with septic shock during a bout of salmonellosis. While a vascular abnormality may become infected with any serotype of *Salmonella, S. cholerae-suis* has an inordinately greater likelihood of being the infecting agent in aortic endovasculitis.[100,103] The probable mechanism of infection of an abdominal aortic aneurysm is either secondary infection of the vessel wall arising from septicemia from a distant portal, including endocarditis, or direct extension of an adjacent inflammatory process, usually lumbar osteomyelitis which has developed secondary to pressure necrosis of the vertebral bodies from transmitted pulsations of the aneurysm.[100,104] It has been suggested that it is possible to differentiate between infection of an aortic aneurysm arising through a hematogenous route of transmission from that arising through direct extension of an adjacent infection by examining the adventitia of the aneurysmal sac.[105] In the case of direct spread, the adventitia is extensively involved, whereas it is usually spared in infection arising from within. In *Salmonella* infection of an aneurysm, not only is there a likelihood of recurrent bacteremia without an associated gastroenteritis, but the aneurysm may rupture, leading to sudden death.[78,100] The major form of therapy is early surgical replacement of the aneurysm with a synthetic prosthesis. Surgery performed late in the process is rarely successful.

Salmonellosis and Schistosomiasis

Chronic *Salmonella* bacteremia has been associated with Manson's schistosomiasis since 1958, while subsequent reports have revealed an association of *Salmonella* urinary tract carriage with *Schistosoma hematobium* infection. Chronic *Salmonella* bacteremia may persist from 2 to 24 months,[106–109] may be due to any serotype of *Salmonella,* and is usually well tolerated by patients affected with schistosomiasis. Others may present with hepatosplenomegaly, abdominal pain, diarrhea, epistaxis, adenopathy, anemia, and eosinophilia. Stool, urine, and bile cultures usually are negative, and Widal's agglutination tests are of little help in diagnosing the problem. Patients generally respond clinically to a course of parenteral ampicillin or oral chloramphenicol, although relapse is common.

In experimental schistosomiasis of mice, susceptibility to *Salmonella* infection appears to be secondary to an impaired mechanism of intracellular killing by cells of the RES.[110] Sera from patients with hepatosplenic schistosomiasis show a decrease in anti-*Salmonella* activity and delayed leukocytic migration as compared to controls, suggesting alternative reasons for enhanced susceptibility to salmonellosis.[111] Indirect evidence was put forth that the site of *Salmonella* multiplication and seeding of the bloodstream in prolonged salmonellosis conceivably may be the *Schistosoma* organisms themselves.[112,113] This could explain the observation that cure of salmonellosis may occur with treatment directed toward the *Schistosoma* infection.[114]

Salmonellosis and Ulcerative Colitis

Both idiopathic ulcerative colitis and salmonellosis are common disorders, and it is not surprising that the two occasionally coexist and produce diagnostic and therapeutic difficulties. It has not been established whether ulcerative colitis actually predisposes patients to salmonella infection. In one study of 175 patients with *Salmonella* gastroenteritis, 64 (37%) had a major underlying disease, 28 of whom had a gastrointestinal disorder,[16] suggesting an association of host disorder with susceptibility to *Salmonella* infection. In a separate study of 153 patients with idiopathic ulcerative colitis, 5% were shown to have developed salmonellosis.[115]

It is known that acute *Salmonella* enteritis may be associated with grossly bloody stools, although it is far less common than in bacillary dysentery. Idiopathic ulcerative colitis should be considered in any patient with *Salmonella* gastroenteritis and bloody stools, especially if the bloody diarrhea persists for two to three weeks. One of the diagnostic difficulties is that acute *Salmonella* enteritis may produce colonic mucosal changes which mimic idiopathic ulcerative colitis. From a therapeutic standpoint, the problem is unsettling in view of the indication of corticosteroids for treatment of ulcerative colitis and the potentiation of intestinal salmonellosis and even death following initiation of corticosteroid therapy.[116] Systemic antimicrobial agents probably should be given to patients with a positive stool culture for *Salmonella* who receive corticosteroids for treatment of their ulcerative colitis.

DIAGNOSIS

Nontyphoid *Salmonella* Infection

Salmonella gastroenteritis should be suspected in any febrile patient with diarrhea. Other findings which further support the diagnosis include the identification of multiple cases of diarrhea 8–36 hr after a common poultry meal and the presence of leukocytes in stool examined microscopically. The diagnosis is confirmed by identification of a *Salmonella* strain from stool culture. In nontyphoid *Salmonella* bacteremia, the diagnosis is made by recovering the causative agent from blood culture. Serologic procedures are of no practical value in diagnosing nontyphoid salmonellosis in view of the diverse serotypes responsible for illness and because of cross-antigenicity between *Salmonella* strains and other gram-negative bacilli.

Typhoid Fever

Typhoid fever should be suspected in any patient with characteristic clinical features, especially if the infection is acquired in an area of typhoid endemicity, such as Latin America, Egypt, or India. The diagnosis is established only by recovering the causative agent from stool, blood, or other body tissue. Blood cultures are positive in approximately 80% of patients with typhoid fever; however, it may be more difficult to culture the organism from blood of patients who have received an antimicrobial agent. Gilman *et al.*[117] demonstrated that bone marrow cultures and skin biopsy cultures of rose spots were more often positive for *S. typhi* than blood cultures.

Widal's reaction is a tube dilution test measuring agglutinating antibodies against somatic O, flagellar H, and occasionally envelope Vi antigens. A fourfold rise in titer of O agglutinins or a single titer of 1:160 or higher during the first two to three weeks of illness is suggestive of typhoid fever. Serologic diagnosis of typhoid fever is useful in parts of the world where the illness is endemic due to the relative importance of *S. typhi.* On the other hand, in areas where typhoid fever is unusual, such as the United States, serologic evidence of infection (elevation of O or H agglutinins) more likely represents an exposure to cross-reacting gram-negative rods (including nontyphoid *Salmonella*) than to the typhoid bacillus, at a ratio of approximately 3:1.[39] At least 290 serotypes of *Salmonella* share one or more of the three antigens of *S. typhi.* Typhoid immunization produces transiently elevated O antibody levels, while H agglutinins may be persistently elevated for many years, limiting the usefulness of measuring the titer of flagellar agglutinins in diagnosing typhoid fever. Vi (envelope) agglutinins rise late in the evolution of the infection, usually after clinical symptoms have disappeared. There is no evidence that chloramphenicol interferes with the formation of agglutinin antibodies to typhoid antigens.[118]

ANTIMICROBIAL RESISTANCE AMONG *SALMONELLA* ORGANISMS: RELATIONSHIP OF HUMAN AND ANIMAL STRAINS

Salmonella organisms are widely distributed in domestic animals and animals raised for meat production. They are found in milk, milk products, poultry, beef, pork, and lamb. Subtherapeutic levels of various antimicrobials are routinely used as growth promoters in animal feed. Currently, the Food and Drug Administration is evaluating the hazards to human health of the routine use of antibiotics for this purpose. There is little doubt that animals maintained on low doses of antimicrobial agents will develop an intestinal flora which is resistant to the drug in the feed. While *Salmonella* resistance may occur,[119] the more profound and predictable effects are upon the intestinal *E. coli*, which rapidly become resistant to the drug used.[120,121] The resistant enteric flora then serves as a reservoir of antibiotic resistance, which may be important if the animal is subsequently placed on therapeutic levels of the drug to treat infection. In studies of resistance among animal bacteria, it is difficult to separate the effects of selective pressure due to use of subtherapeutic levels of an antimicrobial agent in feed from those of therapeutic use of drugs in diseased animals. It is of interest that antibiotic resistance among bacterial flora occurs in animal species such as horses, cats, and dogs[122] where there is no exposure to antibiotic agents.

If animals contribute significantly to either bacterial or plasmid reservoirs of human bacterial strains, one would expect that farm workers or families with direct contact with livestock might show different patterns of resistance when compared to those without regular contact with animals. A study of poultry farmers showed acquisition of tetracycline-resistant *E. coli* among the farmers' intestinal flora when animal feed contained the drug in subtherapeutic levels.[123] The resistance disappeared once the drug was removed from animal feed. This transfer of resistant bacteria from animals to humans requires an intense and recurrent exposure such as would occur on farms. Those less intensively exposed, such as meat eaters, do not appear to become colonized by resistant bacteria when compared to vegetarians.[121] On rare occasions, an antibiotic-resistant *Salmonella* strain is important in an outbreak of salmonellosis among farm personnel. In 1965, Anderson and Lewis[124] described such an outbreak which was due to *S. typhimurium*, phage type 29. The strain was resistant to sulfonamide, streptomycin, ampicillin, tetracycline, and the furans. The *Salmonella* strain was acquired by calves during a time when antibiotic was being used in animal feed and was spread from diseased animals to farm workers, producing human fatality. However, there were several other conditions present which undoubtedly contributed to this unusual outbreak. Poor sanitation and inappropriate therapeutic use of antibiotics were noted during the serious and generalized outbreak. Each probably contributed to the spread of the agent. A second, less dramatic outbreak of human illness on a farm was reported. The causative agent was a multiply resistant *Salmonella* strain which was traced to unpasteurized milk.[125] A prospective study was conducted among children residing on commercial poultry farms to determine the relative importance of contact with poultry as a contributor to diarrhea and *Salmonella* infection.[126] The occurrence of diarrhea and *Salmonella* infection among the farm children did not differ over the one-year period of surveillance as compared to a matched group of children without animal contact.

Resistance among *Salmonella* isolates probably is becoming a more important problem,[127,128] although there is a lack of total agreement on this point.[129] It does appear that tetracycline resistance among *Salmonella* of animal origin is becoming more common, while ampicillin resistance is more important among human isolates.[128,130] This apparently reflects the common use of tetracycline as a growth promoter in animal feed and the frequent prescribing of ampicillin for humans with a variety of minor infections. The contribution of antibiotic resistance among animal *Salmonella* to human medicine is unknown. An important relationship is suggested by the finding that antibiograms of human and animal strains are similar for the major *Salmonella* serotypes[128] and by the results of bacterial genetic studies indicating that R factors of enteric bacteria of animals and humans frequently are the same.[131] Chloramphenicol resistance among animal strains of *Salmonella*[122,132] has been associated with increasing resistance among human isolates in certain geographic areas.[133] However, other studies have shown that susceptibility patterns of *Salmonella* isolates of human origin commonly differ from patterns of resistance for animal strains.[134] Independence of resistance among human and animal strains was shown for ampicillin. Whereas resistance of *S. typhimurium* strains to ampicillin has become a problem in human illness, only recently has resistance to ampicillin become a problem among animal strains.[130] Finally, the importance of human-to-human spread of salmonellosis may have been underestimated.[36]

More work needs to be conducted to evaluate the importance to human medicine of resistance among animal bacteria. It is surprising that little research has been carried out to examine the problem in a careful prospective fashion in spite of the vast amount of money spent each year for antibiotic-enriched feed. The lack of research may reflect the meat-production industry's strong view that routine use of antibiotic agents in feed is associated with profound savings in production costs due to the resultant enhanced animal growth and reduced number of deaths from infection. The complexity of this issue is becoming apparent as further studies are being conducted. We are finding that a high degree of species specificity exists among enteropathogens, particularly in the colonizing potential of the agent. Also, the biologic characteristics of plasmids may explain a barrier to spread of resistance among bacteria of different species origin. R factors are usually transferred at 37°C or 28°C or both. Those that transfer at 28°C but not 37°C are considered to be heat-sensitive R factors.[135,136] Heat-sensitive R factors are more common among animal strains of *S. typhimurium*[122] and may be expected to readily transfer outside the body. Tetracycline resistance most often is controlled by heat-sensitive R factors, perhaps related to the widespread use of this antibiotic in animal feed. These plasmids, being associated with transfer outside the body, could lead to resistance in the gut of animals recurrently ingesting large numbers of bacteria containing R factors. However, *in vivo* spread of the heat-sensitive R factors should be unusual. This may explain the difficulty of showing *in vivo* transfer of resistance from animal bacteria to resident flora in humans.[137] No such difficulty should exist for R factors that transfer at 37°C. Ampicillin appears to select non-heat-sensitive factors, which may explain the rapid emergence of antibiotic resistance among *Salmonella* in persons taking ampicillin.[41] Undoubtedly, *Salmonella* can efficiently acquire the non-heat-sensitive R factors from other enteric bacteria under the selective force of an antibiotic.

Future studies in this field need to be focused in two major directions. The first is to design and implement careful prospective studies among farming communities to examine the biologic events which surround routine use of antibiotics in animal feed. Colonization of humans with antibiotic-resistant strains of animal origin should be sought, but, more importantly, human illness must be carefully studied to determine the occurrence of animal strains as infecting agents. Primary or secondary spread of animal strains must be sought among persons not having direct contact with animals. The other major focus should be on the laboratory investigation of comparisons of common mechanisms of action of resistance among animal and human strains and the determination of the similarities among plasmids of differing origins. Plasmid biologists, who have done so much with genetic engineering, must be encouraged to tackle the problem of antibiotic resistance mechanisms. In the meantime, antibiotics that are important in human medicine, including ampicillin, chloramphenicol, tetracycline, aminoglycosides, penicillins, and cephalosporins, should not be employed in veterinary medicine as food additives or as therapeutic agents. Practitioners of animal medicine should consider alternative antimicrobials and select those with little importance to humans for use in animal feeds and as therapeutic agents.

ANTIMICROBIAL THERAPY

Salmonella Gastroenteritis

Since the discovery that *Salmonella* strains were inhibited by antimicrobial agents *in vitro*, these drugs have been employed in the treatment of human salmonellosis. There was initial enthusiasm about chloramphenicol in the treatment of infantile diarrhea when it appeared to reduce morbidity and mortality.[138] A study soon followed which included a greater number of infants observed over a 17-month period. It failed to demonstrate a favorable effect of chloramphenicol on pediatric gastoenteritis due to *Salmonella* as compared to an untreated control group.[139] Two studies in the late 1960s demonstrated that children and adults with *Salmonella* gastroenteritis who were treated with oral ampicillin, chloramphenicol, or neomycin paradoxically excreted *Salmonella* longer than those left untreated.[41,140] Therapy also led to *in vivo* resistance of the *Salmonella* strains to the employed drug.[41] A case report showed that severe diarrhea was induced in an asymptomatic *Salmonella* carrier by oral ampicillin.[141] TMP plus SMX has been employed in the treatment of *Salmonella* gastroenteritis. In one study, it appeared to influence clinical and bacteriologic findings, especially when combined with polymyxin,[142] while in a second study, it did not appear to favorably alter the intestinal carriage of the infecting strain during the postconvalescent stage.[143] In a third study, TMP–SMX and ampicillin were ineffective in modifying clinical features and in influencing rates of intestinal excretion of the *Salmonella* strain in children.[144]

While it is not entirely clear why the condition is not more responsive to antimicrobial agents that show *in vitro* activity, the data thus far published suggest that antibiotics should be withheld from patients with uncomplicated gastroenteritis and those who are asymptomatic carriers of nontyphoid *Salmonella*. As previously discussed, bacteremia may occur in *Salmonella* gastroenteritis in just under 10% of cases. While an insufficient number of such patients have been well studied, it is the opinion of most authorities that patients with nontyphoid *Salmonella* bacteremia should receive an antimicrobial agent and be treated as if they have typhoid fever with chloramphenicol, ampicillin, or TMP-SMX (see Table 10.4, Chapter 10, for dosages). Our policy is to treat with antibiotics any patient with salmonellosis who has evidence of a progressive infection: systemic toxicity, hypotension, renal failure, etc. Practically speaking, this usually includes any patient ill enough to be admitted to the hospital.

Typhoid (Enteric) Fever

Antimicrobial agents play an indisputable role in the treatment of enteric fever, whether the infection is due to *S. typhi, S. cholerae-suis, S. paratyphi,* or other *Salmonella* serotypes. In selecting the agent for therapy, it is important to realize that *in vitro* inhibition of *Salmonella* cannot be used as sufficient evidence of a drug's effectiveness. The polypeptide antimicrobials (polymyxin), aminoglycosides (gentamicin), and cephalosporins are all bactericidal to *Salmonella* organisms *in vitro* at low concentrations, yet each is ineffective in treating typhoid.[145] On the other hand, *in vitro* resistance is correlated with *in vivo* resistance. During 1972, a large epidemic of typhoid fever in Mexico was caused by a single chloramphenicol-resistant *S. typhi* strain. *In vitro* resistance[146] and *in vivo* resistance[147] were confirmed. Fortunately, only a small number of strains identified in this outbreak were demonstrated to be resistant to ampicillin.[146] Since that outbreak, chloramphenicol-resistant *S. typhi* strains have been identified throughout the world.[148-151]

The first report of successful therapy of typhoid fever with chloramphenicol was published by Woodward *et al.*[152] in 1948; however, chloramphenicol was not an ideal drug, since relapses of illness were twice as common as previously reported for untreated disease, and carriers were not eliminated. Also, the rare development of bone marrow aplasia was of concern. In the 1960s, ampicillin was shown to have antityphoid activity, and in the 1970s the fixed-combination drug TMP–SMX[143,147,153-162] and a drug related to ampicillin, amoxicillin,[163-165] were found to be effective. The only other agent with some usefulness in the therapy of typhoid fever is furazolidone. A number of excellent clinical trials have been carried out comparing the available forms of therapy. These studies do not allow definitive statements to be made about the relative value of the preparations. In comparing oral ampicillin with chloramphenicol, investigators indicated that defervescence occurred more rapidly with chloramphenicol.[166,167] Others found the drugs equal with regard to fever response.[168,169] In one of these studies, it appeared that relapses and *Salmonella* carriage might have been more favorably reduced by ampicillin therapy.[167] While there is a feeling among investigators that ampicillin must be given parenterally, and there are case reports supporting this notion, evidence would suggest that the drug is effective when given orally.[168,169]

Similar confusion exists regarding the relative usefulness of chloramphenicol and TMP–SMX. In one study, TMP–SMX produced a more rapid reduction in systemic toxicity of typhoid illness but not a greater fever response than chloramphenicol,[156] another showed an impressive advantage for TMP–SMX in reduction of toxemia and number of relapses, although again defervescence was equal,[160] and a third indicated that fewer relapses and typhoid carriers were seen in the group treated with TMP–SMX.[158] Another study indicated that systemic toxicity was more rapidly reduced by chloramphenicol, although reduction of fever was equal and carrier rates may actually have been increased by TMP–SMX.[159] Studies comparing TMP–SMX and chloramphenicol showed an advantage for TMP–SMX when this drug combination was employed in a higher dose (240–320 mg TMP plus 1200–1600 mg SMX b.i.d. in adults early in illness), while other studies showed chloramphenicol to be superior (when 160 mg TMP plus 800 mg SMX were given b.i.d.). Investigations need to be carried out to determine if a higher dose of TMP–SMX does offer advantages over the more traditional dosage regimen.

Amoxicillin given orally appears to be well tolerated and produces favorable results in the therapy of typhoid fever.[163] It was found to be equal to chloramphenicol in all respects in one comparative study[164] and to be better than chloramphenicol (more rapid defervescence, lower relapse and carrier rate) in another,[165] while it appeared to be equal to TMP–SMX in a third.[162] In the treatment of chloramphenicol-resistant strains of *S. typhi*, ampicillin, TMP–SMX, and furazolidone, but not chloramphenicol, have been found to be helpful.[157,162]

Table 5.4 compares the four major forms of antityphoid therapy. Chloramphenicol probably will remain the standard form of therapy for typhoid fever throughout most of the world, since it is predictably successful against sensitive strains and is significantly less expensive than the other drugs. Chloramphenicol is available for oral administration in capsules containing chloramphenicol base and as a suspension of palmitate ester suitable for use by infants and children. Chloramphenicol is mar-

TABLE 5.4
Comparison of Antityphoid Antimicrobials

Antimicrobial	Method of administration		Advantages
	Oral	Parenteral	
Chloramphenicol	+	+	Significantly lower cost; predictable response for sensitive strains
Ampicillin	+	+	Effective against chloramphenicol-resistant strains; more effective in treating and probably reducing *Salmonella typhi* carriage
Amoxicillin	+	0^a	Same as ampicillin, plus more predictable blood levels following oral therapy
TMP–SMX	+	0	Effective against rare chloramphenicol/ampicillin-resistant strains

^{a}Will be available in the future.

keted for parenteral use as a succinate ester, which should be administered intravenously, since low levels of biologically active drug in serum are achieved after intramuscular administration.[170] Both the palmitate and succinate esters must be hydrolyzed into an active form *in vivo*. Oral administration of chloramphenicol in the palmitate form produces serum concentrations and areas under the dissappearance curve similar to those achieved after intravenous administration of the same dose.[171] We do not believe that there is sufficient evidence to allow the often-made statement that aplastic anemia is a complication of oral and not parenteral therapy. In the past, it has been unusual to administer chloramphenicol solely by the parenteral route. It is our recommendation that chloramphenicol be given orally whenever possible. The preferred oral form of chloramphenicol for older children and adults is the free drug prepared in capsules; however, the pediatric suspension of chloramphenicol palmitate is adequate for small children. The drug should be given intravenously to patients unable to take an oral drug because of toxemia, obtundation, severe ileus, intestinal perforation, etc. Ampicillin or amoxicillin probably should be the treatment of choice for typhoid fever in the United States, where the cost of the drug is relatively less important and in view of the occasional occurrence of chloramphenicol-resistant strains. At this time, the main value of TMP–SMX is in the treatment of chloramphenicol/ampicillin-resistant strains. If future studies show that higher doses of TMP–SMX are more effective than other treatment groups, these recommendations may be altered. (See Table 10.4 in Chapter 10 for drugs and dosages used in the treatment of typhoid fever.)

Typhoid Carriers

Carriers of *S. typhi* are the major source of endemic and epidemic typhoid fever. A person is considered a carrier if stools are consistently positive for *S. typhi* for one year or longer. Before the availability of antimicrobial agents, cholecystectomy was the only means of therapy.[172] In an occasional patient, large doses of penicillin were found to be effective,[44,173] yet chloramphenicol was ineffective. Ampicillin was found to be useful, perhaps because of its bactericidal activity, its high concentration in biliary secretions, and the high doses in which it could be given. Initially, it was felt that large doses of ampicillin could eliminate the carrier state if there were no coexistent gallbladder disease but that it was ineffective in the presence of cholelithiasis.[174,175] It was urged that cholecystectomy be performed on patients with biliary disease in addition to administering ampicillin therapy. Other studies evaluating prolonged oral ampicillin therapy[176–178] and shorter courses of ampicillin given intravenously[179] demonstrated that intestinal carriage of *S. typhi* could be interrupted, in many cases even in the face of documented cholelithiasis. Although not as well studied, amoxicillin should be just as effective and may be better tolerated by patients.[180] A few studies have shown the value of treatment of carriers with TMP–SMX.[181–183]

Children who carry *S. typhi* probably should receive ampicillin 100 mg/kg/day (p.o.) in four divided doses plus probenecid 30 mg/kg/day (p.o.) in four divided doses or amoxicillin 40 mg/kg/day (p.o.) in three divided doses for four to six weeks. Adult carriers should receive ampicillin 1 g (p.o.) q.i.d. for four to six weeks or an intensive hospital course of 1 g (i.v.) every 6 hr for 15 days. Amoxicillin may be effective in adult carriers when given in a dosage of 2 g (p.o.) t.i.d. for 28 days.[184] If cholelithiasis is documented, cholecystectomy should complement therapy unless there are medical contraindications for surgery.

IMMUNOPROPHYLAXIS

Immunity in *Salmonella* infection is serotype-specific. Therefore, due to the heterogeneity of the various serotypes of *Salmonella* responsible for gastroenteritis, an immunizing agent is not a feasible means of controlling infection. On the other hand, due to the antigenic homogeneity of typhoid strains, the propensity for epidemic spread of typhoid fever, and the general seriousness of infection, an effective *S. typhi* vaccine would have profound public health usefulness.

In experimental salmonellosis, there are at least two different types of immune response. Cellular immunity generally is induced by living organisms, natural infection, or administering killed cells in Freund's complete adjuvant, whereas humoral immunity is primarily elicited by immunization with killed cells and LPS.[185–189] Although both O and Vi antigens are associated with virulence of *S. typhi* strains, O and Vi serum agglutinin titers are not correlated with typhoid immunity.[185] Flagellar (H) antibody levels are more closely associated with resistance to infection.

Typhoid fever occurs among the vaccinated[185] and those who have recovered from active infection.[190,191] Immunity induced by parenteral administration of commercially available killed vaccine has been quantitated in previously unexposed volunteers and in field areas where disease is hyperendemic. In volunteers, immunity is partial and related to the dose of ingested bacteria,[3] while the same immunizing agents are highly effective for prolonged periods under field conditions. Undoubtedly, the differences in vaccine efficacy relate to the disparity in the prevaccination immune status of the groups under study. In areas where disease is endemic, repeated exposure to live typhoid or related *Salmonella* antigens under natural conditions probably leads to a level of resistance which is enhanced by immunization. The volunteers probably represent unexposed, highly susceptible persons for whom the sole typhoid exposure is the parenterally administered immunizing agent. The commercial vaccine is not entirely satisfactory, therefore, in view of its relative ineffectiveness in protecting previously unexposed persons such as those from industrialized parts of the world who are traveling to areas of typhoid endemicity. Also, there is a high percentage of local and systemic reactions to the preparation and a need for sterile conditions for preparation, preservation, and administration of the vaccine. Studies are being conducted in an attempt to improve the immunizing agent, either through development of an oral live vaccine or by identifying subunit or ribosomal elements which are immunogenic.

Parenteral Typhoid Vaccines

One of the available typhoid fever vaccines is monovalent heat–phenol preserved and dried Ty2v strain of *S. typhi* (vaccine L). In producing a killed typhoid vaccine by heat–formalin or phenol inactivation, cell-wall antigens are not destroyed, but Vi antigen is made less antigenic. An acetone-inactivated vaccine (vaccine K) has been developed which more effectively preserves the Vi antigen. Both vaccines L and K, administered in two or three subcutaneous or intramuscular doses, have been extensively field tested in Guyana, Poland, the Soviet Union, and Yugoslavia, and protective immunity resulted which was most impressive in children.[192-196] The only serologic indicator of superiority of vaccine K over L was the titer of H agglutinins and not antibody to O or Vi antigens.[185,193] Active mouse protection correlated to some degree with field trial results,[97,198] but a better laboratory assay of potency and immunogenicity is needed. In areas of endemicity, one dose of vaccine was as protective as two.[194,195] The local and systemic reactions to vaccination were less commonly seen with the second dose of vaccine as compared to the first.[196] In most of the published field studies, both L and K vaccines were approximately 80% protective during the first year, and the rate of protection remained constant for vaccine K for three years but fell to 55% for vaccine L (see Figure 5.4). In a large study of Guyanese school children, two doses of either vaccine gave even more striking protection which did not fall until the fifth year, and they were still protective (65% for L and 88% for K) into the seventh year.[194] The improved protection of acetone-inactivated vaccine (K) is attributed to fixation by acetone of the Vi antigen to the bacteria.[199] As Vi antigen has been associated with virul-

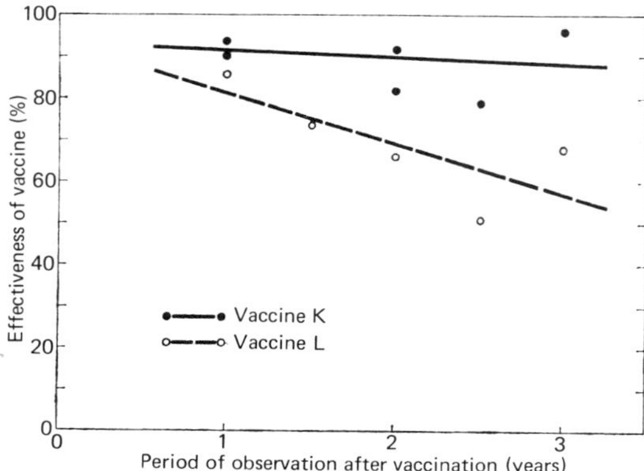

Figure 5.4. Effectiveness of typhoid fever vaccines K and L in field trials conducted in Guyana, Poland, the Soviet Union, and Yugoslavia. From Cvjetanović and Uemura.[192]

ence of *S. typhi*, and since vaccine K which spared the antigen is more protective against typhoid illness than L, a number of investigators have worked with purified Vi antigen in attempting to clarify its role in human disease and to determine its immunizing potential.[200–202] Purified Vi antigen was not found to induce protective typhoid immunity in experimental animals[203] or humans.[3]

Other approaches have been to employ an LPS or ribosome-rich fractions of bacteria as an immunizing agent.[204–209] Preliminary studies indicated that a nonliving ribosomal vaccine was comparable to a living vaccine in stimulating immunity,[204,205] apparently through a cell mediated host immune response.[206,207] Protective immunity might have been related to purified ribonucleic acid fraction,[204] ribosomal protein,[208] or contaminating LPS.[205,209] A whole-ribosomal vaccine (not purified component) was compared as an immunizing agent to purified LPS, acetone-killed whole-cell vaccine, and living cells in an experimental animal model.[205] Ribosomes were not superior to acetone-killed cells, and both were almost as effective as the living vaccine. LPS was by far the least protective.

Oral Typhoid Vaccines

The concept of intestinal immunization in typhoid fever was first supported by Metchnikoff and Besredka in 1911 while studying infection in monkeys.[210] An oral vaccine would have certain advantages over a parenteral preparation, since the oral route of administration would probably minimize local and systemic postvaccinal reactions found with parenteral vaccines and might also directly stimulate local intestinal immune mechanisms.

Oral killed typhoid antigen has been tried in a volunteer model[191] and field tested in areas of endemicity.[211,212] Significant protection did not occur in any of the studies, although in volunteers, the killed vaccine did appear to confer a limited "intestinal immunity" whereby intestinal multiplications and isolation of virulent *S. typhi*, employed to test vaccine efficacy, were inhibited by prior oral immunization.[191]

Living attenuated oral vaccines also have been tested, including genetic recombinations employing different bacterial species,[213,214] streptomycin-dependent (SMD) mutants,[215–217] uridine-diphosphate–galactose-4-epimerase (UDP) deficient mutants,[4,218–220] and temperature-sensitive *Salmonella* mutants.[221,222] Reitman has tested an SMD mutant of *S. typhi* in mice and found it to be safe, stable, and immunogenic.[216] When fed to volunteers in multiple high doses, with and without streptomycin, the SMD vaccine was well tolerated and *in vivo* reversion was not found.[215] Intestinal biopsy was performed in a number of volunteers receiving multiple oral doses of SMD vaccine, and in each case an increase in the number of plasma cells was noted in the lamina propria (see Figure 5.5). The immunized volunteers resisted active infection when subsequently challenged with virulent *S. typhi*, and a profound influence on inhibition of intestinal proliferation of the typhoid strain was documented in those immunized. A similar SMD *S. typhi* vaccine was evaluated in chimpanzees and found to be protective.[217] Problems with SMD vaccine are its potential for reversion to virulence, which occurs only rarely,[223] and possible inactivation of potency by lyophilization.[220]

UDP mutants have incomplete cell-wall LPS structures and remain rough and avirulent. In the presence of low concentrations of galactose, as is the case *in vivo*, a phenotypic curing occurs, allowing biosynthesis of smooth-like LPS, thereby explaining the strain's immunogenicity.[219] However, galactose uptake induces bacteriolysis preventing reversion to virulence.[224] This strain is protective in mice,[218] and preliminary data in volunteers suggest that it may serve as a satisfactory immunizing agent in humans.[225]

A temperature-sensitive mutant is avirulent, as it is unable to proliferate at 37°C.[221] Such a strain may be protective, since it has been shown to induce an immune response in a mouse model. In this model, a reduction in multiplication of virulent organisms in Peyer's patch was demonstrated which was not dependent upon development or presence of specific humoral antibody.[222]

Figure 5.6 summarizes results of volunteer studies designed to determine the efficacy of various antityphoid vaccines and to compare the level of immunity which was seen following recovery from active typhoid fe-

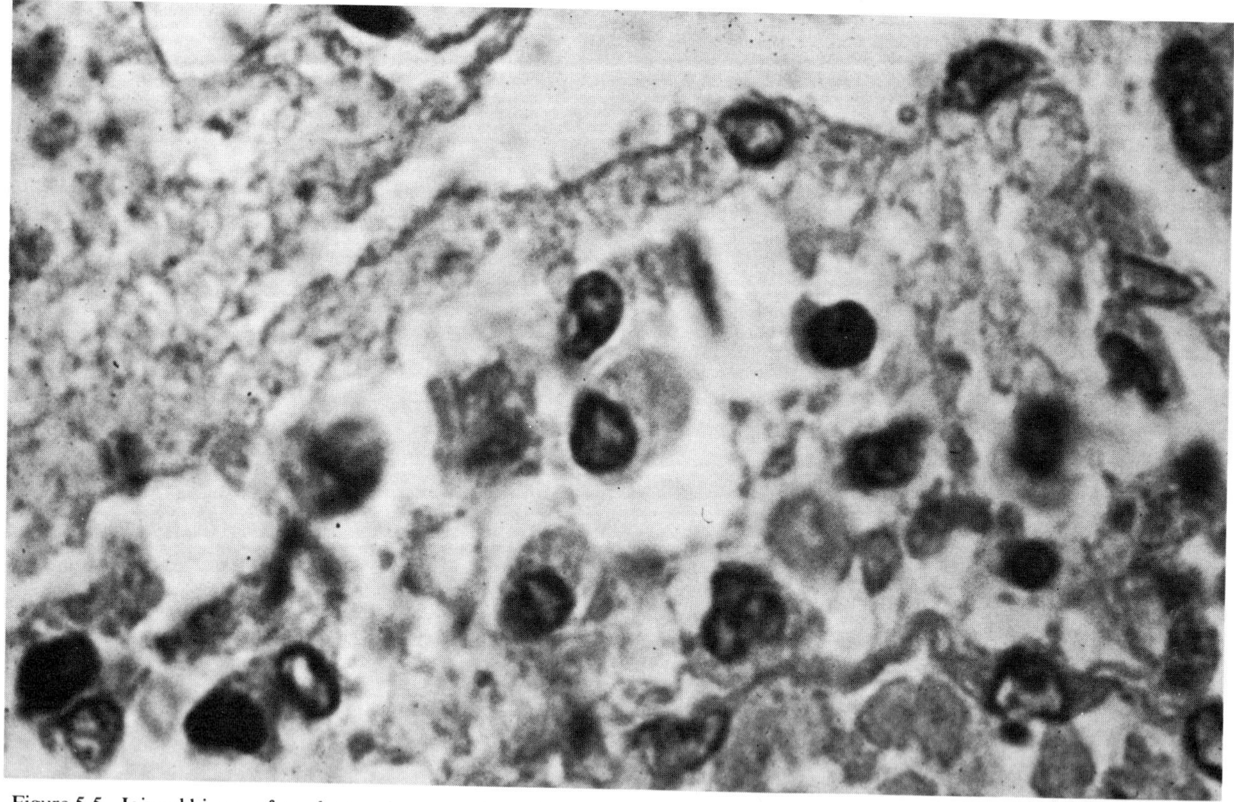

Figure 5.5. Jejunal biopsy of a volunteer immunized with four oral doses of SMD *Salmonella typhi*. Numerous plasma cells are noted (hematoxylin and cosin, ×1000). *From H.L. DuPont, R.B. Hornick, T.E. Woodward, University of Maryland School of Medicine.

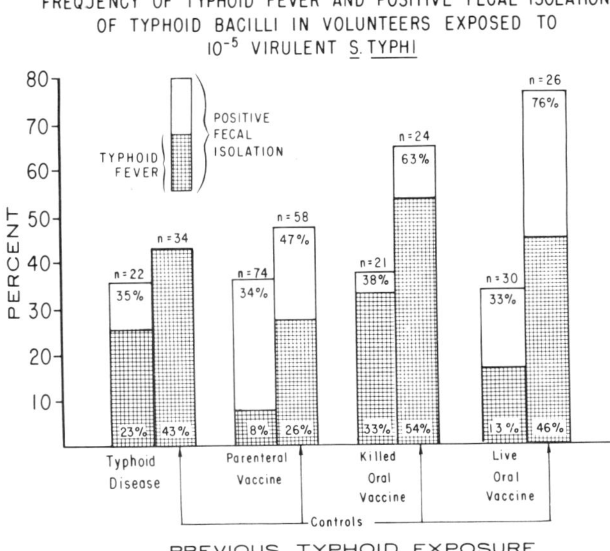

Figure 5.6. Typhoid fever immunity in volunteers. Previous disease and administration of parenteral (killed) vaccine led to protection from illness; oral vaccines (killed and live) produced protective immunity, whereby illness rates were lowered and intestinal proliferation of the virulent challenge strain was also inhibited (intestinal immunity). From DuPont.[226]

ver. Protective typhoid immunity was seen in volunteers after recovery from illness and following administration of commercially available parenteral typhoid vaccine or a live orally administered SMD vaccine. A striking difference, however, was that the stool excretion of virulent *S. typhi* differed in the various groups. Oral vaccines (both live and killed) were associated with an antibacterial effect at the gut level, whereby *S. typhi* was less commonly isolated from stool in those immunized as compared to the control groups, to those recovering from active disease, or to those administered parenteral vaccine.

REFERENCES

1. Edwards, P. R., Ewing, W. H. *Identification of Enterobacteriaceae*, 3rd ed. Burgess, Minneapolis, 1972.
2. Felix, A., Pitt, R. M. The pathogenic and immunogenic activities of *Salmonella typhi* in relation to its antigenic constituents. *J. Hyg. (Cambridge)* **49**:92–110, 1951.
3. Hornick, R. B., Greisman, S. E., Woodward, T. E., *et al.* Typhoid fever: Pathogenesis and immunologic control. *N. Engl. J. Med.* **283**:686–691, 739–746, 1970.

4. Germanier, R., Füer, E. Isolation and characterization of *gal* E mutant Ty 21a of *Salmonella typhi*. A candidate strain for a live, oral typhoid vaccine. *J. Infect. Dis.* **131:**553–558, 1975.

5. Speck, W. T., Wlodkowski, T. J., Rosenkranz, H. S. Decreased virulence of chlorate-resistant *Salmonella typhimurium*. *J. Infect. Dis.* **134:**90–92, 1976.

6. DuPont, H. L., Formal, S. B., Hornick, R. B., *et al.* Pathogenesis of *Escherichia coli* diarrhea. *N. Engl. J. Med.* **285:**1–9, 1971.

7. Giannella, R. A., Formal, S. B., Dammin, G. J., *et al.* Pathogenesis of salmonellosis: Studies of fluid secretion, mucosal invasion, and morphologic reaction in the rabbit ileum. *J. Clin. Invest.* **52:**441–453, 1973.

8. Taylor, J., Wilkins, M. P., The effect of *Salmonella* and *Shigella* on ligated loops of rabbit gut. *Indian J. Med. Res.* **49:**544–549, 1961.

9. Koupal, L. R., Deibel, R. H. Assay, characterization, and localization of an enterotoxin produced by *Salmonella*. *Infect. Immun.* **11:**14–22, 1975.

10. Sandefur, P. D., Peterson, J. W. Isolation of skin permeability factors from culture filtrates of *Salmonella typhimurium*. *Infect. Immun.* **14:**671–679, 1976.

11. Miller, R. M., Garbus, J., Hornick, R. B. Lack of enhanced oxygen consumption by polymorphonuclear leukocytes on phagocytosis of virulent *Salmonella typhi*. *Science* **175:**1010–1011, 1972.

12. D'Aoust, J. Y., Pivnick, H. Small infectious doses of salmonella. *Lancet* **1:**866, 1976.

13. Lipson, A., Infecting dose of salmonella (letter). *Lancet* **1:**969, 1976.

14. Waddell, W. R., Kunz, L. J. Association of *Salmonella enteritis* with operations on the stomach. *N. Engl. J. Med.* **255:**555–559, 1956.

15. Garrod, L. P. The susceptibility of different bacteria to destruction in the stomach (abstract). *J. Pathol. Bacteriol.* **45:**473–474, 1937.

16. Hook, E. W. Salmonellosis: Certain factors influencing the interaction of salmonella and the human host. *Bull. N.Y. Acad. Med.* **37:**499–512, 1961.

17. Nordbring, F. Contraction of salmonella gastroenteritis following previous operation on the stomach. *Acta Med. Scand.* **171:**783–790, 1962.

18. Giannella, R. A., Broitman, S. A., Zamcheck, N. *Salmonella enteritis:* I. Role of reduced gastric secretion in pathogenesis. *Am. J. Dig. Dis.* **16:**1000–1006, 1971.

19. Giannella, R. A., Broitman, S. A., Zamcheck, N. *Salmonella enteritis:* II. Fulminant diarrhea in and effects on the small intestine. *Am. J. Dig. Dis.* **16:**1007–1013, 1971.

20. Kent, T. H., Formal, S. B., LaBrec, E. H. *Salmonella* gastroenteritis in rhesus monkeys. *Arch. Pathol.* **82:**272–279, 1966.

21. Rout, W. R., Formal, S. B., Dammin, G. J., *et al.* Pathophysiology of salmonella diarrhea in the rhesus monkey: Intestinal transport, morphological, and bacteriological studies. *Gastroenterology* **67:**59–70, 1974.

22. Sprinz, H., Gangarosa, E. J., Williams, M., *et al.* Histopathology of the upper small intestines in typhoid fever: Biopsy study of experimental disease in man. *Am. J. Dig. Dis.* **11:**615–624, 1966.

23. Gaines, S., Sprinz, H., Tully, J. G., *et al.* Studies on infection and immunity in experimental typhoid fever: VII. The distribution of *Salmonella typhi* in chimpanzee tissue following oral challenge, and the relationship between the numbers of bacilli and morphologic lesions. *J. Infect. Dis.* **118:**293–306, 1968.

24. Gaines, S., Tully, J. G., Tigertt, W. D. Studies on infection and immunity in experimental typhoid fever: VIII. Intravenous and intra-lymph node challenge of chimpanzees with *Salmonella typhi*. *J. Infect. Dis.* **118:**393–401, 1968.

25. Edsall, G., Gaines, S., Landy, M., *et al.* Studies on infection and immunity in experimental typhoid fever: I. Typhoid fever in chimpanzees orally infected with *Salmonella typhosa*. *J. Exp. Med.* **112:**143–166, 1960.

26. Takeuchi, A. Penetration of intestinal epithelium by various microorganisms. *Curr. Top. Pathol.* **54:**1–27, 1971.
27. Harris, J. C., DuPont, H. L., Hornick, R. B. Fecal leukocytes in diarrheal illness. *Ann. Intern. Med.* **76:**697–703, 1972.
28. Aleekseev, P. A., Berman, M. I., Korneeva, E. P. Clinical and histological picture of *Salmonella typhimurium* infection in children. *Zh. Mikrobiol. Epidemiol. Immunobiol.* **31:**111–116, 1960.
29. Mandal, B. K., Mani, V. Colonic involvement in salmonellosis. *Lancet* **1:**887–888, 1976.
30. Radsel-Medvescek, A., Zargi, R., Acko, M., *et al.* Colonic involvement in salmonellosis (Letter). *Lancet* **1:**601, 1977.
31. Appelbaum, P. C., Scragg, J., Schonland, M. M. Colonic involvement in salmonellosis. *Lancet* **2:**102, 1976.
32. Greisman, S. E., Hornick, R. B., Wagner, H. N., *et al.* The integrity of the endotoxin tolerance mechanisms during typhoid fever in man. *Trans. Assoc. Am. Physicians* **80:**250–258, 1967.
33. Schroeder, S. A., Aserkoff, B., Brachman, P. S. Epidemic salmonellosis in hospitals and institutions: A five-year review. *N. Engl. J. Med.* **279:**674–678, 1968.
34. Cohen, M. L., Fontaine, R. E., Pollard, R. A., *et al.* An assessment of patient-related economic costs in an outbreak of salmonellosis. *N. Engl. J. Med.* **299:**459–460, 1978.
35. Wilder, A. N., MacCready, R. A. Isolation of salmonella from poultry, poultry products and poultry processing plants in Massachusetts. *N. Engl. J. Med.* **274:**1453–1460, 1966.
36. Cherubin, C. E., Fodor, T., Denmark, L., *et al.* The epidemiology of salmonellosis in New York City. *Am. J. Epidemiol.* **90:**112–125, 1969.
37. Greenburg, B., Kowalski, J. A., Klowden, M. J. Factors affecting the transmission of *Salmonella* by flies: Natural resistance to colonization and bacterial interference. *Infect. Immun.* **2:**800–809, 1970.
38. Feldman, R. E., Baine, W. B., Nitzkin, J. L., *et al.* Epidemiology of *Salmonella typhi* infection in a migrant labor camp in Dade County, Florida. *J. Infect. Dis.* **130:**335–342, 1974.
39. *Annual Salmonella Surveillance Report.* United States Department of Health, Education and Welfare, Public Health Service, National Communicable Disease Center, Atlanta, 1967.
40. Musher, D. M., Rubenstein, A. D. Permanent carriers of nontyphosa salmonellae. *Arch. Intern. Med.* **132:**869–872, 1973.
41. Aserkoff, B., Bennett, J. V. Effect of antibiotic therapy in acute salmonellosis on the fecal excretion of salmonellae. *N. Engl. J. Med.* **281:**636–640, 1969.
42. Watson, K. C. Intravascular *Salmonella typhi* as a manifestation of the carrier state. *Lancet* **2:**332–334, 1967.
43. Huckstep, R. L. Recent advances in the surgery of typhoid fever. *Ann. R. Coll. Surg. Engl.* **26:**207–230, 1960.
44. Woodward, T. E., Smadel, J. E. Management of typhoid fever and its complications. *Ann. Intern. Med.* **60:**144–157, 1964.
45. Archampong, E. Q. Operative treatment of typhoid perforation of the bowel. *Br. Med. J.* **3:**273–276, 1969.
46. Angorn, I. B., Pillay, S. P., Hegarty, M., *et al.* Typhoid perforation of the ileum: A therapeutic dilemma. *S. Afr. Med. J.* **49:**781–784, 1975.
47. Strate, R. W., Bannayan, G. A. Typhoid fever causing massive lower gastrointestinal hemorrhage: A reminder of things past. *J. Am. Med. Assoc.* **236:**1979–1980, 1976.
48. Ramachandran, S., Godfrey, J. J., Perera, M. V. F. Typhoid hepatitis. *J. Am. Med. Assoc.* **230:**236–240, 1974.

49. Faierman, D., Ross, F. A., Seckler, S. G. Typhoid fever complicated by hepatitis, nephritis, and thrombocytopenia. *J. Am. Med. Assoc.* **221**:60–61, 1972.
50. Sitprija, V., Pipatanagul, V., Boonpucknavig, V., *et al.* Glomerulitis in typhoid fever. *Ann. Intern. Med.* **81**:210–213, 1974.
51. Rheingold, O. J., Greenwald, R. A., Hayes, P. J., *et al.* Myoglobinuria and renal failure associated with typhoid fever. *J. Am. Med. Assoc.* **238**:341, 1977.
52. Allen, N., Nomanbhoy, Y., Green, D., *et al.* Typhoid fever with consumption coagulopathy. *J. Am. Med. Assoc.* **208**:689–690, 1969.
53. Van Diem, L., Arnold, K. Typhoid fever with myocarditis. *Am. J. Trop. Med. Hyg.* **23**:218–221, 1974.
54. Rowland, H. A. K. The complications of typhoid fever. *J. Trop. Med. Hyg.* **64**:143–152, 1961.
55. Briem, H., Evengard, B., Jonsson, M. Reiter's syndrome complicating *Salmonella enteritidis* infection. *Lancet* **2**:112, 1978.
56. Siasoco, R. E., Chen, C., Chang, T. Tuberculin reaction in typhoid fever. *Ann. Intern. Med.* **81**:400, 1974.
57. Baine, W. B., Gangarosa, E. J., Bennett, J. V., *et al.* Institutional salmonellosis. *J. Infect. Dis.* **128**:357–360, 1973.
58. McCall, C. E., Collins, R. N., Jones, D. B., *et al.* An interstate outbreak of salmonellosis traced to a contaminated food supplement. *Am. J. Epidemiol.* **84**:32–39, 1966.
59. Komarmy, L. E., Oxley, M. E., Brecher, G. Hospital-acquired salmonellosis traced to carmine dye capsules. *N. Engl. J. Med.* **276**:850–852, 1967.
60. Lang, D. J., Kunz, L. J., Martin, A. R., *et al.* Carmine as a source of nosocomial salmonellosis. *N. Engl. J. Med.* **276**:829–832, 1967.
61. Rhame, F. S., Root, R. K., MacLowry, J. D. Salmonella septicemia from platelet transfusions: Study of an outbreak traced to a hematogenous carrier of *Salmonella cholerae-suis. Ann. Intern. Med.* **78**:633–641, 1973.
62. *Salmonella Surveillance Report* No. 59. United States Department of Health, Education and Welfare, Public Health Service, National Communicable Disease Center, Atlanta, 1967, p. 8.
63. Ryder, R. W., Crosby-Ritchie, A., McDonough, B., *et al.* Human milk contaminated with *Salmonella kottbus:* A cause of nosocomial illness in infants. *J. Am. Med. Assoc.* **238**:1533–1534, 1977.
64. Rubenstein, A. D., Fowler, R. N. Salmonellosis of the newborn with transmission by delivery room resuscitators. *Am. J. Public Health* **45**:1109–1114, 1955.
65. Edgar, W. M., Lacey, B. W. Infection with *Salmonella heidelberg:* An outbreak presumptively not foodborne. *Lancet* **1**:161–163, 1963.
66. Epstein, H. C., Hochwald, A., Ashe, R. Salmonella infections of the newborn infant. *J. Pediatr.* **38**:723–731, 1951.
67. Pearson, H. E., Grant, W. J. Presumed transmission of salmonella by sigmoidoscope. *Calif. Med.* **112**:23–25, 1970.
68. Watt, J., Wegman, M. E., Brown, O. W., *et al.* Salmonellosis in a premature nursery unaccompanied by diarrheal disease. *Pediatrics* **22**:689–705, 1958.
69. Bate, J. G., James, U. *Salmonella typhimurium* infection dust-borne in a children's ward. *Lancet* **2**:713–715, 1958.
70. Mushin, R. An outbreak of gastroenteritis due to *Salmonella derby. J. Hyg. (Cambridge)* **46**:151–157, 1948.
71. Szmuness, W. Infections hospitalières par *Salmonella enteritidis* chez les enfants. *Rev. Hyg. Méd. Soc.* **13**:531–548, 1965.
72. Sanders, E., Sweeney, F. J., Jr., Friedman, E. A., *et al.* An outbreak of hospital-associated infections due to *Salmonella derby. J. Am. Med. Assoc.* **186**:984–986, 1963.

73. Hirsch, W., Sapiro-Hirsch, R., Berger, A., *et al. Salmonella edinburg* infection in children: A protracted hospital epidemic due to a multiple-drug-resistant strain. *Lancet* 2:828–830, 1965.
74. Leeder, F. S. An epidemic of *Salmonella panama* infections in infants. *Ann. N.Y. Acad. Sci.* 66:54–60, 1956.
75. Abroms, I. F., Cochran, W. D., Holmes, L. B., *et al.* A *Salmonella newport* outbreak in a premature nursery with a 1-year follow-up: Effect of ampicillin following bacteriologic failure of response to kanamycin. *Pediatrics* 37:616–623, 1966.
76. Szanton, V. L. Epidemic salmonellosis—a 30-month study of 80 cases of *Salmonella oranienburg* infection. *Pediatrics* 20:794–808, 1957.
77. Cherubin, C. E., Neu, H. C., Imperato, P. J., *et al.* Septicemia with nontyphoid salmonella. *Medicine* 53:365–376, 1974.
78. Black, P. H., Kunz, L. J., Swartz, M. N. Salmonellosis: A review of some unusual aspects. *N. Engl. J. Med.* 262:811–817, 864–870, 921–927, 1960.
79. Angrist, A., Mollov, M. Bacteriologic, clinical and pathological experience with 86 sporadic cases of salmonella infection. *Am. J. Med. Sci.* 212:336–346, 1946.
80. Harvey, A. M. *Salmonella suipestifer* infection in human beings: Review of the literature and report of twenty-one new cases. *Arch. Intern. Med.* 59:118–135, 1937.
81. Griffiths, P. W. W. Atypical cases of salmonellosis in hospital. *Lancet* 2:958–960, 1961.
82. Kaye, D., Gill, F. A., Hook, E. W. Factors influencing host resistance to salmonella infections: The effects of hemolysis and erythrophagocytosis. *Am. J. Med. Sci.* 254:205–215, 1967.
83. Bennett, I. L., Jr., Hook, E. W. Infectious diseases: Some aspects of salmonellosis. *Annu. Rev. Med.* 10:1–20, 1959.
84. Anderson, T. R., Zimmerman, L. E. Relapsing fever in Korea: Clinicopathologic study of eleven fatal cases with special attention to association with *Salmonella* infections. *Am. J. Pathol.* 31:1083–1109, 1955.
85. Ricketts, W. E. Intercurrent infections of Carrion's disease observed in Peru. *Am. J. Trop. Med. Hyg.* 28:437–451, 1948.
86. Hand, W. L., King, N. L. Serum opsonization of salmonella in sickle cell anemia. *Am. J. Med.* 64:388–395, 1978.
87. Field, R., Overturf, G. D. Defective opsonization of salmonella lipopolysaccharide in sickle cell disease. *Pediatr. Res.* 12:491, 1978.
88. Cooper, M. R., DeChatelet, L. R., McCall, C. E., *et al.* Complete deficiency of leukocyte glucose-6-phosphate dehydrogenase with defective bactericidal activity. *J. Clin. Invest.* 51:769–778, 1972.
89. Iron and resistance to infection (editorial). *Lancet* 2:325–326, 1974.
90. Rodey, G. E., Park, B. H., Windhorst, D. B., *et al.* Defective bactericidal activity of monocytes in fatal granulomatous disease. *Blood* 33:813–820, 1969.
91. Davis, W. C., Huber, H., Douglas, S. D., *et al.* A defect in circulating mononuclear phagocytes in chronic granulomatous disease of childhood. *J. Immunol.* 101:1093–1095, 1968.
92. Van Furth, R., Cohn, Z. A. The origin and kinetics of mononuclear phagocytes. *J. Exp. Med.* 128:415–435, 1968.
93. Moellering, R. C., Jr., Weinberg, A. N. Persistent salmonella infection in a female carrier for chronic granulomatous disease. *Ann. Intern. Med.* 73:595–601, 1970.
94. Barker, L. F., Sladen, F. J. A small epidemic of jaundice with symptoms of gastrointestinal catarrh. *Bull. Johns Hopkins Hosp.* 20:310–314, 1909.
95. Han, T., Sokal, J. E., Neter, E. Salmonellosis in disseminated malignant diseases: A seven-year review (1959–1965). *N. Engl. J. Med.* 276:1045–1052, 1967.
96. Shechmeister, I. L., Paulissen, L. J., Fishman, M. Sublethal total body x-radiation and

susceptibility of mice to *Salmonella enteritidis* and *Escherichia coli. Proc. Soc. Exp. Biol. Med.* **83:**205–209, 1953.

97. Bowen, S. T., Gowen, J. W., Tauber, O. E. Cortisone and mortality in mouse typhoid: I. Effect of hormone dosage and times of injection. *Proc. Soc. Exp. Biol. Med.* **94:**476–479, 1957.

98. Hammond, C. W., Tompkins, M., Miller, C. P. Occurrence of generalized infection of enteric origin in mice poisoned with nitrogen mustard. *Proc. Soc. Exp. Biol. Med.* **82:**137–140, 1953.

99. Lewis, J. F., Warshauer, S. E. Mycotic aneurysm of the abdominal aorta: A case due to *Salmonella cholerae-suis* var. Kunzendorf. *South. Med. J.* **62:**597–598, 1969.

100. Kanwar, Y. S., Malhotra, V., Andersen, B. R., *et al.* Salmonellosis associated with abdominal aortic aneurysm. *Arch. Intern. Med.* **134:**1095–1098, 1974.

101. Ten Eyck, F. W., Wellman, W. E. Salmonellosis associated with abdominal aortic aneurysm and edema of lower extremities: A case report. *Postgrad. Med.* **26:**334–339, 1959.

102. Zak, F. G., Strauss, L., Saphra, I. Rupture of diseased large arteries in the course of enterobacterial (salmonella) infections. *N. Engl. J. Med.* **258:**824–828, 1958.

103. Dixon, R. H., Lowicki, E. M. Salmonellosis associated with abdominal aortic aneurysm. *South. Med. J.* **59:**1403, 1408, 1966.

104. Crane, A. R. Primary multilocular mycotic aneurysm in the aorta. *Arch. Pathol.* **24:**634–641, 1937.

105. Dehlinger, K. R. Salmonella osteomyelitis of the spine associated with abdominal aortic aneurysm: Report of a case. *N. Engl. J. Med.* **238:**728–732, 1948.

106. Teixerira, R. Typhoid fever of protracted course. *Rev. Inst. Med. Trop. Sao. Paulo* **2:**56–70, 1960.

107. Tai, T. Y., Hsu, C. Y., Chang, H. C., *et al.* Typhoid and paratyphoid fevers occurring in cases of schistosomiasis. *Chin. Med. J.* **76:**426–435, 1958.

108. Neves, J., Martins, N. R. Long duration of septicaemic salmonellosis: 35 cases with 12 implicated species of salmonella. *Trans. Soc. Trop. Med. Hyg.* **61:**541–552, 1967.

109. Rocha, H., Kirk, J. W., Hearey, C. D., Jr. Prolonged *Salmonella bacteremia* in patients with *Schistosoma mansoni* infection. *Arch. Intern. Med.* **128:**254–257, 1971.

110. Rocha, H., Magnavita, M., Teles, E. da S., *et al.* Atividade antibacteriana do sôro de pacientes com forma hepatesplénica de esquistóssomose mansônica. *Rev. Inst. Med. Trop. São Paulo* **10:**364–370, 1968.

111. Fernandes, D. J., Rocha, H. Características de reacão inflamatória em pacientes com forma hepatesplénica da esquistóssomose mansônica e calazar. *Rev. Inst. Med. Trop. São Paulo* **9:**129–134, 1967.

112. Ottens, H., Dickerson, G. Bacterial invasion of schistosomes. *Nature (London)* **223:**506–507, 1969.

113. Biological control of schistosomiasis? *Lancet* **2:**477–478, 1969.

114. Neves, J., Marinho, R. P., Martins, N. R. L. L., *et al.* Prolonged septicemic salmonellosis: Treatment of intercurrent schistosomiasis with niridazole. *Trans. R. Soc. Trop. Med. Hyg.* **63:**79–84, 1969.

115. Lindeman, R. J., Weinstein, L., Levitan, R., *et al.* Ulcerative colitis and intestinal salmonellosis. *Am. J. Med. Sci.* **254:**855–861, 1967.

116. Dronfield, M. W., Fletcher, J., Langman, M. J. S. Coincident salmonella infections and ulcerative colitis: Problems of recognition and management. *Br. Med. J.* **1:**99–100, 1974.

117. Gilman, R. H., Terminel, M., Levine, M. M., *et al.* Relative efficacy of blood, urine, rectal swab, bone-marrow, and rose-spot cultures for recovery of *Salmonella typhi* in typhoid fever. *Lancet* **1:**1211–1213, 1975.

118. Robertson, R. P., Abdel Wahab, M. F. A. Influence of chloramphenicol and ampicillin on antibody response in typhoid–paratyphoid fever. *Ann. Intern. Med.* **72**:219–221, 1970.

119. Kobland, J. D., Gustafson, R. H., Langner, P. H. Antibiotic sensitivity of *Salmonella* isolated from healthy market hogs (abstract No. A57). In *Abstracts of the Annual Meeting of the American Society for Microbiology*, Atlantic City, N.J., May 7, 1976.

120. Siegel, D., Huber, W. G., Enloe, F. Continuous non-therapeutic use of antibacterial drugs in feed and drug resistance of the gram-negative enteric florae of food-producing animals. *Antimicrob. Agents Chemother.* **6**:697–701, 1974.

121. Guinée, P., Ugueto, N., VanLeeuwen, N. *Escherichia coli* with resistance factors in vegetarians, babies, and nonvegetarians. *Appl. Microbiol.* **20**:531–535, 1970.

122. Timoney, J. F. The epidemiology and genetics of antibiotic resistance of *Salmonella typhimurium* isolated from diseased animals in New York. *J. Infect. Dis.* **137**:67–73, 1978.

123. Levy, S. B., Fitzgerald, G. B., Macone, A. B. Changes in intestinal flora of farm personnel after introduction of a tetracycline-supplemented feed on a farm. *N. Engl. J. Med.* **295**:583–588, 1976.

124. Anderson, E. S., Lewis, M. J. Drug resistance and its transfer in *Salmonella typhimurium*. *Nature* **206**:579–583, 1965.

125. United States Department of Health, Education and Welfare, Center for Disease Control. *Morbid. Mortal. Week. Rep.*, July 22, 1977.

126. Marx, M. B. The effect of interspecies contact upon diarrhea morbidity and salmonellosis in children. *J. Infect. Dis.* **120**:202–209, 1969.

127. Neu, H. C., Winshell, E. B., Winter, J., *et al.* Antibiotic resistance of *Salmonella* in the northeastern United States 1968–1969. *N.Y. State J. Med.* **71**:1196–1200, 1971.

128. Neu, H. C., Cherubin, C. E., Longo, E. D., *et al.* Antimicrobial resistance and R-factor transfer among isolates of *Salmonella* in the northeastern United States: A comparison of human and animal isolates. *J. Infect. Dis.* **132**:617–622, 1975.

129. Finland, M., Garner, C., Wilcox, C., *et al.* Salmonellosis and shigellosis at Boston City Hospital: Part 2. Susceptibility of strains of salmonellae and shigellae to antibacterial agents. *J. Am. Med. Assoc.* **229**:1309–1312, 1974.

130. Pocurull, D. W., Gaines, S. A., Mercer, H. D. Survey of infectious multiple drug resistance among *Salmonella* isolated from animals in the United States. *Appl. Microbiol.* **21**:358–362, 1971.

131. Anderson, E. S., Threlfall, E. J. The characterization of plasmids in the enterobacteria. *J. Hyg. (Cambridge)* **72**:471–487, 1974.

132. Hariharan, H., Barnum, D. A., Mitchell, W. R. Drug resistance among pathogenic bacteria from animals in Ontario. *Can. J. Comp. Med.* **38**:213–221, 1974.

133. Grant, R. B., Bannatyne, R. M., Shapley, A. J. Resistance to chloramphenicol and ampicillin of *Salmonella typhimurium* in Ontario, Canada. *J. Infect. Dis.* **134**:354–361, 1976.

134. Saad, A. F., Farrar, W. E. Antimicrobial resistance and R factors in *Salmonella* isolated from humans and animals in Georgia and South Carolina. *South. Med. J.* **70**:305–308, 1977.

135. Smith, H. W. Thermosensitive transfer factors in chloramphenicol-resistant strains of *Salmonella typhi*. *Lancet* **2**:281–282, 1974.

136. Anderson, E. S. The problem and implications of chloramphenicol resistance in the typhoid bacillus. *J. Hyg. (Cambridge)* **74**:289–299, 1975.

137. Smith, H. W. Transfer of antibiotic resistance from animal and human strains of *Escherichia coli* to resident *E. coli* in the alimentary tract of man, *Lancet* **1**:1174–1176, 1969.

138. Fison, D. C., Singer, E. Treatment of gastro-enteritis in infants with "chloromycetin." *Med. J. Aust.* **2:**957–959, 1950.
139. Macdonald, W. B., Friday, F., McEacharn, M. The effect of chloramphenicol in *Salmonella* enteritis of infancy. *Arch. Dis. Child.* **29:**238–241, 1954.
140. Rosenstein, B. J. Salmonellosis in infants and children: Epidemiologic and therapeutic considerations. *J. Pediatr.* **70:**1–7, 1967.
141. Rosenthal, S. J. Exacerbation of *Salmonella* enteritis due to ampicillin. *N. Engl. J. Med.* **280:**147–148, 1969.
142. Münnich, D. The treatment of salmonellosis with trimethoprim/sulphamethoxazole and their combination with polymyxin B in adult patients. *Chemotherapy (Basel)*, **18:**119–129, 1973.
143. Geddes, A. M., Fothergill, R., Goodall, J. A. D., *et al.* Evaluation of trimethoprim-sulphamethoxazole compound in treatment of salmonella infections. *Br. Med. J.* **3:**451–454, 1971.
144. Kazemi, M., Gumpert, T. G., Marks, M. I. A controlled trial comparing sulfamethoxazole-trimethoprim, ampicillin, and no therapy in the treatment of *Salmonella gastroenteritis* in children. *J. Pediatr.* **83:**646–650, 1973.
145. Dawkins, A. T., Jr., Hornick, R. B. Evaluation of antibiotics in a typhoid model. *Antimicrob. Agents Chemother.*—1966, 6–10, 1967.
146. Olarte, J., Galindo, E. *Salmonella typhi* resistant to chloramphenicol, ampicillin, and other antimicrobial agents: Strains isolated during an extensive typhoid fever epidemic in Mexico. *Antimicrob. Agents Chemother.* **4:**597–601, 1973.
147. Vázquez, V., Calderón, E., Rodríguez, R. S. Chloramphenicol-resistant strains of *Salmonella typhosa.* *N. Engl. J. Med.* **286:**1220, 1972.
148. Brown, J. D., Mo, D. H., Rhoades, E. R. Chloramphenicol-resistant *Salmonella typhi* in Saigon. *J. Am. Med. Assoc.* **231:**162–166, 1975.
149. Lawrence, R. M., Goldstein, E., Hoeprich, P. D. Typhoid fever caused by chloramphenicol-resistant organisms. *J. Am. Med. Assoc.* **224:**861–863, 1973.
150. Overturf, G., Marton, K. I., Mathies, A. W., Jr. Antibiotic resistance in typhoid fever: Chloramphenicol resistance among clinical isolates of *Salmonella typhosa* in Los Angeles, 1972—epidemiologic and bacteriologic characteristics. *N. Engl. J. Med.* **280:**463–465, 1973.
151. Paramasivan, C. N., Subramanian, S., Shanmugasundaram, N. Antimicrobial resistance and incidence of R factor among *Salmonella* isolated from patients with enteric fever and other clinical conditions in Madras, India (1975–1976). *J. Infect. Dis.* **136:**796–800, 1977.
152. Woodward, T. E., Smadel, J. E., Ley, H. L., Jr., *et al.* Preliminary report on the beneficial effect of chloromycetin in the treatment of typhoid fever. *Ann. Intern. Med.* **29:**131–134, 1948.
153. Dammermann, R., Freitag, V. Die Behandlung des Typhos abdominalis mit Trimethoprim–Sulfamethoxazol. *Dtsch. Med. Wochenschr.* 98:1251–1253, 1973.
154. Stamps, T. J., Wicks, A. C. B. Trimethoprim–sulphamethoxazole (Bactrim) in the treatment of typhoid fever. *S. Afr. Med. J.* **46:**652–655, 1972.
155. Farid, Z., Hassan, A., Wahab, M. F. A., *et al.* Trimethoprim–sulphamethoxazole in enteric fevers. *Br. Med. J.* **3:**323–324, 1970.
156. Kamat, S. A. Evaluation of therapeutic efficacy of trimethoprim–sulphamethoxazole and chloramphenicol in enteric fever. *Br. Med. J.* **3:**320–322, 1970.
157. Gutiérrez, G., Serafín, F., Sánchez, R., *et al.* Evaluación de cuatro antimicrobianos en el tratamiento de tifoidea por *Salmonella typhi* resistente a chloramfénicol. *Bol. Méd. Hosp. Infant. Méx. (Span. Ed.)* 31:597–606, 1974.
158. Salcedo, M., Borgoño, J. M., Greiber, R., *et al.* Tratamiento de la fiebre tifoidea y paratifus con trimétoprim y sulfametóxazol. *Rev. Méd. Chile* **100:**1064–1067, 1972.

159. Snyder, M. J., Perroni, J., Gonzalez, O., *et al.* Trimethoprim–sulfamethoxazole in the treatment of typhoid and paratyphoid fevers. *J. Infect. Dis.* **128**:S734–S737, 1973.

160. Sardesai, H. V., Karandikar, R. S., Harshe, R. G. Comparative trial of cotrimoxazole and chloramphenicol in typhoid fever. *Br. Med. J.* **1**:82–83, 1973.

161. Hassan, A., Hathout, S., Safwat, Y., *et al.* A comparative evaluation of the treatment of typhoid fevers with co-trimoxazole and chloramphenicol in Egypt. *J. Trop. Med. Hyg.* **78**:50–53, 1975.

162. Gilman, R. H., Terminel, M., Levine, M. M., *et al.* Comparison of trimethoprim-sulfamethoxazole and amoxicillin in therapy of chloramphenicol-resistant and chloramphenicol-sensitive typhoid fever. *J. Infect. Dis.* **132**:630–636, 1975.

163. Farid, Z., Bassily, S., Mikhail, I. A., *et al.* Treatment of chronic enteric fever with amoxicillin. *J. Infect. Dis.* **132**:698–701, 1975.

164. Scragg, J. N., Rubidge, C. J. Amoxycillin in the treatment of typhoid fever in children. *Am. J. Trop. Med. Hyg.* **24**:860–865, 1975.

165. Scragg, J. N. Further experience with amoxycillin in typhoid fever in children. *Br. Med. J.* **2**:1031–1033, 1976.

166. Hoffman, T. A., Ruiz, C. J., Counts, G. W., *et al.* Waterborne typhoid fever in Dade County, Florida: Clinical and therapeutic evaluation of 105 bacteremic patients. *Am. J. Med.* **59**:481–487, 1975.

167. Robertson, R. P., Wahab, M. F. A., Raasch, F. O. Evaluation of chloramphenicol and ampicillin in salmonella enteric fever. *N. Engl. J. Med.* **278**:171–176, 1968.

168. Hardy, G., Padfield, C. J., Chadwick, P., *et al.* Typhoid outbreak in Kingston, Ontario: Experience with high-dose oral ampicillin. *Can. Med. Assoc. J.* **116**:761–764, 767, 1977.

169. Mikhail, I. A., Kent, D. C., Sorensen, K., *et al.* Concentrations of ampicillin and chloramphenicol in the serum of patients with acute salmonella enteric fever. *Antimicrob. Agents Chemother.* **2**:336–339, 1972.

170. DuPont, H. L., Hornick, R. B., Weiss, C. F., *et al.* Evaluation of chloramphenicol acid succinate therapy of induced typhoid fever and Rocky Mountain spotted fever. *N. Engl. J. Med.* **282**:53–57, 1970.

171. Pickering, L. K., Hoecker, J. L., Kramer, W. G., *et al.* Clinical pharmacology of two chloramphenicol preparations in children: Sodium succinate (IV) and palmitate (oral) esters. *J. Pediatr.* **96**:757-761, 1980.

172. Main, R. G. Treatment of the chronic alimentary enteric carrier. *Br. Med. J.* **1**:328–333, 1961.

173. Jersild, T., Neukirch, E., Raun, J., *et al.* Typhoid carriers treated with high dosages of penicillin. *Antibiot. Med.* **6**:292–294, 1959.

174. Perkins, J. C., Devetski, R. L., Dowling, H. F. Ampicillin in the treatment of *Salmonella* carriers. *Arch. Intern. Med.* **118**:528–533, 1966.

175. Dinbar, A., Altmann, G., Tulcinsky, D. B. The treatment of chronic biliary salmonella carriers. *Am J. Med.* **47**:236–242, 1969.

176. Simon, H. J., Miller, R. C. Ampicillin in the treatment of chronic typhoid carriers: Report on fifteen treated cases and a review of the literature. *N. Engl. J. Med.* **274**:807–815, 1966.

177. Phillips, W. E. Treatment of chronic typhoid carriers with ampicillin. *J. Am. Med. Assoc.* **217**:913–915, 1971.

178. Johnson, W. D., Jr., Hook, E. W., Lindsey, E., *et al.* Treatment of chronic typhoid carriers with ampicillin. *Antimicrob. Agents Chemother.* **3**:439–440, 1973.

179. Scioli, C., Fiorentino, F., Sasso, G. Treatment of *Salmonella typhi* carriers with intravenous ampicillin. *J. Infect. Dis.* **125**:170–173, 1972.

180. Nolan, C. M., White, P. C., Jr. Treatment of typhoid carriers with amoxicillin: Correlates of successful therapy. *J. Am. Med. Assoc.* **239**:2352–2354, 1978.

181. Brodie, J., Macqueen, I. A., Livingstone, D. Effect of trimethoprim–sulphamethoxazole on typhoid and salmonella carriers. *Br. Med. J.* **3:**318–319, 1970.

182. Clementi, K. J. Treatment of *Salmonella* carriers with trimethoprim–sulfamethoxazole. *Can. Med. Assoc. J.* **122**(Spec. No. 13):28–32, 1975.

183. Freerksen, E., Rosenfeld, M., Freerksen, R., *et al.* Treatment of chronic salmonella carriers: Study with 40 cases of *S. typhi*, 19 cases of *S. paratyphi B* and 28 cases of *S. enteritidis* strains. *Chemotherapy* **23:**192–210, 1977.

184. Nolan, C. M., White, P. C. Treatment of typhoid carriers with amoxicillin. *J. Am. Med. Assoc.* **239:**2352–2354, 1978.

185. Benenson, A. S. Serological responses of man to typhoid vaccines. *Bull. W.H.O.* **30:**653–662, 1964.

186. Mackaness, G. B., Blanden, R. V., Collins, F. M. Host–parasite relations in mouse typhoid. *J. Exp. Med.* **124:**573–583, 1966.

187. Ushiba, D. Two types of immunity in experimental typhoid: "Cellular immunity" and "humoral immunity." *Keio J. Med.* **14:**45–61, 1965.

188. Mackaness, G. B. Resistance to intracellular infection. *J. Infect. Dis.* **123:**439–445, 1971.

189. Collins, F. M. Effect of specific immune mouse serum on the growth of *Salmonella enteritidis* in mice preimmunized with living or ethyl alcohol-killed vaccines. *J. Bacteriol.* **97:**676–683, 1969.

190. Marmion, D. E., Naylor, G. R. E., Stewart, I. O. Second attacks of typhoid fever. *J. Hyg. (London)* **51:**260–267, 1953.

191. DuPont, H. L., Hornick, R. B., Snyder, M. J., *et al.* Studies of immunity in typhoid fever: Protection induced by killed oral antigens or by primary infection. *Bull. W.H.O.* **44:**667–672, 1971.

192. Cvjetanović, B., Uemura, K. The present status of field and laboratory studies of typhoid and paratyphoid vaccines: With special reference to studies sponsored by the World Health Organization. *Bull. W.H.O.* **32:**29–36, 1965.

193. Hejfec, L. B., Salmin, M. Z., Lejtman, M. L., *et al.* A controlled field trial and laboratory study of five typhoid vaccines in the USSR. *Bull. W.H.O.* **34:**321–339, 1966.

194. Ashcroft, M. T., Singh, B., Nicholson, C. C., *et al.* A seven-year field trial of two typhoid vaccines in Guyana. *Lancet* **2:**1056–1059, 1967.

195. Hejfec, L. B., Levina, L. A., Kuzminova, M. L., *et al.* A controlled field trial to evaluate the protective capacity of a single dose of acetone-killed agar-grown and heat-killed broth-grown typhoid vaccines. *Bull. W.H.O.* **40:**903–907, 1969.

196. Hejfec, L. B., Levina, L. A., Kuzminova, M. L., *et al.* Controlled field trial with dried sorbed parathyphoid B and typhoid vaccines. *Bull. W.H.O.* **45:**787–794, 1971.

197. Spaun, J., Uemura, K. International reference preparations of typhoid vaccine: A report on international collaborative laboratory studies. *Bull. W.H.O.* **31:**761–791, 1964.

198. Pittman, M., Bohner, H. J. Laboratory assays of different types of field trial typhoid vaccines and relationship to efficacy in man. *J. Bacteriol.* **91:**1713–1723, 1966.

199. Wong, K. H., Feeley, J. C., Pittman, M., *et al.* Adhesion of Vi antigen and toxicity in typhoid vaccines inactivated by acetone or by heat and phenol. *J. Infect. Dis.* **129:**501–506, 1974.

200. Wong, K. H., Feeley, J. C., Northrup, R. S., *et al.* Vi antigen from *Salmonella typhosa* and immunity against typhoid fever: I. Isolation and immunologic properties in animals. *Infect. Immun.* **9:**348–353, 1974.

201. Levin, D. M., Wong, K. H., Reynolds, H. Y., *et al.* Vi antigen from *Salmonella typhosa* and immunity against typhoid fever: II. Safety and antigenicity in humans. *Infect. Immun.* **12:**1290–1294, 1975.

202. Landy, M. Studies on Vi antigen: VI. Immunization of human beings with purified Vi antigen. *Am. J. Hyg.* **60**:52–62, 1954.
203. Diena, B. B., Ryan, A., Wallace, R., *et al.* Ineffectiveness of Vi and chemically treated endotoxins as typhoid vaccines in mice challenged with a *Salmonella typhosa–Salmonella typhimurium* hybrid. *Infect. Immun.* **12**:1470–1471, 1975.
204. Venneman, M. R. Purification of immunogenically active ribonucleic acid preparations of *Salmonella typhimurium:* Molecular-sieve and anion-exchange chromatography. *Infect. Immun.* **5**:269–282, 1972.
205. Angerman, C. R., Eisenstein, T. K. Comparative efficacy and toxicity of a ribosomal vaccine, acetone-killed cells, lipopolysaccharide, and a live cell vaccine prepared from *Salmonella typhimurium. Infect. Immun.* **19**:575–582, 1978.
206. Venneman, M. R., Berry, L. J. Cell-mediated resistance induced with immunogenic preparations cf *Salmonella typhimurium. Infect. Immun.* **4**:381–387, 1971.
207. Smith, R. A., Bigley, N. J. Detection of delayed hypersensitivity in mice injected with ribonucleic acid–protein fractions of *Salmonella typhimurium. Infect. Immun.* **6**:384–389, 1972.
208. Johnson, W., Ribosomal vaccines: II. Specificity of the immune response to ribosomal ribonucleic acid and protein isolated from *Salmonella typhimurium. Infect. Immun.* **8**:395–400, 1973.
209. Eisenstein, T. K. Evidence for O antigens as the antigenic determinants in "ribosomal" vaccines prepared from *Salmonella. Infect. Immun.* **12**:364–377, 1975.
210. Metchnikoff, E., Besredka, A. Recherches sur la fièvre typhoïde expérimentale. *Ann. Inst. Pasteur Paris* **25**:193–221, 1911.
211. Chuttani, C. S., Prakash, K., Vergese, A., *et al.* Effectiveness of oral killed typhoid vaccine. *Bull. W.H.O.* **45**:445–450, 1971.
212. Chuttani, C. S., Prakash, K., Vergese, A., *et al.* Ineffectiveness of an oral killed typhoid vaccine in a field trial. *Bull. W.H.O.* **48**:754–755, 1973.
213. Kiefer, W., Gransow, P., Schmidt, G., *et al.* Salmonellosis in mice: Immunization experiments with *Salmonella–Escherichia coli* hybrids. *Infect. Immun.* **13**:1517–1518, 1976.
214. Diena, B. B., Ryan, A., Wallace, R., *et al.* Effectiveness of parenteral and oral typhoid vaccination in mice challenged with a *Salmonella typhi–Salmonella typhimurium* hybrid. *Infect. Immun.* **15**:997–998, 1977.
215. DuPont, H. L., Hornick, R. B., Snyder, M. J., *et al.* Immunity in typhoid fever: Evaluation of live streptomycin-dependent vaccine. *Antimicrob. Agents Chemother.* **10**:236–239, 1970.
216. Reitman, M. Infectivity and antigenicity of streptomycin-dependent *Salmonella typhosa. J. Infect. Dis.* **117**:101–107, 1967.
217. Cvjetanović, B., Mel, D. M., Felsenfeld, O. Study of live typhoid vaccine in chimpanzees. *Bull. W.H.O.* **42**:449–507, 1970.
218. Germanier, R. Immunity in experimental salmonellosis: I. Protection induced by rough mutants of *Salmonella typhimurium. Infect. Immun.* **2**:309–315, 1970.
219. Germanier, R., Fürer, E. Immunity in experimental salmonellosis: II. Basis for the avirulence and protective capacity of *gal* E mutants of *Salmonella typhimurium. Infect. Immun.* **4**:663–673, 1971.
220. Levine, M. M., DuPont, H. L., Hornick, R. B., *et al.* Attenuated, streptomycin-dependent *Salmonella typhi* oral vaccine: Potential deleterious effects of lyophilization. *J. Infect. Dis.* **133**:424–429, 1976.
221. Fahey, K. J., Cooper, G. N. Oral immunization against experimental salmonellosis: I. Development of temperature-sensitive mutant vaccines. *Infect. Immun.* **1**:263–270, 1970.

222. Fahey, K. J., Cooper, G. N. Oral immunization in experimental salmonellosis: II. Characteristics of the immune response to temperature-sensitive mutants given by oral and parenteral routes. *Infect. Immun.* **2:**183–191, 1970.
223. Vladoianu, I. R., Dubini, R., Bolloli, A. Contribution to the study of live streptomycin-dependent salmonella vaccines: The problem of reversion to a virulent form. *J. Hyg. (Cambridge)* **75:**203–214, 1975.
224. Fukasawa, T., Nikaido, H. Galactose-sensitive mutants of *Salmonella:* II. Bacteriolysis induced by galactose. *Biochim. Biophys. Acta* **48:**470–483, 1961.
225. Gilman, R. H., Hornick, R. B., Woodward, W. E., *et al.* Evaluation of 2 UDP-glucose-4-epimeraseless mutant of *Salmonella typhi* as a live oral vaccine. *J. Infect. Dis.* **136:**717–723, 1977.
226. DuPont, H. L. Recent developments in immunization against diarrhea diseases. *South. Med. J.* **68:**1027–1034, 1975.

6

Cholera and *Escherichia coli* Diarrhea

INTRODUCTION

Few diseases have been characterized more clearly than cholera and enterotoxigenic *E. coli* (ETEC) diarrhea. During the 1960s, a number of landmark studies helped to elucidate the mechanisms of disease production in naturally acquired and laboratory induced cholera, and cholera toxin was purified and characterized. In the 1970s, research interest turned to the study of diarrhea produced by ETEC. Success with *E. coli* has stimulated renewed interest in cholera research. Many workers in these areas remain optimistic that both cholera and ETEC diarrhea may one day be controlled by immunoprophylactic measures.

Other enteropathogens produce cholera- and *E. coli*- like enterotoxins which appear to play a role in disease pathogenesis. Such agents include nonagglutinable vibrios, *V. parahemolyticus*, *Aeromonas* species, *Y. enterocolitica*, *Clostridium perfringens*, and *Staphylococcus aureus*. This chapter will focus on developments in enteric infection due to *V. cholerae* and ETEC. Enteropathogenic *E. coli* as determined by serotype will be discussed as an etiologic agent of diarrhea. For information on the importance of enterotoxigenic and enteropathogenic *E. coli* as causes of diarrhea see Chapters 8 and 9.

CHOLERA

Cholera Toxin

The two major serotypes of *V. cholerae* are termed Inaba and Ogawa and belong to either classical or El Tor biotypes. Distinction between them is made by slide agglutination with type-specific antisera. Cholera strains belonging to either of these serotypes produce an immunologically identical toxin[1,2] which has been purified and characterized.[3–7] It is a protein of 84,000 daltons and, like diphtheria toxin, is composed of two types of noncovalently linked subunits: an active fragment, A, and a binding portion, B. The A fragment appears to consist of a subunit of approximately 28,000 daltons, while the B fragment has a molecular weight of 56,000 and consists of six subunits. The B fragment, referred to as choleragenoid, is a naturally occurring fermentation product of entero-toxigenic *V. cholerae* and is devoid of toxin activity in most study systems. The B subunit is responsible for the binding of cholera toxin to G M1 ganglioside cell receptors.[4,8] Subunit A, unique to cholera toxin and not part of choleragenoid, is composed of two chains held together by a disulfide bridge.[9,10] This subunit stimulates the action of adenyl cyclase.

Pathogenesis of Cholera

As with other infectious diseases, the development of cholera will depend upon a productive interaction between host and microbial factors. Table 6.1 summarizes host defense mechanisms and microbial virulence properties which are important in the pathogenesis of cholera. In the upper intestine, saliva[11] and gastric acidity inhibit the intestinal transit of viable organisms. Patients who have developed clinical cholera in areas where disease is endemic have been shown to frequently suffer from achlorhydria or hypochlorhydria.[12,13] Fasting and postprandial stomach acid production is lower in these patients, and their gastric juice will not kill vibrios *in vitro*.[13] A fivefold log reduction in dose of *V. cholerae* necessary to induce illness is seen when volunteers are first given sodium bicarbonate,[14] demonstrating the importance of the gastric acid trap in the pathogenesis of clinical cholera. It appears that idiopathic tropical hypochlorhydria is a major factor contributing to the level of endemicity of cholera in the world. Additional host defense mechanisms include intestinal peristalsis,[15] which limits local bacterial proliferation; nonspecific antibacterial factors,[16,17] such as lactic acid and short-chain fatty acids, which are produced by the indigenous microflora; the physical barrier imposed by the intestinal mucus layer[18–22]; and intestinal immunoglobulins which reflect prior exposure to *V. cholerae* antigens.[23]

The pathogenic potential of a *V. cholerae* strain depends upon a number of microbial factors (Table 6.1). Virulence of *V. cholerae* may depend upon motility of the organism[19,24,26]; nonmotile strains have been shown to be unable to adhere to the intestinal lining.[26] Strains show a variable propensity for localizing in the toxin-sensitive upper

TABLE 6.1
Host And Microbial Factors in the Pathogenesis of Cholera

Host defense mechanisms	*Microbial virulence factors*
Saliva	Motility
Gastric acidity	Ability to localize in upper gut
Intestinal peristalsis	Smooth lipopolysaccharide structures
Antibacterial catabolites of enteric flora	Extracellular proteins
Mucus barrier	Enterotoxin
Intestinal immunoglobulins	Toxoid
	Hemagglutinin
	Enzymes
	Neuraminidase
	Mucinase
	Protease

intestine.[27,28] Virulent strains also produce extracellular proteins, including smooth lipopolysaccharide structures, enterotoxin, toxoid, hemagglutinin, endotoxin, and enzymes.[29,30,31] The enzymes produced by *V. cholerae* play a role in penetrating the mucus barrier (mucinases)[19,22] or relate to pathogenicity by poorly characterized mechanisms, as is the case for neuraminidases[32,33] and proteases.[21,34] Mutant strains lacking one or more of these virulence properties have to be administered in higher (at least 100-fold) doses to induce experimental cholera infection in animals.[35]

Mechanism of Action of Cholera Toxin

The first event in the action of cholera toxin on intestinal cells is a rapid, tight binding to the cell membrane. Prompted by the observation that a crude mixture of gangliosides could inactivate cholera toxin,[36] it was found that pure monosialosyl ganglioside GM_1 (galactosyl-*N*-acetyl-galactosaminy[sialosyl]lactosyl ceramide) would bind and inactivate cholera toxin at a 1:1 molar ratio, whereas no other glycolipid reacted in a specific manner with the toxin.[37] Further studies demonstrated that the number of binding sites for cholera toxin on different cells was correlated directly to the amount of GM_1 in cell membranes.[38] Chemical modification of various amino acid residues in cholera toxin concomitantly affected binding to cells and to matrix-coupled GM_1.[39] GM_1 could be incorporated into the membrane of intestinal cells, thereby increasing the number of binding sites for cholera toxin in the intestine and leading to an enhanced susceptibility of the intestine to the diarrheogenic potential of the toxin.[38] It has been proposed that GM_1 is the natural receptor in the intestine, and perhaps in other, nonintestinal tissue, for the enterotoxin of

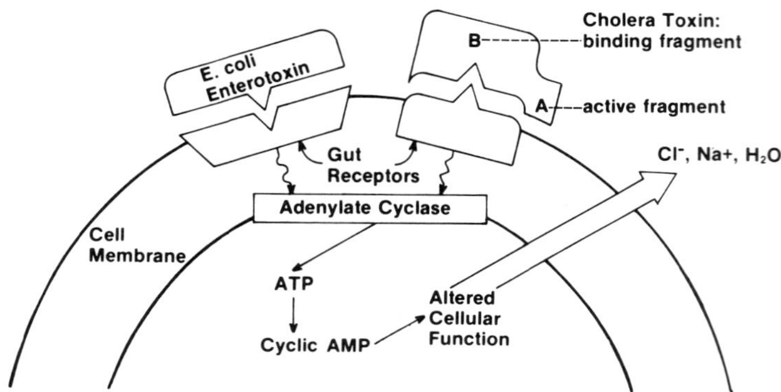

Figure 6.1. Schematic representation of intestinal binding of cholera toxin and heat-labile *Escherichia coli* toxin (LT) leading to intestinal secretion of fluid and electrolytes.

V. cholerae, based on the relative degrees of inactivation of the toxins by GM_1 ganglioside.[40–43]

Studies using cholera toxin labeled with radioactive iodine have demonstrated that it binds rapidly and has a high affinity for cell mem branes.[38,44–47] Subunit B mediates the binding of toxin on the cell membrane but is not involved in the activation of adenyl cyclase. The role of the B subunit is to facilitate productive interaction of the active subunit A with the cell (Figure 6.1).[45] Minutes after the rapid reversible binding of toxin to the receptor on the cell surface, the toxin becomes irreversibly associated with the cell, probably by penetration into the cell membrane.[39] Cholera vibrios produce neuraminidase, which can hydrolyze oligosialosylgangliosides (primarily GD_1 [disialosyl-galactosyl-*N*-acetyl-galactosaminyllactosyl ceramide] and GT_1 [trisialosyl-galactosyl-*N*-acetyl-galactosaminyllactosyl ceramide]) to GM_1. Neuraminidase may play a role in the pathogenesis of cholera by increasing the number of receptors on intestinal cells for interaction with toxin, although there is no direct evidence for such an effect.[38]

GM_1 ganglioside has been considered to be a potentially useful agent for the prevention or treatment of cholera. Prior exposure of subunit B (choleragenoid) to GM_1 ganglioside can effectively protect a cell against subsequent exposure to the toxin,[41,42] with binding inhibited and stimulation of adenyl cyclase and cyclic AMP-(cAMP)-associated events prevented. The possibility is being pursued that the specific binding peptides of subunit B are identifiable and might be tested as a practical prophylactic agent.

The mechanisms whereby adenyl cyclase is stimulated by subunit A remain largely undefined.[48] Unless binding of toxin to the intestinal surface is prevented by prior mixing of the toxin with antitoxin[49] or with ganglioside,[36] the characteristic secretory response begins after a lag period ranging from 10 min[50] to 1 hr.[51] The lag probably relates to the time needed by the toxin to activate adenyl cyclase.[51,52] The massive secretion of fluid and electrolytes from the small bowel in *V. cholerae* infection is known to result when the enterotoxin is applied to the mucosal but not the serosal surface[53,54] or when it is administered by the intravenous route.[55,56] Although binding of toxin is strongly associated with the brush border of the apical portion of the epithelial cell, the basal and lateral portions of cells also contain high concentrations of adenyl cyclase.[57] Pharmacologically significant concentrations of toxin can be absorbed rapidly despite the large size of the toxin molecule and its affinity for brush-border binding.[58] Absorption of the toxin explains how the basal and lateral areas of the cell develop high concentrations of adenyl cyclase,[57] leading to the process of hypersecretion. Activated adenyl cyclase appears to further activate protein kinases, leading to hypersecretion.[59] Some evidence has been offered to suggest that the crypt epithelium is the important site of fluid and electrolyte secretion.[59,61]

The effects of cholera toxin on intestinal secretion can be mimicked by administering cAMP directly to the mucosal surface of the intestine[61] or by applying other compounds that stimulate cAMP or interfere with cAMP degradation.[62,63] Theophylline, which causes cAMP to accumulate by inhibiting the breakdown of phosphodiesterase, produces changes in ion movement which are similar in magnitude and direction to those induced by cholera toxin.[64] The action of cholera toxin resembles that of cAMP and theophylline, offering presumptive evidence that cholera toxin and cAMP influence the transport of ions through similar pathways. Additional evidence that cholera toxin is operative through adenyl cyclase mechanisms is furnished by the finding that toxin accelerates lipolysis in rat epididymal fat cells[65] which are known to be responsive to cAMP.[66]

Normally, a healthy intestinal mucosa absorbs salt and water by a mechanism that requires expenditure of metabolic energy. The driving force of water absorption in the normal intestine is an active transport of electrolytes, particularly sodium and chloride.[67] In membranes treated with filtrates containing cholera or *E. coli* enterotoxin, the net movement of sodium is inhibited and the direction of chloride flux is reversed,[62,68] with increased cell surface glycoprotein turnover.[69] The net effect is that chloride is secreted and sodium is no longer absorbed.[70] Sodium no longer acts as a driving force (the net movement is zero), and chloride is actively moved from blood to lumen, pulling cations and water with it into the gut lumen for maintenance of an osmotic equilibrium with blood plasma. Isotonic fluid low in protein, with bicarbonate concentrations twice and potassium concentrations four times that of normal plasma,[71] is lost rapidly from all segments of the small bowel.[72,73] The loss of fluid may exceed 1 liter/hr.

The time course of secretory response has been established in Thiry–

Vella jejunal canine loops.[74] Isotonic fluid production begins within seconds after contact with the toxin, with a maximum rate occurring during the fourth hour and fluid output being maintained at near maximum levels through the tenth hour after inoculation. This decreases gradually and stops completely within 24 hr. Although cholera toxin causes all segments of the small intestine to secrete, there is a decreasing gradient from duodenum to ileum.[75] In a rat model, cholera toxin led to cecal transport of water and electrolytes, but *E. coli* and *S. dysenteriae* toxins did not.[76] There is no major histologic damage to the gastrointestinal tract in cholera[77–79]; minimal changes include depletion of mucus in goblet cells, dilatation of crypts, and edema in the lamina propria.[79]

Prostaglandin E_1 (PGE_1), like cholera toxin, increases mucosal cAMP and stimulates intestinal secretion.[63,81] Pretreatment of animals with aspirin or indomethacin,[81–83] each of which is known to inhibit prostaglandin synthesis,[84] has been shown to produce an inhibitory effect on cholera-toxin-induced secretion. A study was conducted whereby rabbit ileal loops were stimulated with cholera toxin and cAMP and PGE_1 concentrations were measured by radioimmunoassay.[85] cAMP accumulation and intestinal secretion were independent of PGE_1 synthesis, providing some evidence against a specific role of prostaglandins in mediating the cholera toxin effects. Further efforts have been directed toward determining whether agents known to decrease intracellular cAMP may block the secretion of fluid caused by enterotoxin. The loop diuretic ethacrynic acid, a known inhibitor of adenyl cyclase, will cause a reduction in fluid volume from the small bowel secondary to cholera toxin challenge[86]; however, there is no therapeutic value for ethacrynic acid, since renal fluid loss exceeds the decrease in loss due to a block in secretion.

The value of intravenous fluids in the therapy of cholera was known as early as 1832.[87] Intestinal glucose absorption and glucose-enhanced sodium absorption are not impaired in cholera.[88,89] Glucose-mediated transport of sodium and water has been utilized in oral therapy of cholera[90,91] and of colibacillosis of swine.[92] In studies conducted in Pakistan and India,[88,90] orally administered glucose-containing electrolyte solutions were shown to be adequate in maintaining electrolyte balance in patients with actively purging cholera. Glucose-, sucrose-, and glycine-containing electrolyte solutions have each been used with success.

Cholera Immunity

It has been observed in cholera-endemic areas that there is a drastic fall in the incidence of cholera with age, that there is a low frequency of reinfection in those convalescing from cholera, and that there is a reduction of disease following immunization, each suggesting that acquired immunity does occur.[93] Clinical cholera gives rise to serum antibodies to both bacteria and toxin. A protective role for both types of antibodies has been shown in experimental animals. These antibodies have their protective effects at the intestinal level, although they may be produced outside of the gut. It is known that there is a significant influx of serum immunoglobulins into the small intestine and that an inverse correlation exists between vibriocidal antibodies in serum and incidence of cholera in cholera-endemic areas.[93] Furthermore, after parenteral immunization, there is a direct correlation between titers of antitoxin–serum antibody and protection against experimental cholera in dogs[94] and rabbits.[95] The importance of local intestinal formation of antibodies in cholera was first noted by Burrows *et al.*[96] Protective immunity against experimental cholera was documented in the absence of significant titers of antibody in serum after immunization using killed vibrios. Intestinal installation of antigen was shown to be a means of eliciting a protective immunization response in experimental cholera.[95]

Antibacterial Immunity

Purified lipopolysaccharide (LPS) of *V. cholerae* has been found to induce significant protection against cholera in animals and humans, where antibody to LPS correlated with protectiveness.[97] The LPS of Ogawa and Inaba serotypes of *V. cholerae* cross-reacts immunologically through an antigenic determinant. In field studies, monovalent vaccines (Inaba or Ogawa) have induced a higher degree of protection against infection from the homologous as compared to the heterologous strain. The degree of protection corresponded to a higher titer of type-specific antibody, as compared to cross-reactive antibody. Protection with these vaccines lasts only a few months. The mechanism of cholera immunity following vaccination is unclear, since neither bactericidal nor opsonizing antibody in serum completely explains the resultant protective immunity. Freter[23] provided evidence that antibacterial antibody works by inhibiting the adhesion of *V. cholerae* to the mucosal surface, thus preventing the action of toxin. This proposal was based on the finding that passive immunization with specific antibacterial serum instilled intraluminally, as well as active oral immunization with killed vibrios, led to a decrease in the number of vibrios adsorbed to the mucosa in experimental animal loops challenged with *V. cholerae.* The number of intraluminal cholera organisms was not affected. IgG, IgA, and IgM classes of immunoglobulins directed against *V. cholerae* have all been shown to be equally effective in preventing experimental cholera in the mouse model.[98]

Antitoxic Immunity

The limited efficacy of killed vibrio vaccine and knowledge of the role of enterotoxin in pathogenesis of cholera have prompted development of vaccines based on production of a toxoid. Since neither the vibrio nor the toxin appears to necessarily penetrate the intestinal mucosa, antibacterial or antitoxic antibodies probably act at the mucosal surface. Antitoxic immunity appears to be mediated by antibodies to subunit B, indicating that protective antibodies to toxin probably act by preventing the binding of subunit B of the toxin to GM_1 ganglioside receptors in the intestinal epithelium rather than by interacting with the active A subunit. IgG antibodies have much greater neutralizing effect.[99] A protective role of IgA antibodies with toxin-neutralizing capacity, from crypts of intestinal mucosa, also has been demonstrated in immunized rabbits.[100]

Intestinal immune response to cholera toxoid has been studied in dogs and rats. Using a toxin-specific immunofluorescence technique in a rat model, Pierce and Gowans[101] observed that repeated local administration of formalin-prepared cholera toxoid gave rise to specific antibody-containing cells in the lamina propria of the small intestine. Antitoxin antibodies found in the small bowel may be derived from serum or produced locally.[101,102] Peyer's patches contain the precursors of IgA-secreting plasma cells which are capable of responding to antigens present within the intestinal lumen.[103] These precursor cells do not begin this activity until they travel through the mesenteric lymph nodes and enter the systemic circulation by way of the thoracic duct.[102,104,105] Many of these cells return to the lamina propria area of the intestine as fully differentiated IgA-producing lymphocytes or plasma cells. Oral or intraperitoneal priming followed by duodenal boosting with toxoid resulted in antitoxin-containing plasma cells in jejunal lamina propria of rats.[102] Priming and boosting by the intraperitoneal route alone induced almost no jejunal response. Protection in dog jejunal Thiry–Vella loops repeatedly challenged with cholera toxin appeared to be due to locally produced antitoxin antibody. The toxin-neutralizing antibodies appeared in jejunal washings in amounts far exceeding those expected if the antibodies had been derived from serum; based on the small rise in titer of serum antitoxin antibodies.

Repeated subcutaneous or intramuscular immunization with toxin or toxoid antigens has been shown to protect dogs against oral challenge with viable *V. cholerae.* The antigens employed in these studies included toxins in Freund's complete adjuvant, fluid formalinized toxoid, and glutaraldehyde toxoid precipitated with aluminum phosphate.[106,107] Protection after repeated parenteral immunization with toxin or toxoid preparations probably was related to intestinal concentrations of serum-derived antitoxin antibody, in contrast to the immunologic changes following oral vaccination.

Holmgren and Svennerholm[108,109] quantitated local and systemic antibody formation to cholera antigen after various routes of immunization. Two subcutaneous immunizations with *V. cholerae* LPS and enterotoxin led to synthesis of antibodies to both antigens in spleen, intestinal tissue, and Peyer's patches. Repeated installation of antigen into the intestinal lumen induced synthesis of similar amounts of antibodies as occurred after parenteral immunization, but smaller amounts were produced in the spleen and serum titers were lower than after subcutaneous vaccination. Enzyme-linked immunosorbent assay (ELISA) studies of antibody production showed IgG to be predominant in spleen, regardless of route of administration of vaccine.[99]

Combined use of toxoid plus somatic antigen, possibly given by both oral and parenteral routes, may be an excellent means of obtaining effective immunoprophylaxis.[110] In one study, *V. cholerae* toxin plus LPS antigens induced a 100-fold greater degree of immunity in the rabbit against challenge with live vibrios than did immunization with either antigen alone.[108] Interference with two separate events in the pathogenesis of cholera probably occurred. With regard to the toxoid component of a combined vaccine, traditional methods of inactivation, such as treatment with formalin or glutaraldehyde, have met with limited success because of reversion to toxicity and/or extensive destruction of antigenicity. Purified subunit B may be the ideal toxoid, since elimination of subunit A will exclude the potential for reversion to toxicity without significant loss of protective antigenic determinant. Alternatively, selective chemical modification of the toxic site by amino-acid-specific reagents may be useful. Arginyl-specific reagents completely abolished the biologic activity without inhibiting the antibody-fixing capacity of cholera toxin.[111] Purified bacterial LPS would probably be as effective as whole vibrios. It may be possible to synthesize the immunodeterminant fragments of the LPS molecule. Such fragments, free of endotoxic activity, may be coupled to a carrier in order to be immunogenic; perhaps a toxoid could be employed as the carrier for a somatic-antigen component.[108]

ETEC DIARRHEA

Enterotoxins of *E. coli*

Taylor *et al.*[112] reported in 1961 that *E. coli* isolated from stool specimens of a number of children with diarrhea gave a positive rabbit intestinal loop response, whereas strains from stools of healthy infants, from well water, or from the urine of individuals with urinary tract infections invariably were negative. Two enterotoxins were later shown to be produced by strains of *E. coli* pathogenic for swine: one antigenic and heat-labile (LT) and the other nonantigenic and heat-stable (ST). Both toxins were identified by their ability to dilate ligated segments of pig intestine. The dilating effects of LT were neutralized by antisera, while ST was not neutralizable.[113] Colostrum-deprived piglets often were found to become infected with ETEC by day 4 of life.[114] Positive enterotoxic responses were observed in mice given filtrates of feces or intestinal contents infected with ETEC known to produce ST. These studies, as well as another,[115] indicated that ST was important in diarrhea of swine.

Both toxins (LT and ST) from porcine *E. coli* were shown to be controlled by a transmissible plasmid often referred to as Ent. Among strains of *E. coli* known to be pathogenic for domestic animals, a number of additional properties have been shown to be plasmid-mediated.[113,116] A large proportion of enterotoxigenic strains pathogenic for swine carry the plasmids for production of hemolysin and K88 antigen. Other factors under plasmid control include colicin production and antibiotic resistance (R factors). ETEC that produce similar, if not identical, toxins (both ST and LT) have been shown to be important as causative agents in diseases of calves and humans.

Although plasmids are independent units of replication and transmission, the total plasmid complex has important implications for the ability of the organism to persist and to produce diarrhea.[117,118] At least one transmissible plasmid was present in 90% of 96 enterotoxigenic strains in one study compared to a frequency of 36% among 204 nontoxigenic strains; Ent plasmids were demonstrated in 17% of the enterotoxigenic strains and often appeared to be self-transmissible.[119] Clones bearing a single species of DNA whose presence was associated with ST or with ST plus LT were isolated. Ent plasmids that determine the production of ST plus LT were reported to be homogeneous and to consist of a single DNA species of approximately 6.0×10^7 daltons. The Ent plasmid that codes for ST only was shown to be heterogeneous and to consist of a single species of DNA that ranged from 2.1 to 8.0×10^7 daltons.[119] Studies of the LT DNA region revealed it to be of 1.2×10^6 daltons, and the genetic map was found to consist of two cistrons encoding for two LT proteins, one of 11,500 daltons, the other 25,500 daltons.[120] The gene encoding ST was found to be a transposon.[121] The transposability of the ST gene explains the heterogeneity of ST plasmids.

Strains belonging to different serotypes show variable stability for ST and LT production. Some have been shown to be completely stable, while others are very unstable.[122] ST+LT+ strains belonging to certain specific serotypes possess one of two colonization factor antigens which are discussed later. These serotypes are remarkably stable for ST and LT production. ST⁺LT⁻ and ST⁻LT⁺ strains may represent variations in the molecular biology of Ent plasmids with or without common parents, showing variable loss or repression of the properties of toxigenicity.

Ørskov *et al.*[123] reported a study of 106 ETEC strains isolated from adults and children from various parts of the world. Similar O:H types among ETEC were found repeatedly in this study as well as in other reports,[122,124] including O6:H16, O8:H9, O15:H11, O25:H42, O78:H11, and O78:H12. Similarly, four serotypes, O6:H16, O6:H⁻, O25:H42, and O20:H⁻, represented 38% of the ETEC isolated from students with diarrhea at a Mexican university.[122] The *E. coli* polysaccharide K antigens can be determined by countercurrent immunoelectrophoresis,[125] which eventually will allow a refinement of the serologic analysis of *E. coli* when the techniques are readily available. Enterotoxigenic strains from a variety of locations were examined for K antigens, and the following were identified: O6:K15:H16, O8:K40:H9, O25:K7:H42, and O25:K98:H⁻.[126] Also, characteristic fermentation patterns were associated with specific K patterns. The demonstration that stability of enterotoxin production is related to serotype of *E. coli* suggests that serotyping will play an important role in the future in the screening of *E. coli* isolates for pathogenicity.

Purification of Enterotoxins

Although LT was described more than ten years ago,[127] attempts at purifying this toxin have been inhibited by the inability to produce large amounts of biologically active, cell-free enterotoxin and by a considerable heterogeneity in size of active molecules.[128–133] Trypsin-treated cell-free filtrates from toxigenic *E. coli* exhibited a fourfold or greater increase in vascular permeability factor and a tenfold or greater increase in ability to stimulate secretion of growth hormone by rat pituitary cells.[34] These findings suggest that activation of *E. coli* LT by host enzymes may play a role in the development of pathogenic effects.

Studies with crude products have established immunologic and biologic similarities between LT and the purified enterotoxin of *V. cholerae*.[135–138] LT preparations, like cholera toxin, increase adenyl cyclase activity,[139,140] produce increased capillary permeability in rabbit skin,[141,142] show biologic effects in cultured cells[143–145] and may interact with the same GM_1 ganglioside receptor as cholera toxin on whole-cell membranes,[40] although there is additional evidence that GM_1 does not serve as the LT receptor.[41,42]

In the various laboratories attempting purification of *E. coli* toxin, molecular weights have range from 20,000 to approximately 1,000,000.[128,146–151] Earlier efforts at LT purification resulted in the isolation of high-molecular-weight complexes containing significant amounts of LPS.[129,130] It was possible to isolate from a human enterotoxigenic strain a homogeneous protein as determined by disc electrophoresis and sodium dodecyl sulfate gel electrophoresis with activity in skin tests and Chinese hamster ovary cells.[149] Toxins identified in these studies differed in immunologic and physicochemical properties depending on the strain and growth medium employed. The products were single polypeptide chains with molecular weights ranging from 35,000 to over 100,000. In a separate laboratory, affinity chromatography was used to purify *E. coli* LT where an immunoadsorbent column was prepared with antiserum to toxin of *V. cholerae* for the specific isolation of *E. coli* LT.[150] Chromatography and preparative isotachophoresis yielded a pure preparation according to immunoelectrophoretic, disc electrophoretic, ultracentrifugal, and immunologic criteria.[151] The molecular weight was 102,000, and the preparation retained secretory activity in rabbit and piglet intestine. There was an increase in adenyl cyclase activity in broken-cell preparations of cat heart tissue, and a dissociation of enterotoxin material from endotoxin or capsular material containing the polysaccharide structure was demonstrated. A separate attempt employed a polymyxin-B-induced release of *E. coli* LT from strain H-10407 (an ST⁺LT⁺, O78:H11 strain).[128] The molecular weight was approximately 20,000 (estimated by the gel filtration technique). This lower-molecular-weight enterotoxin possessed vascular permeability factor and diarrheogenic properties in animal assays. Both the permeability factor and rabbit loop dilatation effect were neutralized by homologous antisera. Another study employed the affinity gel technique to identify the LT of H10407.[147] A single precipitin band was produced in the presence of several different antisera against the crude preparation of the toxin. The antigen produced a precipitin band in the presence of both cholera antitoxin and choleragenoid antisera. Chromatographic separation has been difficult, since enterotoxic activity is associated with a wide spectrum of molecular sizes.[129,130] ETEC produce toxin molecules which vary in subunit structure, showing a close antigenic interrelationship[131] but differing in toxic effects in tissue culture.[132] LT(s) from *E. coli* is related immunologically to both subunits A and B of cholera enterotoxin, as determined by immunodiffusion and neutralization.[152]

ST was partially purified 13-fold by ultrafiltration and gel filtration chromatography.[153] The molecular weight of ST was between 1000 and 10,000, and it was shown to be resistant to heat, trypsin, and pronase. An ST preparation from an ST-only porcine strain was purified to homogeneity by sequential ultrafiltration, acetone fractionation, preparative gel electrophoresis, diethylaminoethyl Bio-Gel A ion exchange chromotography, and Bio-Gel P-10 gel filtration.[154] The ST was purified more than 1500-fold and showed molecular weights ranging from 4400 to 5100. Antiserum produced in rabbits immunized with ST neutralized the enterotoxic activity in suckling mice, although passive hemagglutination and hemolysis titer assays supported the previous notion that ST is a poor antigen. Problems with purification of ST include the complexity of various growth media used for toxin production, the low levels of toxin made by ST-producing *E. coli* strains, and the presence of nonactive solids and cyclic AMP in culture media.[154,155] It may be that several STs are produced by ETEC which differ in reactivity in suckling mice and in methanol solubility.[156]

Assays for *E. coli* Enterotoxin

Assay for LT

Animal Models. The ligated rabbit loop model for assaying *V. cholerae* toxin was described in 1953.[53] This model was used later to show that *E. coli* isolates from stool of infants and calves with diarrhea produced dilatation of rabbit intestinal loops, while those strains isolated from patients with urinary tract infection did not.[112] Smooth strains of *E. coli* were shown to be more active in rabbit loops than rough variants. In 1970, broth culture supernatant of strains of *E. coli* enterotoxigenic for swine were tested in ligated rabbit loops and pig jejunal loops, thereby enabling quantitation of toxin. While bacteria-free filtrates were more frequently reactive in the rabbit loop when compared to the pig loop model, whole organisms were not always positive in the rabbit model.[157] The amount of toxin produced by *E. coli* isolates was increased by using agitation during bacterial growth.[157] *E. coli* strains isolated from the homologous animal species have been studied successfully for enterotoxin production by injecting whole *E. coli* into ligated pig intestinal loops.[158]

The isolated rabbit ileal loop preparation is the standard model for testing strains for enterotoxigenicity. Twelve to 18 hr after injection of LT-containing bacteria-free filtrates into sausage-shaped intestinal segments tied by suture, the loop will show swelling from the transudation of fluid and electrolytes (Figure 6.2).

A skin permeability assay for detection of *E. coli* toxin was developed in rabbits. LT injected intradermally into rabbits produced local vascular permeability which was visible after intravenous injection of Evans blue dye. Permeability activity of various strains of ETEC, as well as of cholera toxin, is neutralized by LT antiserum prepared against the enterotoxin of *E. coli* strain H-10407.[142]

Tissue Culture Techniques. LT-containing cell-free culture filtrates

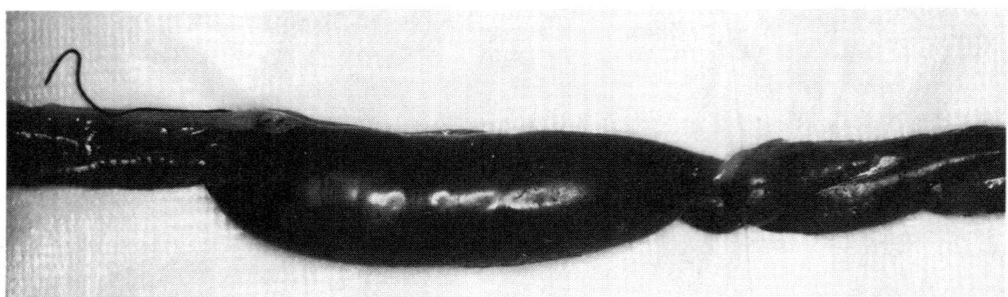

Figure 6.2. Rabbit intestinal loop reaction to heat-labile *Escherichia coli* enterotoxin (LT). Dilated loop of rabbit ileum 18 hr after injection of filtrate containing the toxin.

of *E. coli* caused morphologic changes and enhanced steroidogenesis in cultures of Y1 rat adrenal sarcoma cells[159] (Figures 6.3 and 6.4). A rapid test employing Y1 adrenal cells in tissue miniculture was adapted for routine testing of potentially enterotoxigenic isolates.[160] A continuous cell line of African green monkey (vero) cells[161] and a Chinese hamster ovary (CHO) tissue culture system[162] also were developed for detection of LT. Because of their reproducibility and suitability for assaying large numbers of strain filtrates, the tissue culture assays (particularly the adrenal and CHO cell assays) were instrumental to our being able to conduct field studies employing large number of isolates.

Serologic Procedures. Sheep erythrocytes sensitized with *E. coli* LT exhibited passive immune hemolysis when exposed to specific antitoxin and complement.[163] LT+ isolates can be detected in a standard test-tube or microtiter system by determining hemoglobin release spectrophotometrically. The major requirement for the procedure is anti-LT serum. The development of an ELISA for detection of IgG and IgM antibody to LT has allowed the characterization of these specific immunoglobulins.[164]

Assay for ST

The mechanism of action of ST differs from that of LT.[165] Two whole-animal models have been used to detect ST: the adult (ligated) rabbit ileal loop assay[165] and the suckling mouse assay.[166] The suckling mouse assay is the only current method which has been adopted for routine screening of large numbers of isolates. It generally is required that between five and ten *E. coli* isolates be tested from a stool sample to establish a reasonable probability of detecting the presence of the agent. Test materials are supernatant fluids obtained by high-speed centrifugation of *E. coli* grown in CYE broth[141,167,168] at 37°C for 16–18 hr. Aeration is provided by mechanical shaking. To control for variation among individual animals, approximately six mice per test specimen are used in

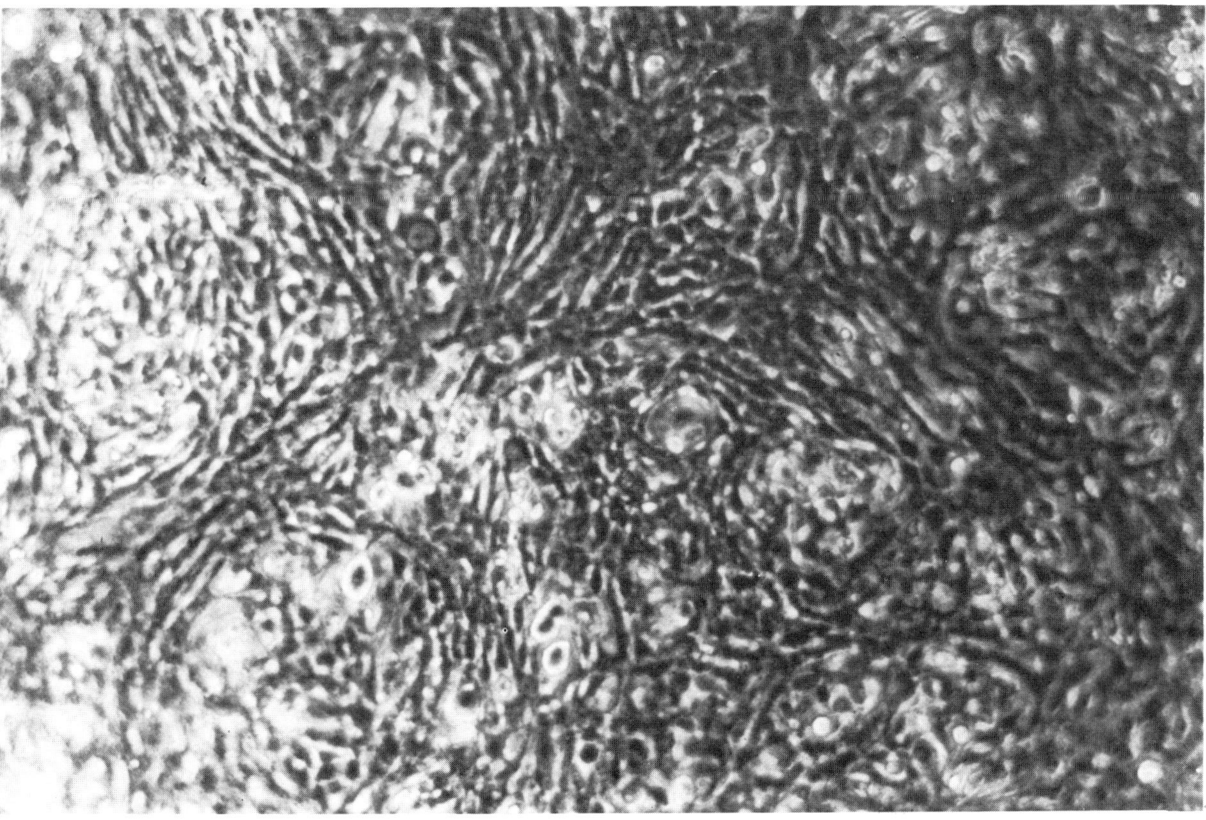

Figure 6.3.   Y1 adrenal cell monolayer culture control (×375).

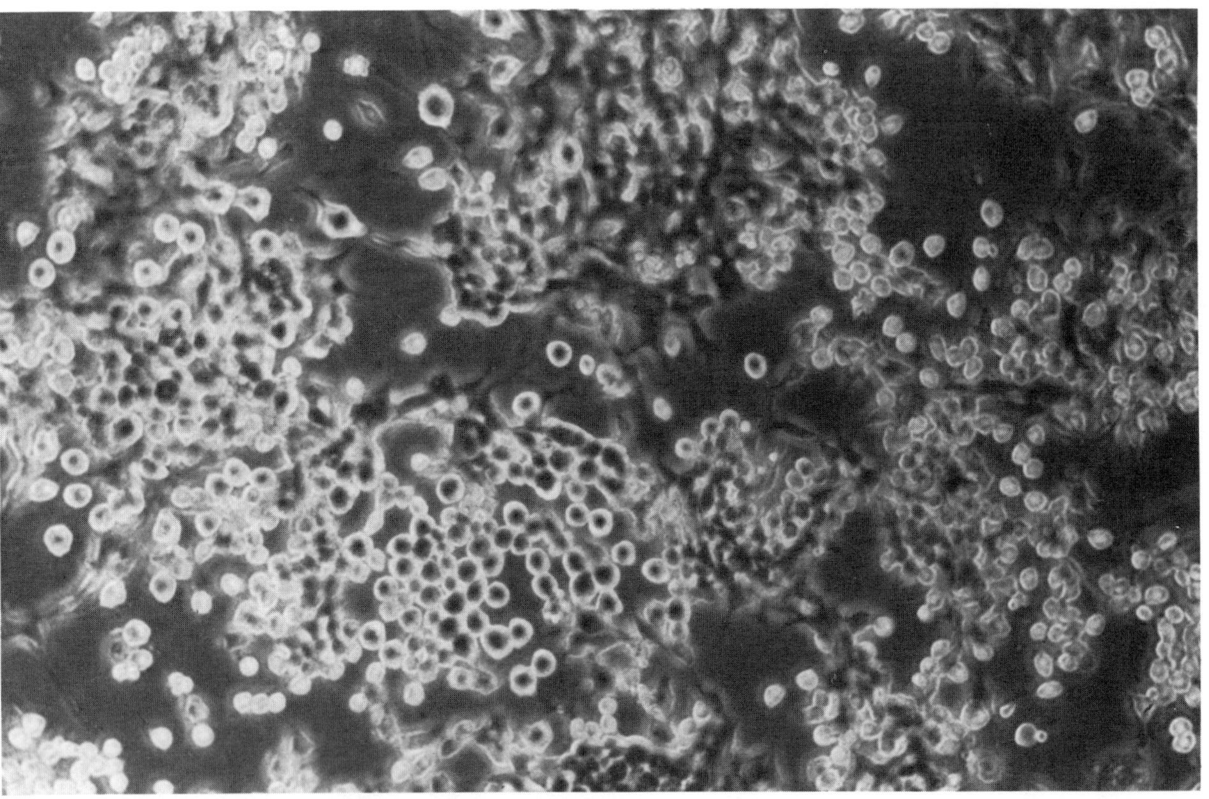

Figure 6.4. Y1 adrenal cell monolayer culture 24 hr after the addition of filtrate containing *Escherichia coli* enterotoxin (LT). Characteristic rounding of the cells is shown. (×375).

the assay. Newborn mice (one to four days old) are injected immediately after removal from the mother when the presence of milk allows localization of the stomachs. Mice are maintained at a constant temperature of 28°C in plastic beakers in a low-level water bath for 2–4 hr. After ether sacrifice, the intestines but not the stomachs of animals corresponding to test isolates are pooled and weighed, and the remaining bodies (with stomachs but without intestines) are pooled and weighed (see Figure 6.5). A ratio of gut weight to remaining body weight for the two pools of equal to or greater than 0.090 is considered positive, indicating ST activity. Up to five individually grown colonies may be pooled for determining ST activity in suckling mice. This should improve the efficiency of the assay when testing large numbers of isolates in field studies.[168] The 6-hr rabbit loop reaction is useful to verify ST^+ strains in selected instances.[165] Due to the cumbersome nature of the assay, however, it is not a suitable screening test for ST.

Pathogenesis of ETEC Diarrhea

ETEC strains produce illness in a host by colonizing the toxin-sensitive upper intestine prior to releasing the secretory enterotoxins. An adhesive interaction between a microbial pathogen and epithelium of a target organ is a primary prerequisite for infection by a number of agents. The mechanism of adhesion is not always clear, but microbial pathogens usually show a degree of host and organ specificity for colonization. For ETEC, the colonizing or adhesive property appears to lie in surface fimbriae which serve as ligands in an intestinal binding process (Figure 6.6). These structures have been termed "colonization factor antigens" (CFAs).[169]

Intestinal Colonization by ETEC

ETEC show a high degree of host specificity which is related to the propensity of the organism to proliferate in the small bowel and not to any known differences in the enterotoxins produced.

The importance of adhesion of _E. coli_ to small-intestinal villi as a prelude to porcine diarrhea has been verified.[170–172] In the small bowel of piglets, the K88 antigen appears to bind to a receptor on the villous epithelial cells.[117,171,173] K88 antigen was shown to be a plasmid-mediated nonflagellar, filamentous surface-protein appendage resembling bacterial fimbriae which differed from the common type 1 _E. coli_ pilus structure.[174] It is of particular interest that attachment of ETEC to the upper gut of the piglet not only depends upon their possessing K88, but

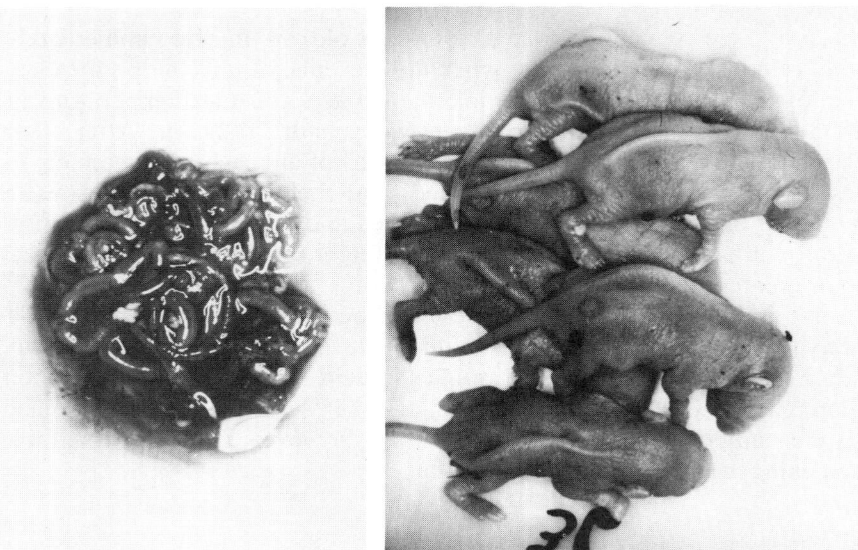

Figure 6.5. Suckling mouse assay for heat-stable *Escherichia coli* enterotoxin (ST). Two to four hours after intragastric injection of filtrate containing ST, the intestines of six mice are weighed and the ratio of intestinal weight to remaining body weight determined.

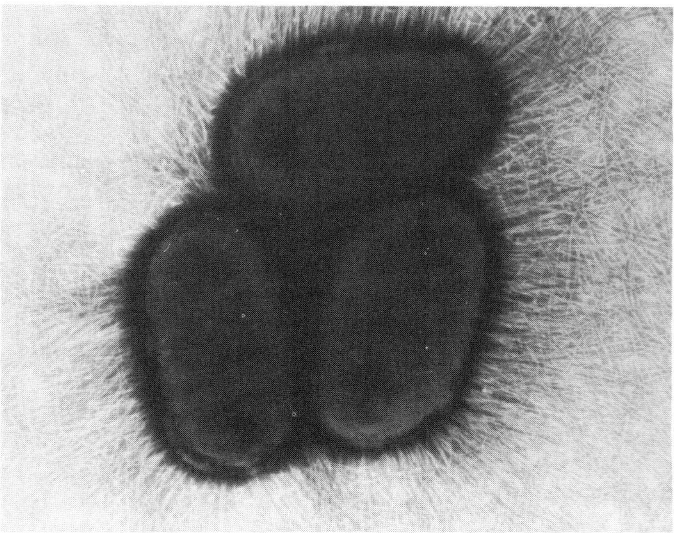

Figure 6.6 Enterotoxigenic *Escherichia coli* (ETEC) as visualized by electron microscopy (negative staining technique). The surface-colonization fimbriae are shown (×35,000). From Evans *et al.*[185]

TABLE 6.2
ETEC Adhesion Fimbriae and Susceptible Animal Hosts

Surface antigen	Natural host	Other susceptible animal
K88	Piglet	Suckling mouse
K99	Calf, lamb	Piglet
987-type	Piglet	Unknown
Type 1 (common pili)	Unknown	Unknown
CFA/I	Human	Infant rabbit
CFA/II	Human	Infant rabbit

the genetic phenotype of the animal is also important in the adhesive interaction of the organism and intestinal brush border.[175] Table 6.2 lists the characterized adhesion fimbriae according to natural host, as well as other animal species found to be susceptible to each adhesion property. A K88 strain of ETEC, highly virulent for swine, was fed to adult volunteers in a dose of 10^{10} viable cells. Gut colonization did not occur, and illness failed to develop.[176] The possession of K99 is an important virulence property of ETEC strains pathogenic for calves, lambs, and newborn piglets.[177–180] A non-K88, non-K99 fimbrial antigen also has been shown to be responsible for the property of intestinal colonization by porcine ETEC, with the production of naturally occurring illness.[181,182] This is referred to as a 987-type fimbrial antigen, named after the strain number. The antigenically different fimbriae, K88, K99, 987-type, and type 1 pili, adhere equally to porcine epithelium.[183] The various ligands appear to bind to different receptors, in view of a lack of competitive inhibition of bacterial cell attachment to procine intestinal epithelium *in vitro* using purified antigens.[183] Human ETEC strains isolated from patients with diarrhea often possess CFA/I or CFA/II. The colonizing capability has been documented in the upper gut of infant rabbits[184] and confirmed by immunofluorescence.[185]

The surface-associated adhesion fimbriae can be detected by determining their hemagglutination properties utilizing erythrocytes derived from different animal species and by determining mannose sensitivity (inhibition) of the reaction.[126,174,186,187] To determine hemagglutination of the various adhesion fimbriae, it is necessary to grow the strains in solid agar medium or liquid medium to allow the expression of CFA or type 1 pilus formation [169,187–189] Table 6.3 outlines the human-adapted CFAs and the associated *E. coli* serogroups. CFA/I mediates mannose-resistant hemagglutination (MRH) of human (group A) and bovine erythrocytes,[189,190] while CFA/II mediates MRH of bovine but not human erythrocytes, which is accelerated at 4°C.[191] Type 1 pili mediate hemag-

TABLE 6.3
Human-Adapted CFAs

CFA	Mannose-resistant hemagglutination (MRH)	*Escherchia coli* serogroup[a]
I	Human and bovine red blood cells	O15:H11, O15:H$^-$, O25:H42, O25:H$^-$, O63:H12, O63:H$^-$, O78:H11, O78:H12,
II	Bovine red blood cells	O6:H16, O6:H$^-$, O8:H9, O8:H$^-$

[a]It is necessary to determine K antigenicity for complete serotyping.

glutination of human, chicken, and guinea pig erythrocytes, and the reaction in each instance is inhibited by (sensitive to) mannose (MSH). Such a mannose-specific ligand on the surface of *E. coli* may be important to their binding to mannose residues on human intestinal epithelial cells.[192,193] Animal-adapted strains of ETEC may adhere through properties other than MRH or MSH.[181,182]

We have employed a slide hemagglutination procedure with human and animal red blood cells in addition to determining resistance to mannose in order to screen large numbers of *E. coli* for surface-adhesion factors in field studies. Strains showing a characteristic reaction may be verified as CFA$^+$ with specific CFA antibody or with the staphylococcal coagglutination test utilizing staphylococci coupled to CFA-specific antibody.[126,191] Presence of fimbriae may be demonstrated by electron microscopy (Figure 6.6).

Relationships of CFA, Enterotoxin Production, and Serotype

Production of ST and LT has been associated with transmissible plasmids.[174,194] Strains producing one factor or the other occur in nature and are usually designated as ST-only or LT-only. When we have detected CFA/I on *E. coli*, they invariably have been ST$^+$, and most have produced both ST and LT.[185] CFA/I and ST production have been shown by Smith *et al.*[195] to be determined by a simple plasmid. These workers were able to transfer to *E. coli* K12 the plasmid coding for both CFA/I and ST production. Although ETEC strains from humans and animals with diarrhea show a wide variation in O and H serotypes, there is an apparent relationship between the virulence properties (CFA, ST/LT) and serotype. Table 6.3 indicates that many strains of ETEC belonging to

O15, O25, O63, and O78 serogroups are also positive for CFA/I, and those with O6 and O8 antigens generally possess CFA/II. Approximately half of the ETEC isolated from diverse regions of the world belong to serotypes associated with CFA/I and CFA/II.[123,194]

Virulence of CFA/I and CFA/II

Both CFA/I and CFA/II show similar biologic properties, including electron microscopic appearance as filamentous appendages from the cell surface (Figure 6.6), capacity to colonize the upper gut of the infant rabbit, heat lability at 65°C for 1 hr, neutralization by specific antibody, MRH, spontaneous loss of colonizing ability during laboratory transfer, and a relationship to O–H–K serotypes. A series of volunteer studies were carried out to determine the importance of CFA as a prerequisite for human illness produced by an ETEC strain.[196,197] Table 6.4 summarizes the results of these studies. Illness occurred only in those volunteers ingesting 10^8 viable CFA/I$^+$ cells. The importance of CFA is seen, in that excretion of the organism in stool and development of humoral antibodies to CFA and LT all were dependent upon CFA production by the challenge strain. This study confirms and extends the observations employing an animal model[184] which showed the importance of CFA in the pathogenesis of ETEC diarrhea. CFA/I was a necessary prerequisite for ETEC to colonize the gut, produce illness, and stimulate antibody-producing cells. The CFA$^-$ strain, despite producing equivalent amounts of LT and possessing type 1 pili, remained avirulent for humans in a dose of 10^8 cells.

TABLE 6.4

Clinical and Laboratory Findings in Adult Volunteers Receiving an Oral Inoculation of
Escherichia coli H-10407 (CFA+LT+) and H-10407-P (CFA−LT+)[a]

Strain	Dose	Number of volunteers	Illness	Stool excretion of challenge strain ≥4 days	Fourfold or greater rise in serum antibody to	
					CFA	LT
H-10407	10^6 cells	7	0	100%	50%	33%
(CFA$^+$LT$^+$)	10^8 cells	7	86%	100%	67%	57%
H-10407-P	10^6 cells	7	0	0	0	0
(CFA$^+$LT$^-$)	10^8 cells	6	0	17%	0	0

[a]Adapted from Satterwhite *et al.*[197]

Mechanism of Action of *E. coli* Enterotoxin

The physiologic changes in the intestine of humans infected with ETEC resemble those seen in cholera. ETEC strains replicate in the upper gut of the infected host, a finding reported by three laboratories in 1971.[176,198,199] The enterotoxins elaborated by *E. coli* produce changes in ion flux across the small-intestinal mucosa which are responsible for the water and electrolyte loss in illness. The driving force for water movement in the intestine is active transport of electrolytes. Ussing and Zerahn[200] described a membrane chamber model which allowed a study of movement (active transport) of individual ions. When the membrane was exposed to *E. coli* (or cholera) enterotoxin, there was an inhibition of the movement of sodium and a reversal of the chloride flux, that is, chloride secretion.[70] Active chloride movement from blood to lumen provides a force by which cations and water move into the lumen of the gut to maintain osmotic equilibrium with blood plasma.

The two major *E. coli* enterotoxins both appear to affect intestinal secretion, probably through different pathways. ST show a more rapid onset of action and an effect of shorter duration as compared to LT.[113,127,135,157,201] LT, which resembles cholera toxin antigenically and physiologically, appears to have similar biochemical effects. LT has been shown to stimulate adenyl cyclase and increase cAMP in a variety of tissues, including rabbit intestine,[139] fat cells,[140] thyroid tissue,[202] Y1 adrenal cells,[159] CHO cells,[162] cultured intestinal epithelial cells,[203] and mouse thymus cells.[204] Until recently, there was little positive information about the mechanism of ST, although it clearly was a virulence property that produced secretory responses in the rabbit loop preparation and the suckling mouse model. Hughes *et al.*[205] demonstrated that ST-producing *E. coli* caused increased guanyl cyclase concentrations in rabbit intestine and that a cyclic GMP (cGMP) analogue mimicked ST-induced secretion in magnitude and timing in both rabbits and suckling mice. A simultaneous report by Field *et al.*[206] also indicated that ST increased cGMP in rabbit ileum. Newsome *et al.*[207] further reported that cGMP accumulated in eight-day-old mice that had been exposed to methanol-soluble ST. Intestinal cGMP probably is localized in the microvilli of the intestinal mucosa, as has been demonstrated in rats.[208,209]

ETEC Immunity

Natural immunity to ETEC infection occurs as persons remain at high risk for infection. In a study of various student groups attending school in Mexico, the rate of attack for diarrhea was inversely related to the length of time the student lived in the area of endemicity.[210] Newly arrived students from the United States suffered from diarrhea at a rate of 40% per month, as compared to an incidence of 20% per month for United States students who remained at the school for approximately a year or longer. A newly arrived group of students from Venezuela did not have an increased frequency of diarrhea, indicating their previous exposure to agents found in Mexico while they had been living in Venezuela. The decreased incidence of illness among Latin American students corresponded to an apparent resistance to ETEC infection. An inverse relationship was found between geometric mean serum antibody titers to LT and the occurrence of diarrhea due to LT-producing *E. coli,* especially among the newly arrived students from the United States.[211]

The titers of IgG and IgM antitoxin antibodies from birth to three years of age among children from the United States and Mexico have been determined by an ELISA.[164] IgG antitoxin antibody declined from birth to three months (presumably from natural decay of maternally acquired IgG) and rose thereafter throughout the study, while IgM antitoxin antibody increased progressively from birth to three years of age, remaining at lower titers than IgG. The titers were significantly higher among Mexican children than among children from the United States. We have found the geometric mean antibody titers of three-year-old children from Houston, Texas, to be essentially the same as those found in adults from various parts of the United States. A lack of exposure to ETEC in the United States appears to explain the low titers of LT antibody and the remarkable susceptibility to infection among persons from the United States who travel to developing countries.

Immunity in ETEC infection may not be related solely to antitoxic antibody. Latin American students rarely excrete the organism in stool asymptomatically, in contrast to the common finding of asymptomatic excretion of ETEC in stool of United States students.[210,212] These data suggest that an antibacterial immunity is operative whereby virulent strains are excluded from gut colonization. This could represent intestinal antibody to adhesion fimbriae or somatic antigens or other factors.

The existence of a small number of antigenic types of adhesion fimbriae identified on human-associated ETEC has encouraged us to attempt immunoprophylaxis with purified CFA. Such vaccine preparations made of pili or CFA fimbriae are particularly attractive, since they are easily produced, are likely to have a diffuse interaction with gut mucosa, and are unlikely to possess inherent toxicity. A number of studies conducted in animal populations have been published in support of an anti-CFA vaccine. Adhesion of a K88+ porcine strain is blocked by specific antibody,[173,213] and piglets nursed by K88-immune dams are passively protected from lethal oral challenge with a K88+ ETEC.[214] When K88 antigen,[215] K99 antigen,[216] and 987-type fimbrial antigen[217] were used to vaccinate gilts, protection against ETEC infection in the neonatal suckling pigs occurred for strains possessing the homologous but not the heterologous fimbrial antigen. The adhesive properties of the virulent ETEC strains appeared to be neutralized by antibody in colostrum and maternal milk, since transplacental transfer of immunoglobulin does not occur in pigs. The nature of protective antiadhesion antibody has yet to be elucidated. Linggood, Ellis, and Porter[218] have shown that a heat-stable antibody directed against an ETEC strain permanently altered the genetic composition of the strain, eliminating the plasmid controlling K88 antigen production. Such a plasmid-curing effect by antibody might prove to be an important mechanism in successful immunoprophylaxis. The proper immunizing agent might stimulate antibody development, which would render virulent ETEC nonadherent. A trivalent K88, K99, and 987-type fimbrial antigen vaccine may have utility in the control of porcine scours due to ETEC strains.

CFA/I and CFA/II antisera neutralize the colonization potential of human ETEC possessing the respective antigen, as tested in an infant rabbit model.[184,185,191] We have initiated studies to examine the safety and immunogenicity of a purified CFA/I vaccine in student volunteers prior to field testing in an area of ETEC endemicity.

ENTEROPATHOGENIC *E. COLI* (SEROTYPE IDENTIFICATION)

A relationship between serotype of *E. coli* and diarrhea was suggested in 1945 when Bray[219] identified an organism with similar antigenic properties in stool specimens obtained from 42 of 44 infants who had acquired diarrhea during a hospital epidemic. In 1949, Giles *et al.*[220] reported a nursery outbreak of diarrhea with a mortality rate of 56% due to a serologically identified *E. coli.* Taylor *et al.*[221] then described four nursery outbreaks wherein a similar *E. coli* serotype, referred to initially as *Bacterium coli* D433 (later serotyped 0111:B4), was recovered from stool specimens of a percentage of those affected.

During the 1950s, serologic schemes were developed to type *E. coli* on the basis of their somatic and flagellar antigens.[222,223] A series of studies then documented the worldwide distribution of certain *E. coli* serotypes, particularly during hospital nursery outbreaks of diarrhea. These strains were designated as enteropathogenic *E. coli* (EPEC). Following these reports, the assumption was made that the recovery of one of the EPEC serotypes from diarrheal stool of a patient with illness was sufficient to indicate an etiologic diagnosis.

Most of the earlier studies focused on outbreaks in hospital nurseries. EPEC disease was shown to be 20 times more common in infants below the age of six months than in older children between one and two years of age.[224] A study employing a fluorescent antibody method to investigate the importance of EPEC strains as causes of diarrhea during a 15-month period at one hospital revealed that 151 of 383 children (40%) hospitalized with diarrhea had an EPEC serotype in stool.[225] In the same report, a single strain, O126:B16:NM, was identified in 39 of 82 cases (48%) localized in three distinct areas of the community during late summer. During a community investigation, half of the households with an index case had one or more asymptomatic pharyngeal carriers of the epidemic strain and a lower rate of intestinal carriage, implicating possible respiratory transmission of the agent. During one outbreak of diarrhea due to an EPEC strain, nursing personnel and family members were shown to be asymptomatic excretors of the epidemic strain, suggesting a possible role for these individuals in the transmission of the agent.[226] In the same study, an EPEC strain was recovered from stool specimens of 36 mothers (13%) just before delivery, with the subsequent isolation of the same serotype of *E. coli* from 40% of their newborn infants. During epidemics of EPEC diarrhea, the epidemic strain has been detected in air, dust, and fomites within a hospital environment. In children with illness due to EPEC, in contrast to those without symptoms, *E. coli* have been found in great numbers in the small intestine as far up as the duodenum, and stool counts have ranged from 10^6 to 10^8 colonies/g.[227] EPEC outbreaks in newborn nurseries were reported more commonly in industrialized as compared to developing countries. This was felt to be due to the lack of breast-feeding among such populations and to the fact that most births in these parts of the world occur within the hospital, where the newborns are more likely to be exposed to an enteropathogen.

In one outbreak of mild gastroenteritis due to an O128:B12 strain at a university hospital nursery, 24 infants became ill over a three-week period without mortality.[228] In that outbreak, clinically inapparent infection was found frequently but abated soon after the institution of strict aseptic techniques, temporary reorganization of the nurseries, and administration of neomycin to all infants and newborns.

A variety of antimicrobial agents have been employed in the treatment of EPEC infection. Neomycin, a nonabsorbable aminoglycoside, was advocated in a number of earlier studies[229–231] in which the organism was eradicated from stool within several days of therapy. However, neomycin resistance among organisms isolated from stool specimens was shown to develop during the course of therapy.[232] Other drugs that have been employed with success include colymycin[233] and gentamicin.[234]

Evidence was offered that spread of EPEC strains also occurred outside the hospital environment. Kessner *et al.*[232] conducted a prospective examination of EPEC in a defined geographic area in Illinois and Indiana. They documented an extensive community epidemic of diarrhea due to *E. coli* O111:B4 during the winters of 1960 and 1961. There were 77 deaths, with a case fatality of 6%. The carrier rates of asymptomatic contacts of index cases ranged from 5 to 10%. Smith *et al.*[235] carried out a separate one-year longitudinal investigation of 40 households and were able to show that EPEC excretion and infection occurred in all age groups studied, with the highest rates of index cases among children in the age range of four to seven months. Infection rates correlated with crowded sleeping arrangements, intimate contact, household pets, and pork and chicken consumption.

Other studies have failed to show a relationship between serotype of *E. coli* and diarrhea. Thomson *et al.*[236] documented that 20 of 111 infants (18%) transiently were infected or colonized with an EPEC strain without symptoms, while another report showed that numerous infants became colonized with an O111 strain during a one-year study in a hospital nursery without the occurrence of an outbreak of illness.[237] Ramos-Alvarez and Sabin[238] performed an investigation during the summer months in Cincinnati, Ohio, and except for *E. coli* O111, they failed to show a relationship of the known EPEC serotypes to diarrhea when controls were compared to those with illness. Ørskov[239] serotyped 581 isolates from infants with diarrhea and 183 healthy asymptomatic children and found a similar distribution of serotyped organisms in the two groups. A two-year study was performed to determine the association of the serogroup of *E. coli* with the occurrence of illness among 1674 persons, with an emphasis on the inclusion of infants and children.[240] Over the two years, 2411 stool specimens and 514 throat cultures were processed, and there were no discernible differences in serogroups between those with diarrhea and those without. A five-year prospective study in Southampton, England, documented cyclic occurrence of O111, O55, and O26 *E. coli* in the population under study without an apparent association with illness.[241] Soloman *et al.*[242] cultured stool specimens from more than 1000 children and found that EPEC strains were more commonly isolated from well children (5%) than from those with diarrhea (1%).

In many clinical situations, however, illness is clearly related to infection by an EPEC strain. This relationship can be demonstrated by isolation of the strain from most patients with diarrhea during an epidemic, by documentation of a fourfold rise in serum antibodies against the strain isolated from diarrheal stools, or by isolation of the infecting strain from blood of affected infants. Future studies are needed to establish the importance of EPEC strains as causes of endemic diarrheal illness. Certain nonenterotoxigenic serotype-identified *E. coli* not previously classed as "enteropathogenic" have been associated with sporadic cases of diarrhea.[243] Strains belonging to these serotypes should be considered as facultatively enteropathogenic *E. coli* (FEPEC).

Serotyping Procedures

Kauffmann[244] reported serologic methods that led to the development of a taxonomic scheme for *E. coli* based on antigenic differences between strains. The somatic or O antigens of the bacteria were shown not to be inactivated by heating at 121°C, while K antigens, found to be somatic antigens occurring as envelopes or as capsules, were shown to inhibit the agglutination of living bacteria in O antisera. This inhibitory effect of K antigens on agglutination could be inactivated by heat. The flagellar or H antigens also were inactivated by heating to 100°C. Complete serotyping of *E. coli* strains isolated from stools of patients with diarrhea is now known to be dependent upon determining each of the antigenic components: O, K, and H types. The amount and type of K antigen a strain possesses relates to the pathogenicity. K antigens may confer virulence to strains of *E. coli* by making them resistant to complement or to phagocytosis, or they may affect the adhesion properties of the organism.

Serotyping is frequently done incorrectly by diagnostic laboratories, where only a screening procedure is carried out using A or B grouping pools to identify O antigen types.[245] It is necessary to do more than O-group typing, in view of the fact that nonpathogenic strains may show similar O groups and the pathogenic serotypes tend to belong to the same O–H groups or O–H–K groups. Much of the misunderstanding about serotyping has resulted from the use of simplified or abbreviated procedures for serotyping *E. coli.* To perform serotyping in the proper manner, three steps must be performed.[245,246]

1. Strains are initially screened using polyvalent group A and B pools (or C, if employed). If the strain is negative, it is not an EPEC.
2. Presumptive identification of O and K antigens is performed, based on agglutination of living and heated antigen with individual typing sera.
3. Titration of O antiserum is undertaken with the presumptive strain to confirm that the strain is an O group of EPEC. This step is the one most frequently omitted by hospital laboratories.

Table 6.5 lists the generally accepted EPEC serotypes.

TABLE 6.5
EPEC Serotypes^{a,b}

O26:B6	O119:B14
O55:B5	O125:B15
O86:B7	O126:B16
O111:B4	O127:B8
O112:B11	O128:B12
112:B13	

[a] Adapted from Edwards and Ewing.[246]
[b] Additional O20, O44, O114, O142, and O158 serotypes may be considered to be EPEC.

Relationship of *E. coli* Serotype and Pathogenicity

Volunteer studies have been performed in an attempt to establish virulence of EPEC. In 1950, Neter and Shumway[247] fed an O111 strain of *E. coli* to an infant and produced diarrhea wherein the causative agent was recovered from stool. Further volunteer studies with this O111 and an O55 strain demonstrated that the virulence characteristics were unstable and that the severity of illness was dose-dependent.[248,249] Adults were shown to be relatively resistant to clinical illness, as determined by volunteer studies in which a dose of 6–9 × 10^9 cells was required to produce the disease.[248] More recent volunteer studies were conducted by Levine *et al.*,[250] where illness was produced in adults after feeding EPEC strains isolated years earlier from stool specimens of patients with diarrhea.

Based on clinical findings, certain O–K EPEC types were shown to produce illness resembling either *Salmonella*-like enteritis or *Shigella*-like dysentery.[251] Bacterial suspensions of EPEC strains were tested in a related study for virulence properties in the guinea pig eye model (Sérény test), ligated rabbit intestinal loops, and HeLa cells. The agents identified with *Shigella*-like illness were usually positive in an assay for invasiveness while the *Salmonella*-like strains were negative in the assays.[252] Only recently have EPEC strains identified in infantile diarrhea been shown to produce a cholera-like enterotoxin.[253] A number of strains of *E. coli* belonging to classic O–K EPEC serotypes identified in colibacillosis of swine have been shown to be enterotoxigenic.[254] In a study of 48 strains of serotype-identified EPEC isolated from infants and children with diarrhea in Houston, Texas, none was found to be invasive or positive for ST production, and only three were found to produce an LT.[255] In a separate study of 167 isolates of EPEC, only one produced an enterotoxin, and none was invasive.[256] These studies confirm the fact that EPEC are not generally pathogenic by production of an enterotoxin detected by routine procedures, nor do the strains commonly show a *Shigella*-like invasive property.

In one study, there did appear to be a difference in clinical features of illness in children with diarrhea associated with recovery of an EPEC compared to children with nonbacterial gastroenteritis (stool cultures were negative) and infants with shigellosis.[256] The duration of diarrhea for the children with EPEC diarrhea was significantly longer than for those with nonbacterial gastroenteritis, and, in that sense, the EPEC group resembled patients with shigellosis. Patients in the EPEC group were younger, and a higher proportion of infants were of rural origin. A small number of EPEC were shown in a pilot study to produce a cytotoxin in a HeLa cell model which was neutralized by antibody prepared against the toxin elaborated by *S. dysenteriae* 1, the Shiga bacillus.[257] Shiga-like toxins should be sought as potential virulence properties of EPEC. In a separate published study, EPEC isolates were shown to produce LT and ST which altered water transport in a rat jejunal model.[258] Additional evidence has been offered to suggest that EPEC may possess transmissible (plasmid) adhesion properties.[259] *E. coli* identified by serotype have been shown to possess previously undescribed virulence properties. An O15 *E. coli* (strain RDEC-1) produced diarrhea in rabbits when administered by the orogastric route.[260] The strain was adherent to the epithelial surface; it was neither invasive nor enterotoxigenic. The strain produced damage to microvilli, terminal web, and glycocalyx.[261] A similar mechanism of adherence and local intestinal damage was shown for an O125ac:H21 *E. coli* strain which produced protracted diarrhea in an infant.[262] Additional laboratory techniques must be applied to EPEC strains to establish the mechanisms of their pathogenicity.

At present, there exists a dilemma for the diagnostic microbiology laboratory. Should serotyping be continued where an association with illness is not always found and where the test, when done properly and routinely, requires an enormous investment in time and effort? We believe that *E. coli* serotyping as it is now performed should be restricted to diarrhea cases during an outbreak (usually a hospital nursery epidemic). In these cases, serotyping becomes an excellent epidemiologic marker of disease transmission. Although we are not now recommending routine analysis of *E. coli* serotypes in endemic diarrhea, we are optimistic that the future will bring better and more refined methods of serotyping. Serotyping may ultimately be employed in the diagnostic laboratory to routinely screen for EPEC and FEPEC strains, as well as for ETEC and enteroinvasive *E. coli*.

REFERENCES

1. Holmgren, J., Lönnroth, I., Ouchterlony, Ö. Immunochemical studies of two cholera toxin-containing standard culture filtrate preparations of *Vibrio cholerae. Infect. Immun.* **3:**747–755, 1971.
2. Finkelstein, R. A. Antitoxic immunity in experimental cholera: Observations with purified antigens and the ligated ileal loop model. *Infect. Immun.* **1:**464–467, 1970.
3. LoSpalluto, J. J., Finkelstein, R. A. Chemical and physical properties of cholera exo-enterotoxin (choleragen) and its spontaneously formed toxoid (choleragenoid). *Biochim. Biophys. Acta* **257:**158–166, 1972.
4. Van Heyningen, S. Cholera toxin: Interaction of subunits with ganglioside GM_1. *Science* **183:**656–657, 1973.
5. Cuatrecasas, P., Parikh, I., Hollenberg, M. D. Affinity chromatography and structural analysis of *Vibrio cholerae* enterotoxin—ganglioside agarose and the biological effects of ganglioside-containing soluble polymers. *Biochemistry* **12:**4253–4264, 1973.
6. Lönnroth, I., Holmgren, J. Subunit structure of cholera toxin. *J. Gen. Microbiol.* **76:**417–427, 1973.
7. Finkelstein, R. A., LoSpalluto, J. J. Pathogenesis of experimental cholera: Preparation and isolation of choleragen and choleragenoid. *J. Exp. Med.* **130:**185–202, 1969.
8. Van Heyningen, S. The subunits of cholera toxin: Structure, stoichiometry, and function. *J. Infect. Dis.* **133:**S5–S13, 1976.
9. Finkelstein, R. A., Boesman, M., Neoh, S. H., *et al.* Dissociation and recombination of the subunits of the cholera enterotoxin (choleragen). *J. Immunol.* **113:**145–150, 1974.
10. Finkelstein, R. A., Boesman, M., Neoh, S. H., *et al.* Separation and recombination of subunits of cholera enterotoxin. *Fed. Proc. Fed. Am. Soc. Exp. Biol.* **33:**763, 1974.
11. Dawson, C. E., Blagg, W. Effect of human saliva on the cholera vibrio *in vitro:* Pilot study. *J. Dent. Res.* **27:**547–552, 1948.
12. Gitelson, S. Gastrectomy, achlorhydria and cholera. *Isr. J. Med. Sci.* **7:**663–667, 1971.
13. Nalin, D. R., Levine, R. J., Levine, M. M., *et al.* Cholera, non-vibrio cholera, and stomach acid. *Lancet* **2:**856–859, 1978.
14. Cash, R. A., Music, S. I., Libonati, J. P., *et al.* Response of man to infection with *Vibrio cholerae:* 1. Clinical, serologic, and bacteriologic responses to a known inoculum. *J. Infect. Dis.* **129:**45–52, 1974.
15. Dixon, J. M. The fate of bacteria in the small intestine. *J. Pathol. Bacteriol.* **79:**131–140, 1960.
16. Meynell, G. G. Antibacterial mechanisms of the mouse gut: II. The role of Eh and volatile fatty acids in the normal gut. *Br. J. Exp. Pathol.* **44:**209–219, 1963.
17. Freter, R. Interactions between mechanisms controlling the intestinal microflora. *Am. J. Clin. Nutr.* **27:**1409–1416, 1974.
18. Florey, H. W. Observations on functions of mucus and the early stages of bacterial invasion of intestinal mucosa. *J. Pathol. Bacteriol.* **37:**283–289, 1933.
19. Freter, R., Jones, G. W. Adhesive properties of *Vibrio cholerae:* Nature of the interaction with intact mucosal surfaces. *Infect. Immun.* **14:**246–256, 1976.
20. Schrank, G. D., Verway, W. F. Distribution of cholera organisms in experimental *Vibrio cholerae* infections: Proposed mechanisms of pathogenesis and antibacterial immunity. *Infect. Immun.* **13:**195–203, 1976.
21. Burnet, F. M., Stone, J. D. Receptor-destroying enzyme of *V. cholerae. Aust. J. Exp. Biol. Med. Sci.* **25:**227–233, 1947.
22. Burnet, F. M., Stone, J. D. Desquamation of intestinal epithelium *in vitro* by *V. cholerae* filtrates: Characterization of mucinase and tissue disintegrating enzymes. *Aust. J. Exp. Biol. Med. Sci.* **25:**219–226, 1947.

23. Freter, R. Studies of the mechanism of action of intestinal antibody in experimental cholera. *Texas Rep. Biol. Med.* **27**(Suppl. 1):299–316, 1969.

24. Guentzel, M. N., Berry, L. J. Motility as a virulence factor for *Vibrio cholerae*. *Infect. Immun.* **11**:890–897, 1975.

25. Yancey, R. J., Willis, D. L., Berry, L. J. Role of motility in experimental cholera in adult rabbits. *Infect. Immun.* **22**:387–392, 1978.

26. Jones, G. W., Freter, R. Adhesive properties of *Vibrio cholerae:* Nature of the interaction with isolated rabbit brush border membranes and human erythrocytes. *Infect. Immun.* **14**:240–245, 1976.

27. Baselski, V. S., Parker, C. D. Intestinal distribution of *Vibrio cholerae* in orally infected infant mice: Kinetics of recovery of radiolabel and viable cells. *Infect. Immun.* **21**:518–525, 1978.

28. Baselski, V. S., Medina, R. A., Parker, C. D. Survival and multiplication of *Vibrio cholerae* in the upper bowel of infant mice. *Infect. Immun.* **22**:435–440, 1978.

29. Gardner, E. W., Lyles, S. T., Lankford, C. E., *et al. Vibrio cholerae* infection in the embryonated egg. *J. Infect. Dis.* **112**:264–272, 1963.

30. Holmes, R. K., Vasil, M. L., Finkelstein, R. A. Studies on toxinogenesis in *Vibrio cholerae:* III. Characterization of nontoxigenic mutants *in vitro* and in experimental animals. *J. Clin. Invest.* **55**:551–560, 1975.

31. Sandvik, O., Dahle, H. K. Enzymoserological relationships between *Vibrio comma* and other gram-negative organisms. *Acta Pathol. Microbiol. Scand. Sect. B* **79**:285–290, 1971.

32. Burnet, F. M., Stone, J. D. Receptor-destroying enzyme of *V. cholerae. Aust. J. Exp. Biol. Med. Sci.* **25**:227–233, 1947.

33. Gottschalk, A. Neuraminidase: The specific enzyme of influenza virus and *Vibrio cholerae. Biochim. Biophys. Acta* **23**:645–646, 1957.

34. Schneider, D. R., Parker, C. D. Isolation and characterization of protease-deficient mutants of *V. cholerae. J. Infect. Dis.* **138**:143–151, 1978.

35. Baselski, V. S., Upchurch, S., Parker, C. D. Isolation and phenotypic characterization of virulence-deficient mutants of *Vibrio cholerae. Infect. Immun.* **22**:181–188, 1978.

36. Van Heyningen, W. E., Carpenter, C. C. J., Jr., Pierce, N. F., *et al.* Deactivation of cholera toxin by ganglioside. *J. Infect. Dis.* **124**:415–418, 1971.

37. Holmgren, J., Lönnroth, I., Svennerholm, L. Tissue receptor for cholera exotoxin: Postulated structure from studies with GM1 ganglioside and related glycolipids. *Infect. Immun.* **8**:208–214, 1973.

38. Holmgren, J., Lönnroth, I., Månsson, J. E., *et al.* Interaction of cholera toxin and membrane GM1 ganglioside of small intestine. *Proc. Natl. Acad. Sci. U.S.A.* **72**:2520–2524, 1975.

39. Holmgren, J., Lönnroth, I. Cholera toxin and the adenylate cyclase activating signal. *J. Infect. Dis.* **133**:S64–S74, 1976.

40. King, C. A., Van Heyningen, W. E. Deactivation of cholera toxin by a sialidase-resistant monosialosylganglioside. *J. Infect. Dis.* **127**:639–647, 1973.

41. Holmgren, J. Comparison of the tissue receptors for *Vibrio cholerae* and *Escherichia coli* enterotoxins by means of gangliosides and natural cholera toxoid. *Infect. Immun.* **8**:851–859, 1973.

42. Pierce, N. F. Differential inhibitory effects of cholera toxoids and ganglioside on the enterotoxins of *Vibrio cholerae* and *Escherichia coli. J. Exp. Med.* **137**:1009–1023, 1973.

43. Cuatrecasas, P. Gangliosides and membrane receptors for cholera toxin. *Biochemistry* **12**:3558–3566, 1973.

44. Cuatrecasas, P. Interaction of *Vibrio cholerae* enterotoxin with cell membranes. *Biochemistry* **12**:3547–3558, 1973.

45. Holmgren, J., Lindholm, L., Lönnroth, I. Interaction of cholera toxin and toxin deriva-

ties with lymphocytes: I. Binding properties and interference with lectin-induced cellular stimulation. *J. Exp. Med.* **139**:801–819, 1974.

46. Boyle, J. M., Gardner, J. D. Sequence of events mediating the effect of cholera toxin on rat thymocytes. *J. Clin. Invest.* **53**:1149–1158, 1974.

47. Walker, W. A., Field, M., Isselbacher, K. J. Specific binding of cholera toxin to isolated intestinal microvillus membranes. *Proc. Natl. Acad. Sci. U.S.A.* **71**:320–324, 1974.

48. Field, M. Mode of action of cholera toxin: stabilization of catecholamine-sensitive adenylate cyclase in turkey erythrocytes. *Proc. Natl. Acad. Sci. U.S.A.* **71**:3299–3303, 1974.

49. Pierce, N. F., Greenough, W. B., III, Carpenter, C. C. J., Jr. *Vibrio cholerae* enterotoxin and its mode of action. *Bacteriol. Rev.* **35**:1–13, 1971.

50. McGonagle, T. J., Serebro, H. H., Iber, F. L., *et al.* Time of onset of action of cholera toxin in dog and rabbit. *Gastroenterology* **57**:5–8, 1969.

51. Greenough, W. B., III, Pierce, N. F., Vaughn, M. Titration of cholera enterotoxin and antitoxin in isolated fat cells. *J. Infect. Dis. (Suppl.)* **121**:S111–S113, 1970.

52. Sharp, G. W. G., Hynie, S. Stimulation of intestinal adenyl cyclase by cholera toxin. *Nature (London)* **229**:266–269, 1971.

53. De, S. N., Chatterje, D. N. Experimental study of action of *Vibrio cholerae* on intestinal mucous membrane. *J. Pathol. Bacteriol.* **66**:559–562, 1953.

54. Benyajati, C. Experimental cholera in humans. *Br. Med. J.* **1**:140–142, 1966.

55. Banwell, J. G., Sherr, H. S. Effect of bacterial enterotoxins on the gastrointestinal tract. *Gastroenterology* **65**:467–497, 1973.

56. Pierce, N. F., Graybill, R. J., Kaplan, M. M., *et al.* Systemic effects of parenteral cholera enterotoxin in dogs. *J. Lab. Clin. Med.* **79**:145–156, 1972.

57. Parkinson, D. K., Ebel, H., DiBona, D. R., *et al.* Localization of the action of cholera toxin on adenyl cyclase in mucosal epithelial cells of rabbit intestine. *J. Clin. Invest.* **51**:2292–2298, 1972.

58. Grady, G. F., Keusch, G. T., Deschner, E. E. Kinetics of absorption of toxin of *Vibrio cholerae. J. Infect. Dis.* **131**:210–216, 1975.

59. Serebro, H. A., Iber, F. L., Yardley, J. H., *et al.* Inhibition of cholera toxin action in the rabbit by cycloheximide. *Gastroenterology* **56**:506–511, 1969.

60. Roggin, G. M., Banwell, J. G., Yardley, J. H., *et al.* Unimpaired response of rabbit jejunum to cholera toxin after selective damage to villus epithelium. *Gastroenterology* **63**:981–989, 1972.

61. Field, M. Intestinal secretion: Effect of cyclic AMP and its role in cholera. *N. Engl. J. Med.* **284**:1137–1144, 1971.

62. Field, M., Fromm, D., Wallace, C. K., *et al.* Stimulation of active chloride secretion in small intestine by cholera exotoxin. *J. Clin. Invest.* **48**:24a, 1969.

63. Pierce, N. F., Carpenter, C. C., Elliott, H. L., *et al.* Effects of prostaglandins, theophylline and cholera exotoxin upon transmucosal water and electrolyte movement in the canine jejunum. *Gastroenterology* **50**:22–32, 1971.

64. Butcher, R. W., Sutherland, E. W. Adenosine 3′,5′-phosphate in biological material: 1. Purification and properties of cyclic 3′,5′-nucleotide phosphodiesterase and use of this enzyme to characterize adenosine 3′,5′-phosphate in human urine. *J. Biol. Chem.* **237**:1244–1250, 1962.

65. Vaughan, M., Pierce, N. F., Greenough, W. B., III. Stimulation of glycerol production in fat cells by cholera toxin. *Nature (London)* **226**:658–659, 1970.

66. Butcher, R. W., Baird, C. E., Sutherland, E. W. Effects of lipolytic and antilipolytic substances on adenosine 3′,5′-monophosphate levels in isolated fat cells. *J. Biol. Chem.* **243**:1705–1712, 1968.

67. Curran, P. F. Ion transport in intestine and its coupling to other transport processes. *Fed. Proc. Fed. Am. Soc. Exp. Biol.* **24**:993–999, 1965.

68. Leitch, G. J., Iwert, M. E., Burrows, W. Experimental cholera in the rabbit ligated ileal loop: Toxin-induced water and ion movement. *J. Infect. Dis.* **116**:303–312, 1966.

69. Forstner, G., Shih, M., Lukie, B. Cyclic AMP and intestinal glycoprotein synthesis: The effect of β-adrenergic agents, theophylline, and dibutyryl cyclic AMP. *Can. J. Physiol. Pharmacol.* **51**:122–129, 1973.

70. Al-Awqati, Q., Wallace, C. K., Greenough, W. B., III. Stimulation of intestinal secretion *in vitro* by culture filtrates of *Escherichia coli*. *J. Infect. Dis.* **125**:300–303, 1972.

71. Watten, R. H., Morgan, F. M., Yachai-Na-Songkhla, V. N., *et al.* Water and electrolyte studies in cholera. *J. Clin. Invest.* **38**:1879–1889, 1959.

72. Sack, R. B., Carpenter, C. C. J. Experimental canine cholera: 1. Development of the model. *J. Infect Dis.* **119**:138–149, 1969.

73. Leitch, G. J., Burrows, W., Stolle, L. C. Experimental cholera in the rabbit intestinal loop: Fluid accumulation and sodium pump inhibition. *J. Infect. Dis.* **117**:197–202, 1967.

74. Carpenter, C. C., Sack, R. B., Feeley, J. C., *et al.* Site and characteristics of electrolyte loss and effect of intraluminal glucose in experimental canine cholera. *J. Clin. Invest.* **47**:1210–1220, 1968.

75. Carpenter, C. C., Greenough, W. B., III. Response of the canine duodenum to intraluminal challenge with cholera exotoxin. *J. Clin. Invest.* **47**:2600–2607, 1968.

76. Donowitz, M., Binder, H. J. Effect of enterotoxins of *Vibrio cholerae*, *Escherichia coli*, and *Shigella dysenteriae* type 1 on fluid and electrolyte transport in the colon. *J. Infect. Dis.* **134**:135–143, 1976.

77. Gangarosa, E. J., Beisel, W. R., Benyajati, C., *et al.* The nature of the gastrointestinal lesion in Asiatic cholera and its relation to pathogenesis: A biopsy study. *Am. J. Trop. Med.* **9**:125–135, 1960.

78. Norris, H. T., Majno, G. On the role of the ileal epithelium in the pathogenesis of experimental cholera. *Am. J. Pathol.* **53**:263–279, 1968.

79. Elliot, H. L., Carpenter, C. C., Sack, R. B., *et al.* Small bowel morphology in experimental canine cholera: A light and electron microscopic study. *Lab. Invest.* **22**:112–120, 1970.

80. Kimberg, D. V., Field, M., Gershon, E., *et al.* Effects of prostaglandins and cholera enterotoxin on intestinal mucosal cyclic AMP accumulation: Evidence against an essential role for prostaglandins in the action of toxin. *J. Clin. Invest.* **53**:941–949, 1974.

81. Jacoby, H. I., Marshall, C. H. Antagonism of cholera enterotoxin by antiinflammatory agents in the rat. *Nature (London)* **235**:163–165, 1972.

82. Finck, A., Katz, R. Prevention of cholera-induced intestinal secretion in the cat by aspirin. *Nature (London)* **238**:273–274, 1972.

83. Gots, R. E., Formal, S. B., Giannella, R. A. Indomethacin inhibition of *Salmonella typhimurium*, *Shigella flexneri*, and cholera-mediated rabbit ileal secretion. *J. Infect. Dis.* **130**:280–284, 174.

84. Vane, J. R. Inhibition of prostaglandin synthesis as a mechanism of action for aspirin-like drugs. *Nature (London) New Biol.* **231**:232–235, 1971.

85. Hudson, N., Hindi, S. E., Wilson, D. E., *et al.* Prostaglandin E in cholera toxin-induced intestinal secretion: Lack of an intermediary role. *Am. J. Dig. Dis.* **20**:1035–1039, 1975.

86. Carpenter, C. C., Curlin, G. T., Greenough, W. B., III. Response of canine Thiry–Vella jejunal loops to cholera exotoxin and its modification by ethacrynic acid. *J. Infect. Dis.* **120**:332–338, 1969.

87. Latta, T. A. Malignant cholera: Documents communicated by the Central Board of Health, London, relative to the treatment of cholera by the copious injection of aqueous and saline fluids into the veins. *Lancet* **2**:274–277, 1832.

88. Hirschhorn, N., Kinzie, J. L., Sachar, D. B., *et al.* Decrease in net stool output in cholera during intestinal perfusion with glucose-containing solutions. *N. Engl. J. Med.* **279**:176–181, 1968.

89. Serebro, H. A., Bayless, T. M., Hendrix, T. R., *et al.* Absorption of *d*-glucose by the rabbit jejunum during cholera-toxin-induced diarrhoea. *Nature (London)* **217**:1272–1273, 1968.

90. Pierce, N. F., Sack, R. B., Mitra, R. C., *et al.* Replacement of water and electrolyte losses in cholera by an oral glucose–electrolyte solution. *Ann. Intern. Med.* **70**:1173–1181, 1969.

91. Nalin, D. R., Cash, R. A., Islam, R., *et al.* Oral maintenance therapy for cholera in adults. *Lancet* **2**:370–373, 1968.

92. Whipp, S. C., Moon, H. W. Modification of enterosorption in experimental enteric colibacillosis of swine inoculated with *Escherichia coli. J. Infect. Dis.* **127**:255–260, 1973.

93. Mosley, W. H. The role of immunity in cholera: A review of epidemiological and serological studies. *Tex. Rep. Biol. Med.* **27**(Suppl. 1):227–241, 1969.

94. Curlin, G. T., Craig, J. P., Subong, A., *et al.* Antitoxic immunity in experimental canine cholera. *J. Infect. Dis.* **121**:463–470, 1970.

95. Holmgren, J., Svennerholm, A. M., Ouchterlony, Ö., *et al.* Antitoxic immunity in experimental cholera: Protection and serum and local antibody responses in rabbits after enteral and parenteral immunization. *Infect. Immun.* **12**:1331–1340, 1975.

96. Burrows, W., Elliot, M. E., Havens, I. Studies on immunity to Asiatic cholera: Excretion of coproantibody in experimental enteric cholera in guinea pig. *J. Infect. Dis.* **81**:261–281, 1947.

97. Svennerholm, A. M. Experimental studies on cholera immunization: 4. The antibody response to formalinized *Vibrio cholerae* and purified endotoxin with special reference to protective capacity. *Int. Arch. Allergy Appl. Immunol.* **49**:434–452, 1975.

98. Steele, E. J., Chaicumpa, N., Rowley, D. Isolation and biological properties of three classes rabbit antibody to *Vibrio cholerae. J. Infect. Dis.* **130**:93–103, 1974.

99. Holmgren, J., Svennerholm, A. M. Enzyme-linked immunosorbent assay for cholera serology. *Infect. Immun.* **7**:759–763, 1973.

100. Kaur, J., McGhee, J. R., Burrows, W. Immunity to cholera: The occurrence and nature of antibody-active immunoglobulins in the lower ileum of the rabbit. *J. Immunol.* **108**:387–395, 1972.

101. Pierce, N. F., Gowans, J. L. Cellular kinetics of the intestinal immune response to cholera toxoid in rats. *J. Exp. Med.* **142**:1550–1563, 1975.

102. Pierce, N. F., Sack, R. B. Immune response of the intestinal mucosa to cholera toxoid. *J. Infect. Dis.* **136**:S113–S117, 1977.

103. Craig, S. W., Cebra, J. J. Peyer's patches: An enriched source of precursors for IgA-producing immunocytes in the rabbit. *J. Exp. Med.* **134**:188–200, 1971.

104. Gowans, J. L., Knight, E. J. The route of re-circulation of lymphocytes in the rat. *Proc. R. Soc. London Ser. B.* **159**:257–282, 1964.

105. Guy-Grand, D., Griscelli, C., Vassalli, P. The gut-associated lymphoid system: Nature and properties of the large dividing cells. *Eur. J. Immunol.* **4**:435–443, 1974.

106. Pierce, N. F., Kaniecki, E. A., Northrup, R. S. Protection against experimental cholera by antitoxin. *J. Infect. Dis.* **126**:606–616, 1972.

107. Pierce, N. F., Sack, R. B., Sircar, B. K. Immunity to experimental cholera: III. Enhanced duration of protection after sequential parenteral–oral administration of toxoid to dogs. *J. Infect. Dis.* **135**:888–896, 1977.

108. Holmgren, J., Svennerholm, A. M. Mechanisms of disease and immunity in cholera: A review. *J. Infect. Dis. Suppl.* **136**:S105–S112, 1977.

109. Svennerholm, A. M., Holmgren, J. Immunoglobulin and specific antibody synthesis *in vitro* by enteral and nonenteral lymphoid tissues after subcutaneous cholera immunization. *Infect. Immun.* **15**:360–369, 1977.

110. Svennerholm, A. M., Holmgren, J. Synergistic protective effect in rabbits of immunization with *Vibrio cholerae* lipopolysaccharide and toxin/toxoid. *Infect. Immun.* **13:** 735–740, 1976.

111. Lönnroth, I., Holmgren, J. Protein reagent modification of cholera toxin: Characterization of effects on antigenic, receptor-binding and toxic properties. *J. Gen. Microbiol.* **91:**263–277, 1975.

112. Taylor, J., Wilkins, M. P., Payne, J. M. Relation of rabbit gut reaction to enteropathogenic *Escherichia coli*. *Br. J. Exp. Pathol.* **42:**43–52, 1961.

113. Smith, H. W., Gyles, C. L. The relationship between two apparently different enterotoxins produced by enteropathogenic strains of *Escherichia coli* of porcine origin. *J. Med. Microbiol.* **3:**387–401, 1970.

114. Whipp, S. C., Moon, H. W., Lyon, N. C. Heat-stable *Escherichia coli* enterotoxin production *in vivo*. *Infect. Immun.* **12:**240–244, 1975.

115. Gyles, C. L. Heat-labile and heat-stable forms of the enterotoxin from *E. coli* strains enteropathogenic for pigs. *Ann. N.Y. Acad. Sci* **176:**314–322, 1971.

116. Smith, H. W., Halls, S. The transmissible nature of the genetic factor in *Escherichia coli* that controls enterotoxin production. *J. Gen. Microbiol.* **52:**319–334, 1968.

117. Smith, H. W., Linggood, M. A. Observations on the pathogenic properties of the K88, Hly and Ent plasmids of *Escherichia coli* with particular reference to porcine diarrhoea. *J. Med. Microbiol.* **4:**467–485, 1971.

118. Smith, H. W., Linggood, M. A. The transmissible nature of enterotoxin production in a human enteropathogenic strain of *Escherichia coli*. *J. Med. Microbiol.* **4:**301–305, 1971.

119. Gyles, C., So, M., Falkow, S. The enterotoxin plasmids of *Escherichia coli*. *J. Infect. Dis.* **130:**40–49, 1974.

120. Dallas, W. S., Gill, D. M., Falkow, S. Cistrons encoding *Escherichia coli* heat-labile toxin. *J. Bacteriol.* **139:**850–858, 1979.

121. So, M., Heffron, F., McCarthy, B. J. The *E. coli* gene encoding heat stable toxin is a bacterial transposon flanked by inverted repeats of IS1. *Nature* **277:**453–456, 1979.

122. Evans, D. J., Jr., Evans, D. G., DuPont, H. L., *et al.* Patterns of loss of enterotoxigenicity by *Escherichia coli* isolated from adults with diarrhea: Suggestive evidence for an interrelationship with serotype. *Infect. Immun.* **17:**105–111, 1977.

123. Ørskov, F., Ørskov, I., Evans, D. J., Jr., *et al.* Special *Escherichia coli* serotypes among enterotoxigenic strains from diarrhoea in adults and children. *Med. Microbiol. Immunol.* **162:**73–80, 1976.

124. Sack, D. A., McLaughlin, J. C., Sack, R. B., *et al.* Enterotoxigenic *Escherichia coli* isolated from patients at a hospital in Dacca. *J. Infect. Dis.* **135:**275–280, 1977.

125. Semjen, G., Ørskov, I., Ørskov, F. K antigen determination of *Escherichia coli* by counter-current immunoelectrophoresis (CIE). *Acta Pathol. Microbiol. Scand. Sect. B* **85B:**103–107, 1977.

126. Ørskov, I., Ørskov, F. Special O:K:H serotypes among enterotoxigenic *E. coli* strains from diarrhea in adults and children: Occurrence of the CF (colonization factor) antigen and of hemagglutinating abilities. *Med. Microbiol. Immunol.* **163:**99–110, 1977.

127. Smith, H. W., Halls, S. Studied on *Escherichia coli* enterotoxin. *J. Pathol. Bacteriol.* **93:**531–543, 1967.

128. Evans, D. J., Jr., Evans, D. G., Gorbach, S. L. Polymyxin B-induced release of low-molecular-weight, heat-labile enterotoxin from *Escherichia coli*. *Infect. Immun.* **10:**1010–1017, 1974.

129. Larivière, S., Gyles, C. L., Barnum, D. A. Preliminary characterization of the heat-labile enterotoxin of *Escherichia coli* F11 (PISS). *J. Infect. Dis.* **128:**312–320, 1973.

130. Jacks, T. M., Wu, B. J., Braemer, A. C., *et al.* Properties of the enterotoxic compo-

nent in *Escherichia coli* enteropathogenic for swine. *Infect. Immun.* **7:**178–189, 1973.
131. Dafni, Z., Sack, R. B., Craig, J. P. Purification of heat-labile enterotoxin from four *Escherichia coli* strains by affinity immunoadsorbent: Evidence for similar subunit structure. *Infect. Immun.* **22:**852–860, 1978.
132. Konowalchuk, J., Dickie, N., Stavric, S., *et al.* Comparative studies of five heat-labile toxic products of *Escherichia coli*. *Infect. Immun.* **22:**644–648, 1978.
133. Clements, J. D., Finkelstein, R. A. Demonstration of shared and unique immunological determinants in enterotoxins from *Vibrio cholerae* and *Escherichia coli*. *Infect. Immun.* **22:**709–713, 1978.
134. Rappaport, R. S., Sagin, J. F., Pierzchala, W. A., *et al.* Activation of heat-labile *Escherichia coli* enterotoxin by trypsin. *J. Infect. Dis.* **133:**S41–S54, 1976.
135. Gyles, C. L., Barnum, D. A. A heat-labile enterotoxin from strains of *Escherichia coli* enteropathogenic for pigs. *J. Infect. Dis.* **120:**419–426, 1969.
136. Smith, N. W., Sack, R. B. Immunologic cross-reactions of enterotoxins from *Escherichia coli* and *Vibrio cholerae*. *J. Infect. Dis.* **127:**164–170, 1973.
137. Gyles, C. L. Relationships among heat-labile enterotoxins of *Escherichia coli* and *Vibrio cholerae*. *J. Infect. Dis.* **129:**277–283, 1974.
138. Gyles, C. L. Immunological study of the heat-labile enterotoxins of *Escherichia coli* and *Vibrio cholerae*. *Infect. Immun.* **9:**564–570, 1974.
139. Evans, D. J., Jr., Chen, L. C., Curlin, G. T., *et al.* Stimulation of adenyl cyclase by *Escherichia coli* enterotoxin. *Nature (London) New Biol.* **236:**137–138, 1972.
140. Hewlett, E. L., Guerrant, R. L., Evans, D. J., Jr., *et al.* Toxins of *Vibrio cholerae* and *Escherichia coli* stimulate adenyl cyclase in rat fat cells. *Nature (London)* **249:**371–373, 1974.
141. Evans, D. J., Jr., Evans, D. G., Gorbach, S. L. Production of vascular permeability factor by enterotoxigenic *Escherichia coli* isolated from man. *Infect. Immun.* **8:**725–730, 1973.
142. Evans, D. G., Evans, D. J., Jr., Gorbach, S. L. Identification of enterotoxigenic *Escherichia coli* and serum antitoxin activity by the vascular permeability factor assay. *Infect. Immun.* **8:**731–735, 1973.
143. Guerrant, R. L., Brunton, L. L., Schnaitman, T. C., *et al.* Cyclic adenosine monophosphate and alteration of Chinese hamster ovary cell morphology: A rapid, sensitive *in vitro* assay for the enterotoxins of *Vibrio cholerae* and *Escherichia coli*. *Infect. Immun.* **10:**320–327, 1974.
144. Kwan, C. N., Wishnow, R. M. *Escherichia coli* enterotoxin-induced steroidogenesis in cultured adrenal tumor cells. *Infect. Immun.* **10:**146–151, 1974.
145. Donta, S. T., Viner, J. P. Inhibition of the steroidogenic effects of cholera and heat-labile *Escherichia coli* enterotoxins by GM1 ganglioside: Evidence for a similar receptor site for the two toxins. *Infect. Immun.* **11:**982–985, 1975.
146. Söderlind, O., Möllby, R., Wadström, T. Purification and some properties of a heat-labile enterotoxin from *Escherichia coli*. *Xentralbl. Bakteriol. Parasitenkd. Infektionskr. Hyg. Abt. 1: Orig. Reihe A* **229:**190–204, 1974.
147. Evans, D. J., Jr., Evans, D. G., Richardson, S. H., *et al.* Purification of the polymyxin-released, heat-labile enterotoxin of *Escherichia coli*. *J. Infect. Dis.* **133:**S94–S102, 1976.
148. Schenkein, I., Green, R. F., Santos, D. S., *et al.* Partial purification and characterization of a heat-labile enterotoxin of *Escherichia coli*. *Infect. Immun.* **13:**1710–1720, 1976.
149. Finkelstein, R. A., LaRue, M. K., Johnston, D. W., *et al.* Isolation and properties of heat-labile enterotoxin(s) from enterotoxigenic *Escherichia coli*. *J. Infect. Dis.* **133:**S120–S137, 1976.
150. Dafni, Z., Robbins, J. B. Purification of heat-labile enterotoxin from *Escherichia coli*

O78:H11 by affinity chromatography with antiserum to _Vibrio cholerae_ toxin. _J. Infect._
Dis. **133**:S138–S141, 1976.

151. Dorner, F., Jaksche, H., Stöckl, W. _Escherichia coli_ enterotoxin purification, partial
characterization and immunological observations. _J. Infect. Dis._ **133**:S142–S156, 1976.

152. Clements, J. D., Finkelstein, R. A. Immunological cross-reactivity between a heat-
labile enterotoxins(s) of _Escherichia coli_ and subunits of _Vibrio cholerae_ enterotoxin.
Infect. Immun **21**:1036–1039, 1978.

153. Jacks, T. M., Wu, B. J. Biochemical properties of _Escherichia coli_ low-molecular-
weight, heat-stable enterotoxin. _Infect. Immun._ **9**:342–347, 1974.

154. Alderete, J. F., Robertson, D. C. Purification and chemical characterization of the
heat-stable enterotoxin produced by porcine strains of enterotoxigenic _Escherichia_
coli. Infect. Immun. **19**:1021–1030, 1978.

155. Mullan, N. A., Burgess, M. N., Newsome, P. M. Characterization of a partially
purified menthanol-soluble heat-stable _Escherichia coli_ enterotoxin in infant mice.
Infect. Immun. **19**:779–784, 1978.

156. Burgess, M. N., Bywater, R. J., Cowley, C. M., _et al._ Biological evaluation of a
methanol-soluble, heat-stable _Escherichia coli_ enterotoxin in infant mice, pigs, rabbits,
and calves. _Infect. Immun._ **21**:526–531, 1978.

157. Moon, H. W., Whipp, S. C., Engstrom, G. W., _et al._ Response of the rabbit ileal loop
to cell-free products from _Escherichia coli_ enteropathogenic for swine. _J. Infect. Dis._
121:182–187, 1970.

158. Moon, H. W., Sorensen, D. K., Sautter, J. H. _Escherichia coli_ infection of the ligated
intestinal loop of the newborn pig. _Am. J. Vet. Res._ **27**:1317–1325, 1966.

159. Donta, S. T., Moon, H. W., Whipp, S. C. Detection of heat-labile _Escherichia coli_
enterotoxin with the use of adrenal cells in tissue culture. _Science_ **183**:334–336, 1974.

160. Sack, D. A., Sack, R. B. Test for enterotoxigenic _Escherichia coli_ using Y1 adrenal
cells in miniculture. _Infect. Immun._ **11**:334–336, 1975.

161. Speirs, J. I., Stavric, S., Konowalchuk, J. Assay of _Escherichia coli_ heat-labile enterotoxin with vero cells. _Infect. Immun._ **16**:617–622, 1977.

162. Guerrant, R. L., Brunton, L. L. Characterization of the Chinese hamster ovary cell
assay for the enterotoxins fo _Vibrio cholerae_ and _Escherichia coli_ and for specific
antisera, and toxoid. _J. Infect. Dis._ **135**:720–728, 1977.

163. Evans, D. J., Jr., Evans, D. G. Direct serological assay for the heat-labile enterotoxin
of _Escherichia coli_, using passive immung hemolysis. _Infect. Immun._ **16**:604–609, 1977.

164. Ruiz-Palacios, G., Evans, D. G., Evans, D. J., Jr., _et al._ Age-related acquisition of IgG
and IgM antibodies to heat-labile enterotoxin of _Escherichia coli_ (abstract). In _Ab-_
stracts of the Annual Meeting of the American Society for Microbiology, Las Vegas,
Nev., May 17, 1978.

165. Evans, D. G., Evans, D. J., Jr., Pierce, N. F. Differences in the response of rabbit
small intestine to heat-labile and heat-stable enterotoxins of _Escherichia coli. Infect._
Immun. **7**:873–880, 1973.

166. Dean, A. G., Ching, Y., Williams, R. G., _et al._ Test for _Escherichia coli_ enterotoxin
using infant mice: Application in a study of diarrhea in children in Honolulu. _J. Infect._
Dis. **125**:407–411, 1972.

167. Giannella, R. A. Suckling mouse model for detection of heat-stable _Escherichia coli_
enterotoxin: Characteristics of the model. _Infect. Immun._ **14**:95–99, 1976.

168. Byers, P. A, DuPont, H. L. Pooling method for screening large numbers of _Escheri-_
chia coli for production of heat-stable enterotoxin, and its application in field studies.
J. Clin. Microbiol. **9**:541–543, 1979.

169. Evans, D. G., Evans, D. J., Jr., DuPont, H. L. Virulence factors for enterotoxigenic
Escherichia coli. J. Infect. Dis. **136**:S118–S123, 1977.

170. Bertschinger, H. U., Moon, H. W., Whipp, S. C. Association of _Escherichia coli_ with

the small intestinal epithelium: 1. Comparison of enteropathogenic and non-enteropathogenic porcine strains in pigs. *Infect. Immun.* **5**:595–605, 1972.

171. Arbuckle, J. B. R. The location of *Escherichia coli* in the pig intestine. *J. Med. Microbiol.* **3**:333–340, 1970.

172. Hohmann, A., Wilson, M. R. Adherence of enteropathogenic *Escherichia coli* to intestinal epithelium *in vivo*. *Infect. Immun.* **12**:866–880, 1975.

173. Jones, G. W., Rutter, J. M. Role of the K88 antigen in the pathogenesis of neonatal diarrhea caused by *Escherichia coli* in piglets. *Infect. Immun.* **6**:918–927, 1972.

174. Strim, S., Ørskov, F., Ørskov, I., *et al.* Episome-carried surface antigen K88 of *Escherichia coli:* III. Morphology. *J. Bacteriol.* **93**:740–748, 1967.

175. Rutter, J. M., Burrows, M. R., Sellwood, R., *et al.* A genetic basis for resistance to enteric disease caused by *E. coli. Nature* **257**:135–136, 1975.

176. DuPont, H. L., Formal, S. B., Hornick, R. B., *et al.* Pathogenesis of *Escherichia coli* diarrhea. *N. Engl. J. Med.* **285**:1–9, 1971.

177. Ørskov, I., Ørskov, F., Smith, H. W., *et al.* The establishment of K99, a thermo-labile, transmissible *Escherichia coli* K antigen, previously called "KCO," possessed by calf and lamb enteropathogenic strains. *Acta Pathol. Microbiol. Scand. Sect. B* **83**:31–36, 1975.

178. Moon, H. W., Nagy, B., Isaacson, R. E., *et al.* Occurrence of K99 antigen on *Escherichia coli* isolated from pigs and colonization of pig ileum by K99$^+$ enterotoxigenic *E. coli* from claves and pigs. *Infect. Immun.* **15**:614–620, 1977.

179. Isaacson, R. E. K99 surface antigen of *Escherichia coli:* Purification and partial characterization. *Infect. Immun.* **15**:272–279, 1977.

180. Moon. H. W., Whipp, S. C., Skartvedt, S. M. Etiologic diagnosis of diarrheal disease of calves: Incidence and methods for detecting enterotoxin and K99 antigen production by *Escherichia coli Am. J. Vet. Res.* **37**:1025–1029, 1976.

181. Isaacson, R. E., Nagy, B., Moon, H. W. Colonization of porcine small intestine by *Escherichia coli:* Colonization and adhesion factors of pig enteropathogens that lack K88. *J. Infect. Dis.* **135**:531–539, 1977.

182. Nagy, R., Moon, H. W., Isaacson, R. E. Colonization of porcine small intestine by enterotoxigenic *Escherichia coli:* Selection of piliated forms *in vivo*, adhesion of piliated forms to epithelial cells *in vitro* and incidence of a pilus antigen among porcine enteropathogenic *E. coli. Infect. Immun.* **16**:344–352, 1977.

183. Isaacson, R. E., Fusco, P. C., Brinton, C. C. *et al. In vitro* adhesion of *Escherichia coli* to porcine small intestinal epithelial cells: Pili as adhesive factors. *Infect. Immun.* **21**:392–397, 1978.

184. Evans, D. G., Silver, R. P., Evans, D. J., Jr., *et al.* Plasmid-controlled colonization factor associated with virulence in *Escherichia coli* enterotoxigenic for humans. *Infect. Immun.* **12**:656–667. 1975.

185. Evans, D. G., Evans, D. J., Jr., Tjoa, W. S., *et al.* Detection and characterization of colonization factor of enterotoxigenic *Escherichia coli* isolated from adults with diarrhea. *Infect. Immun.* **19**:727–736, 1978.

186. Jones, G. W., Rutter, J. M. The association of K88 antigen with hemagglutinating activity in porcine strains of *Escherichia coli. J. Gen. Microbiol.* **84**:135–144, 1974.

187. Burrows, M. R., Sellwood, R. R., Gibbons, R. A. Haemagglutinating and adhesive properties associated with the K99 antigen of bovine strains of *Escherichia coli. J. Gen. Microbiol.* **96**:269–275, 1976.

188. Swaney, L. M., Liu, Y. P., To, C. M., *et al.* Isolation and characterization of *Escherichia coli* phase variants and mutants deficient in type 1 pilus production. *J. Bacteriol.* **130**:495–505, 1977.

189. Evans, D. G., Evans, D. J., Jr., Tjoa, W. Hemagglutination of human group A erythrocytes by enterotoxigenic *Escherichia coli* isolated from adults with diarrhea: Correla-

tion with colonization factor. *Infect. Immun.* **18**:330–337, 1977.

190. Evans, D. J., Jr., Evans, D. G., DuPont, H. L. Hemagglutination patterns of enterotoxigenic *Escherichia coli* determined with human bovine, chicken, and guinea pig
erythrocytes in the presence and absence of mannose. *Infect. Immun.* **23**:336–346,
1979.

191. Evans, D. G., Evans, D. J., Jr. New surface-associated heat-labile colonization factor
antigen (CFA/II) produced by enterotoxigenic *Escherichia coli* of serogroups O6 and
O8. *Infect. Immun.* **21**:638–647, 1978.

192. Ofek, I., Mirelman, D., Sharon, N. Adherence of *Escherichia coli* to human mucosal
cells mediated by mannose receptors. *Nature* **265**:623–625, 1977.

193. Ofek, I., Beachey, E. H. Mannose binding and epithelial cell adherence of *Escherichia
coli*. *Infect. Immun.* **22**:247–254, 1978.

194. Sack, R. B., Human diarrheal disease caused by enterotoxigenic *Escherichia coli*.
Annu. Rev. Microbiol. **29**:233–253, 1975.

195. Smith, H. R., Cravioto, A., Willshaw, G., *et al.* A plasmid coding for the production of
colonization factor antigen I and heat-stable enterotoxin in strains of *Escherichia coli*
of serogroup O78. *Fed. Eur. Med. Soc. Microbiol. Lett.* **6**:255–260, 1979.

196 Evans, D. G., Satterwhite, T. K., Evans, D. J., Jr., *et al.* Differences in serological
responses and excretion patterns of volunteers challenged with enterotoxigenic *Escherichia coli* with and without the colonization factor antigen. *Infect. Immun.* **19**:883–
888, 1978.

197. Satterwhite, T. K., Evans, D. G., DuPont, H. L., *et al.* Role of *Escherichia coli*
colonisation factor antigen in acute diarrhoea. *Lancet* **2**:181–184, 1978.

198. Sack, R. B., Gorbach, S. L., Banwell, J. G., *et al.* Enterotoxigenic *Escherichia coli*
isolated from patients with severe cholera-like disease. *J. Infect. Dis.* **123**:378–385,
1971.

199. Gorbach, S. L., Banwell, J. G., Chatterjee, B. D., *et al.* Acute undifferentiated human
diarrhea in the tropics: I. Alterations in intestinal microflora. *J. Clin. Invest.* **50**:881–
889, 1971.

200. Ussing, H. H. Zerahn, K. Active transport of sodium as the source of electric current
in the short-circuit isolated frog skin. *Acta Physiol. Scand.* **23**:110–127, 1951.

201. Kohler, E. M. Enterotoxic activity of whole cell lysates of *Escherichia coli* in young
pigs. *Am. J. Vet. Res.* **32**:731–737, 1971.

202. Mashiter, K., Mashiter, G. D., Hauger, R. L., *et al.* Effects of cholera and *E. coli*
enterotoxins on cyclic adenosine 3′, 5′-monophosphate levels and intermediary metabolism in the thyroid. *Endocrinology* **92**:541–549, 1973.

203. Kantor, H. S. Tao, P., Wisdom, C. Action of *Escherichia coli* enterotoxin: Adenylate
cyclase behavior of intestinal epithelial cells in culture. *Infect. Immun.* **9**:1003–1010,
1974.

204. Zenser, T. V., Metzger, J. F. Comparison of the action of *Escherichia coli* enterotoxin
on the thymocyte adenylate cyclase–cyclic adenosine monophosphate system to that
of cholera tox n and prostaglandin E_1. *Infect. Immun.* **10**:503–509, 1974.

205. Hughes, J. M., Murad, F., Chang, B., *et al.* Role of cyclic GMP in the action of heat-
stable enterotoxin of *Escherichia coli*. *Nature* **271**:755–756, 1978.

206. Field, M., Graf, L. H., Jr., Laird, W. J., *et al.* Heat-stable enterotoxin of *Escherichia
coli: In vitro* effects on guanylate cyclase activity, cyclic GMP concentration, and ion
transport in small intestine. *Proc. Natl. Acad. Sci. U.S.A.* **75**:2800–2804, 1978.

207. Newsome, P. M., Burgess, M. N., Mullan, N. A. Effect of *Escherichia coli* heat-stable
enterotoxin on cyclic GMP levels in mouse intestine. *Infect. Immun.* **22**:290–291, 1978.

208. Ong, S. H., Whitley, T. H., Stowe, M. W., *et al.* Immunohistochemical localization of
3′:5′-cyclic AMP and 3′:5′-cyclic GMP in rat liver, intestine, and testis. *Proc. Natl.
Acad. Sci. U.S.A.* **72**:2022–2026, 1975.

209. Kimura, H., Murad, F. Subcellular localization of guanylate cyclase. *Life Sci.* **17:**837–843, 1975.

210. DuPont, H. L., Olarte, J., Evans, D. G., *et al.* Comparative susceptibility of Latin American and United States students to enteric pathogens. *N. Engl. J. Med.* **295:**1520–1521, 1976.

211. Evans, D. J., Jr., Ruiz-Palacios, G., Evans, D. G., *et al.* Humoral immune response to the heat-labile enterotoxin of *Escherichia coli* in naturally acquired diarrhea and antitoxin determination by passive immune hemolysis. *Infect. Immun.* **16:**781–788, 1977.

212. Pickering, L. K., DuPont, H. L., Evans, D. G., *et al.* Isolation of enteric pathogens from asymptomatic students from the United States and Latin America. *J. Infect. Dis.* **135:**1003–1005, 1977.

213. Wilson, M. R., Hohman, A. W. Immunity to *Escherichia coli* in pigs: Adhesion of enteropathogenic *Escherichia coli* to isolated intestinal epithelial cells. *Infect. Immun.* **10:**776–782, 1974.

214. Rutter, J. M., Jones, G. W. Protection against enteric disease caused by *Escherichia coli:* A model for vaccination with a virulence determinant? *Nature (London)* **242:**531–532, 1973.

215. Rutter, J. M., Jones, G. W., Brown, G. T. H., *et al.* Antibacterial activity in colostrum and milk associated with protection of piglets against enteric disease caused by K88-positive *Escherichia coli. Infect. Immun.* **13:**667–676, 1976.

216. Morgan, R. L., Isaacson, R. E., Moon, H. W., *et al.* Immunization of suckling pigs against enterotoxigenic *Escherichia coli*-induced diarrheal disease by vaccinating dams with purified 987 or K99 pili: Protection correlates with pilus homology of vaccine and challenge. *Infect. Immun.* **22:**771–777, 1978.

217. Nagy, B., Moon, H. W., Isaacson, R. E., *et al.* Immunization of suckling pigs against enteric enterotoxigenic *Escherichia coli* infection by vaccinating dams with purified pili. *Infect. Immun.* **21:**269–274, 1978.

218. Linggood, M. A., Ellis, M. L., Porter, P. An examination of the O and K specificity involved in the antibody-induced loss of the K88 plasmid from porcine enteropathogenic strains of *Escherichia coli. Immunology* **38:**123–127, 1979.

219. Bray, J., Isolation of antigenically homogeneous strains of *Bact. coli neapolitanum* from summer diarrhea of infants. *J. Pathol. Bacteriol.* **57:**239–247, 1945.

220. Giles, C., Sangster, G., Smith, J. Epidemic gastro-enteritis of infants in Aberdeen during 1947. *Arch. Dis. Child.* **24:**45–53, 1949.

221. Taylor, J., Powell, B. W., Wright, J. Infantile diarrhea and vomiting: A clinical and bacteriological investigation. *Br. Med. J.* **2:**117–125, 1949.

222. Kauffman, F., DuPont, A. J. *Escherichia* strains from infantile epidemic gastroenteritis. *Acta Pathol. Microbiol. Scand.* **27:**552–564, 1950.

223. Ewing, W. H., Tatum, H. W., Davis, B. R. The occurrence of *Escherichia coli* serotypes associated with diarrheal disease in the United States. *Public Health Lab.* **15:**118–135, 1957.

224. Yow, M. D., Melnick, J. L., Blattner, R. J., *et al.* The association of viruses and bacteria with infantile diarrhea. *Am. J. Epidemiol.* **92:**33–39, 1970.

225. Boris, M., Thomason, B. M., Hines, V. D., *et al.* A community epidemic of enteropathogenic *Escherichia coli* O126:B16:NM gastroenteritis associated with asymptomatic respiratory infection. *Pediatrics* **33:**18–25, 1964.

226. Cooper, M. L., Keller, H. M., Walters, E. W., *et al.* Isolation of enteropathogenic *Escherichia coli* from mothers and newborn infants. *AMAJ Dis. Child.* **97:**255–266, 1959.

227. Thomson, S. The numbers of pathogenic bacilli in faeces in intestinal diseases. *J. Hyg. (Cambridge)* **53:**217–224, 1955.

228. Kaslow, R. A., Taylor, A., Jr., Dweck, H. S., *et al.* Enteropathogenic *Escherichia coli* infection in a newborn nursery. *Am. J. Dis. Child.* **128:**797–801, 1974.

229. Wheeler, W. E. Spread and control of *Escherichia coli* diarrheal disease. *Ann. N.Y. Acad. Sci.* **66:**112–117, 1956.

230. Rogers, K. B., Benson, R. P., Foster, W. P., *et al.* Phthalylsulphacetamide and neomycin in the treatment of infantile gastro-enteritis. *Lancet* **2:**599–604, 1956.

231. Neter, E., Enteritis due to enteropathogenic *Escherichia coli*, present-day status and unsolved problems. *J. Pediatr.* **55:**223–239, 1959.

232. Kessner, D. M., Shaughnessy, H. J., Googins, J., *et al.* An extensive community outbreak of diarrhea due to enteropathogenic *Escherichia coli* O111:B4: I. Epidemiologic studies. *Am. J. Hyg.* **76:**27–43, 1962.

233. South, M. A., Yow, M. D., Robinson, N. M., *et al.* Antibiotic sensitivity patterns of strains of enteropathogenic *Escherichia coli* isolated in various areas of the United States and Mexico. *Antimicrob. Agents Chemother.* **3:**402–405, 1963.

234. Riley, H. D., Jr. Antibiotic therapy in neonatal enteric disease. *Ann. N.Y. Acad. Sci.* **176:**360–370, 1971.

235. Smith, M. H. D., Newell, K. W., Sulianti, J. Epidemiology of enteropathogenic *Escherichia coli* infection in nonhospitalized children. *Antimicrob. Agents Chemother.* **5:**77–83, 1965.

236. Thomson, S., Watkins, A. G., Gray, O. P. *Escherichia coli* gastroenteritis. *Arch. Dis. Child.* **31:**340–345, 1956.

237. Payne, A. M. M., Cook, G. T. A specific serological type of *Bact. coli* found in infants' home in absence of epidemic diarrhea. *Br. Med. J.* **2:**192–195, 1950.

238. Ramos-Alvarez, M., Sabin, A. B. Enteropathogenic viruses and bacteria: Role in summer diarrheal disease of infancy and early childhood. *J. Am. Med. Assoc.* **167:**147–156, 1958.

239. Ørskov, F. *Escherichia coli* strains isolated from cases of infantile diarrhoea and from healthy infants: Serological and biochemical study. *Acta Pathol. Microbiol. Scand.* **39:**137–146, 1956.

240. Czírok, E., Madár, J., Budai, J., *et al.* The role in sporadic enteritis of facultatively enteropathogenic *Escherichia coli* serogroups. *Acta Microbiol. Acad. Sci. Hung.* **23:**359–369, 1976.

241. Hutchinson, R. I. *Escherichia coli* (O types 111, 55 and 26) and their association with infantile diarrhea: A five year study. *J. Hyg.* **55:**27–44, 1957.

242. Soloman, P., Weinstein, L., Joress, S. M. Studies of the incidence of carriers of enteropathogenic *Escherichia coli* in a pediatric population. *J. Pediatr.* **58:**716–721, 1961.

243. Ørskov, I., Ørskov, F., Jann, B., *et al.* Serology, chemistry and genetics of O and K antigens of *Escherichia coli*. *Bacteriol. Rev.* **41:**667–710, 1977.

244. Kauffmann, F. The serology of the *coli* group. *J. Immunol.* **57:**71–100, 1947.

245. Farmer, J. J., III, Davis, B. R., Cherry, W. B., *et al.* "Enteropathogenic serotypes" of *Escherichia coli* which really are not. *J. Pediatr.* **90:**1047–1049, 1977.

246. Edwards, P. R., Ewing, W. H. *Identification of Enterobacteriaceae*, 3rd ed. Burgess, Minneapolis, 1972, pp. 1–362.

247. Neter, E., Shumway, C. N. *E. coli* serotype D433: Occurrence in intestinal and respiratory tracts, cultural characteristics, pathogenicity, sensitivity to antibiotics. *Proc. Soc. Exp. Biol. Med.* **75:** 504–507, 1950.

248. Ferguson, W. W., June, R. C. Experiments on feeding adult volunteers with *Escherichia coli* 111,B4, a coliform organism associated with infant diarrhea. *Am. J. Hyg.* **55:**155–169, 1952.

249. June, R. C., Ferguson, W. W., Worfel, M. T. Experiments in feeding adult volunteers

with *Escherichia coli* 55,B5, a coliform associated with infant diarrhea. *Am. J. Hyg.* **57:**222–236, 1953.

250. Levine, M. M., Bergquist, E. J., Nalin, D. R., *et al. Escherichia coli* strains that cause diarrhoea but do not produce heat-labile or heat-stable enterotoxins and are non-invasive. *Lancet* **1:**1119–1122, 1978.

251. Sakazaki, R., Tamura, K., Saito, M. Enteropathogenic *Escherichia coli* associated with diarrhea in children and adults. *Jpn. J. Med. Sci. Biol.* **20:**387–399, 1967.

252. Ogawa, H., Nakamura, A., Sakazaki, R. Pathogenic properties of "enteropathogenic" *Escherichia coli* from diarrheal children and adults. *Jpn. J. Med. Sci. Biol.* **21:**333–349, 1968.

253. Smith, H. W., Gyles, C. L. The effect of cell-free fluids prepared from cultures of human and animal enteropathogenic strains of *Escherichia coli* on ligated intestinal segments of rabbits and pigs. *J. Med. Microbiol.* **3:**403–409, 1970.

254. Sojka, W. J. Enteric diseases in new-born piglets, calves and lambs due to *Escherichia coli* infection. *Vet. Bull.* **41:**509–522, 1971.

255. Goldschmidt, M., DuPont, H. L. Enteropathogenic *Escherichia coli:* Lack of correlation of serotype with pathogenicity. *J. Infect. Dis.* ,**133:**153–156, 1976.

256. Gurwith, M. J., Wiseman, D. A., Chow, P. Clinical and laboratory assessment of the pathogenicity of serotyped enteropathogenic *Escherichia coli. J. Infect. Dis.* **135:**735–743, 1977.

257. O'Brien, A. D., Thompson, M. R., Cantey, J. R., *et al.* Production of a *Shigella dysenteriae*-like toxin by pathogenic *Escherichia coli (abstract no. B103). In Proceedings of the 77th Annual Meeting of the American Society for Microbiology,* New Orleans, La., May 8–13, 1977.

258. Klipstein, F. A., Rowe, B., Engert, R. F., *et al.* Enterotoxigenicity of enteropathogenic serotypes of *Escherichia coli* isolated from infants with epidemic diarrhea. *Infect. Immun.* **21:**171–178, 1978.

259. Williams, P. H., Sedgwick, M. I., Evans, N., *et al.* Adherence of an enteropathogenic strain of *Escherichia coli* to human intestinal mucosa is mediated by a colicinogenic conjugative plasmid. *Infect. Immun.* **22:**393–402, 1978.

260. Cantey, J. R., Blake, R. K. Diarrhea due to *Escherichia coli* in the rabbit: A novel mechanism. *J. Infect. Dis.* **135:**454–462, 1977.

261. Takeuchi, A., Inman, L. R., O'Hanley, P. D., *et al.* Scanning and transmission electron miscroscopic study of *Escherichia coli* (RDEC-1) enteric infection in rabbits. *Infect. Immun.* **19:**686–694, 1978.

262. Ulshen, M. H., Rollo, J. L. Pathogenesis of *Escherichia coli* gastroenteritis in man—another mechanism. *N. Engl. J. Med.* **302:**99–101, 1980.

7

Viral Agents in Diarrhea

INTRODUCTION

Until the early 1970s, little evidence existed to strongly implicate viruses as important causes of human diarrhea. Earlier, there had been an occasional statistical association of enterovirus and adenovirus recovery from infants with diarrhea when compared to recovery rates of well children. In a small number of sporadic cases of illness, these viruses were shown to cause diarrhea, in view of virus isolation and documentation of a specific antibody rise during convalescence. Echovirus occasionally produced laboratory infection in adults[1,2] and epidemic diarrhea in newborn nurseries.[3] Adenoviruses were felt to play a role in wintertime diarrheal illness, where they were isolated from children with diarrhea and respiratory symptoms. Diarrhea was a known complication of measles and chicken pox in malnourished children,[4,5] and inflammatory changes in the intestinal mucosa of such children were reported.[6,7] Acute diarrhea associated with childhood exanthems is not a common problem in the United States, probably reflecting the importance of malnutrition in the evolution of intestinal complications.

Reimann *et al.*[8] demonstrated that a diarrheal illness could be transmitted to volunteers who ingested bacteria-free filtrates of stool suspensions and throat washings from individuals with illness, yet the filtrates contained none of the well-characterized viral agents known at that time. Gordon *et al.*[9] infected persons with the "Marcy agent" after passage through a series of volunteers. Homologous immunity was documented among those recovering from symptoms, yet Marcy-agent-immune volunteers developed illness when exposed to stool filtrates obtained in a separate outbreak,[10] suggesting that more than one virus was responsible for epidemic gastroenteritis.

In 1971 and 1972, a series of collaborative volunteer experiments were initiated by the National Institutes of Health and the University of Maryland which eventually established without doubt that viruses were important causes of gastroenteritis. The stool material employed was obtained from an adult patient with diarrhea acquired during secondary spread of illness at an elementary school in Norwalk, Ohio. The Norwalk agent was shown to produce illness in a high percentage of serologically unselected prison volunteers.[11] Homologous immunity was demonstrated when Norwalk material was again fed to volunteers following recovery from experimentally induced Norwalk disease. Kapikian *et al.*[12] were able to directly visualize the Norwalk agent by immune electron microscopy (IEM) and indicated that it was a 27-nm particle that morphologically resembled a parvovirus.

The most recent major new development in the area of viral etiology of acute diarrhea was presented by Bishop and her associates in 1973[13] when viral particles were identified in the duodenal mucosa of six of nine infants and children with diarrhea acquired in Australia. Since then, these viral agents (now termed "rotaviruses") have been shown to be the most commonly identified diarrheal agents with worldwide distribution. Table 7.1 lists the viral agents that have been associated with gastroenteritis, along with a brief statement of their importance and means of detection. Since the Norwalk-like agents and rotaviruses represent the only known important viral agents in diarrhea, they will be the focal points of this chapter.

NORWALK-LIKE AGENTS

The Norwalk agent was the first well-characterized enteric viral particle to be associated with diarrhea. A rectal swab specimen obtained during an outbreak of diarrhea in an elementary school in Norwalk, Ohio, produced illness in volunteers before and after serial passage through both human intestinal tract and fetal intestinal organ cultures.[11] A spectrum of clinical illness was produced, ranging from protracted vomiting and low-grade fever without diarrhea to mild watery diarrhea without vomiting or detectable fever (see Figure 7.1). Leukocytosis (with leukocyte counts as high as $18,400/mm^3$) was noted in a few volunteers. The viral particles could be visualized by IEM when stool filtrates were incubated with serum obtained during convalescence from induced Norwalk infection.[12] The Norwalk agent was found by IEM to be a 27-nm particle, and both experimentally and naturally infected individuals were shown to develop serologic evidence of infection. Volunteers who recovered from

TABLE 7.1
Viral Agents in Diarrheal Disease of Humans

Viral agent	Role in human illness	Methods of detection
Norwalk-like agents Norwalk Montgomery County Hawaii "W" Ditchling Cockle	Cause of epidemic diarrhea among adults and children	Immune electron microscopy, radioimmunoassay
Rotavirus	Major cause of pediatric diarrhea	Electron microscopy, serology
Coronavirus	Unknown	Electron microscopy, organ culture
Enterovirus	Rare cause of diarrhea	Immune electron microscopy, tissue culture
Astrovirus	Unknown	Electron microscopy
Adenovirus	Rare cause of diarrhea	Electron microscopy, tissue culture
Minirotavirus	Unknown	Electron microscopy
Calicivirus	Unknown	Electron microscopy

Norwalk illness were immune to a second challenge.[14,15] Either acid (to a pH 2.7) or heat treatment (60° for 30 min) failed to inactivate the virus, as determined by infectivity in volunteers.[15]

Bacteria-free stool filtrates obtained from family outbreaks in Honolulu, Hawaii, and Montgomery County, Maryland, reproduced an illness similar to Norwalk disease in volunteers.[14] Cross-challenge studies with the three agents to look for induced immunity indicated that the Norwalk and Hawaii agents were antigenically dissimilar; disease produced by either agent failed to induce immunity to subsequent illness by the other. The Norwalk and Montgomery County agents appeared to be antigenically similar, in view of each agent's cross-resistance to the other following induced disease by either. Virus-like particles 26–27 nm in diameter were seen in stool in IEM after treatment with Genetron and concentration.[16] The particles of the Hawaii and Montgomery County agents were similar in size and buoyant density to the virus-like particles associated with Norwalk illness. As with Norwalk illness, antibody development was detected by IEM in outbreaks due to the Hawaii and Montgomery County agents.[17] These IEM studies supported the earlier volunteer challenge experiments indicating that the Hawaii agent did not share surface

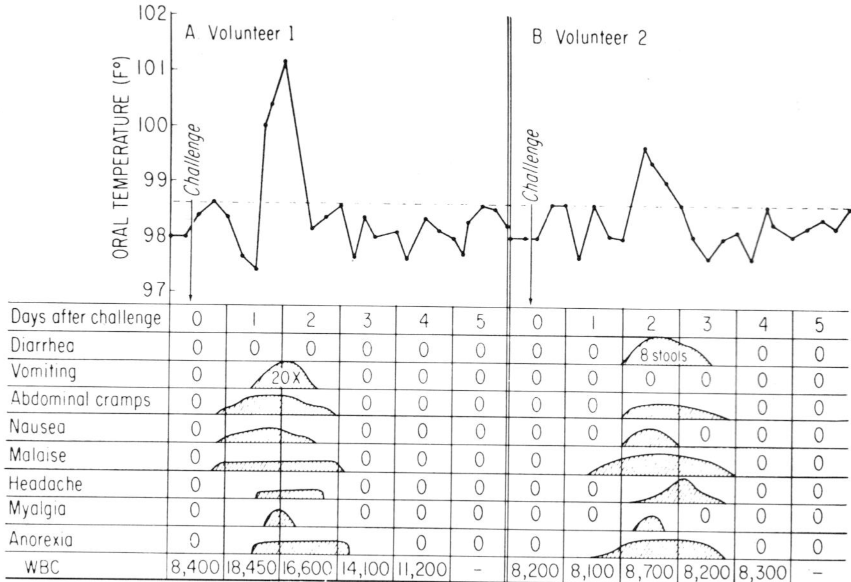

Days after challenge	0	1	2	3	4	5	0	1	2	3	4	5
Diarrhea	0	0	0	0	0	0	0	0	8 stools	0	0	
Vomiting	0	20 X	0	0	0	0	0	0	0	0	0	0
Abdominal cramps	0			0	0	0	0	0		0	0	0
Nausea	0			0	0	0	0	0		0	0	0
Malaise	0			0	0	0	0			0	0	0
Headache	0			0	0	0	0	0		0	0	0
Myalgia	0			0	0	0	0	0		0	0	0
Anorexia	0			0	0	0	0			0	0	0
WBC	8,400	18,450	16,600	14,100	11,200	–	8,200	8,100	8,700	8,200	8,300	–

Figure 7.1. The response of two volunteers experimentally infected with the Norwalk agent. From Blacklow *et al.*[137]

antigens with the Norwalk particle, while the Montgomery County agent did share antigens with the Norwalk agent.[17] Workers in Great Britain offered evidence that a Norwalk-like agent that was distinct antigenically from the Norwalk and Hawaii agents was responsible for an outbreak of winter vomiting disease in a primary school.[17] Six Norwalk-like agents have now been associated with gastroenteritis[15–19]: Norwalk, Hawaii, Montgomery County, "W," Ditchling, and cockle. Each of these agents shows similar ultrastructural and morphologic characteristics: 25-27 nm in diameter, nonenveloped with an apparent cubic symmetry, and a buoyant density in cesium chloride of 1.38-1.40 g/ml. While cross-challenge studies in volunteers and serologic evaluations employing electron microscopy have indicated that the Norwalk agent is antigenically related to the Montgomery County agent and is distinct from the Hawaii particle, the W and Ditchling agents appear to be antigenically related to one another and distinct from the Hawaii or Norwalk agents.[17] The newly described cockle agent appears to be distinct from the other Norwalk-like agents.[19] The relative importance of these infectious particles in causing human illness is unknown. Norwalk infection has been shown to be common in all age groups with worldwide distribution.[20]

Recovery and, therefore, identification of the virus in these cases of gastroenteritis have been difficult. These viral agents have not grown in tissue culture, and humans and chimpanzees appear to be the only naturally susceptible hosts.[21] The virus is present in stools of infected persons in low titer.[22] While IEM is a sensitive test for detecting these viral agents, it is an expensive, tedious procedure requiring a skilled reader and is not adaptable to routine laboratory use. Two other serologic procedures for detection of the Norwalk agent and its antibody have been developed: immune adherence hemagglutination assay (IAHA) and microtiter solid-phase radioimmunoassay (RIA).[20] RIA was found to be more sensitive than IEM and far easier to perform, while IAHA was less sensitive than the other two.

Clinical Aspects

The incubation period of Norwalk illness as induced in volunteers is 18–48 hr, and symptoms persist from one to three days. Viral particles are found in stool specimens during the illness, with the greatest concentration at the onset of illness, and are absent, or present in low titers, just before illness and 60 hr after onset of disease.[22] Intestinal biopsy of volunteers with Norwalk disease[23,24] and illness induced by the Hawaii agent[25] demonstrated histologic changes of the small bowel during infection. These changes included blunting of villi, shortening of microvilli, dilatation of endoplasmic reticulum, increase in the number of intracellular multivesiculate bodies, crypt hypertrophy, increase in the number of epithelial cell mitoses, and mucosal inflammation. Abnormal mucosal findings developed a few hours before clinical illness and persisted for at least four days[24] but less than two weeks.[23] At the time of illness, the brush-border enzymes alkaline phosphatase, sucrase, and trehalase were decreased.[23] Although vomiting is a prominent symptom of illness, a gastric histopathologic lesion is not normally present.[26]

Figure 7.1 shows the clinical response of two volunteers with illness induced by oral inoculation of the Norwalk agent.[11] Note that the first volunteer experienced vomiting and low-grade fever without diarrhea, at which time there was a leukocytosis, while in the second person, watery diarrhea without discernible fever or vomiting characterized the illness. These two cases define the extremes of clinical illness. Vomiting is the most common finding, followed by diarrhea and low-grade fever. A variable degree of abdominal cramps, malaise, anorexia, headache, and myalgias also were reported. In addition to occasional leukocytosis, transient lymphopenia may occur.[27]

Immunity

Experimental infection with the Norwalk agent was shown to result in resistance to reinfection with the same agent for at least 14 weeks.[15] In a separate series of rechallenge studies, certain volunteers were shown to maintain long-term immunity to the Norwalk agent, in view of a lack of symptoms after an initial challenge as well as after a subsequent oral challenge inoculum administered 34 months later, while others who had earlier developed induced clinical illness were immune to clinical illness 27–42 months after recovery from the primary infection.[28] The Norwalk and Hawaii agents are antigenically distinct and do not afford cross-protection, as determined in volunteer studies.[14] Circulating antibody as determined by IEM does not appear to play a major protective role, in view of the lack of a relationship between the level of antibody and susceptibility to infection.[12,28] Studies designed to characterize the local intestinal immune response to infection need to be carried out. Jejunal IgA synthesis occurs during both symptomatic and asymptomatic infection[29]; however, specificity of this intestinal antibody has not been determined. Undoubtedly, delayed hypersensitivity will play a role in susceptibility and immunity.

ROTAVIRUSES (RVs)

The 70-nm particle generally known as rotavirus (RV) because of its morphologic appearance—resembling a wheel with radiating spokes[30]— was first associated with diarrhea in children by Bishop *et al.*[13] It originally was considered to be an orbivirus on morphologic grounds and has been variably called reovirus-like agent, orbivirus, duovirus, rotavirus, and infantile gastroenteritis virus. The virus resembles a reovirus and was shown not to cross-react serologically with a number of orbiviruses or human reoviruses types 1, 2, and 3.[31] Similar RVs have been described as causative agents of diarrhea in the newborn of various animal species,[32] including mice,[33] calves,[34] lambs,[35] monkeys,[36] pigs,[37] and horses.[38]

In the initial report from Melbourne, six of nine infants and children with diarrhea had viral particles detected in duodenal mucosa, while a separate report by the same group published the following year offered evidence that the viral particles could readily be seen by direct examination of stool by electron microscopy.[39] Since these observations, most of the data derived concerning the importance of RV in the etiology of diarrhea and other studies designed to determine the epidemiology of RV gastroenteritis have relied upon the electron microscope for detection of virus.

The organism belongs to the family Reoviridae on the basis of morphologic, biologic, and biochemical properties as well as the presence of double-stranded RNA. RVs are visualized by electron microscopy as particles 60 nm (without an outer shell) and 75 nm (with a double-shelled capsid) in diameter.[40] The virus contains a hexagonal inner core which is approximately 37–38 nm in diameter. The surface in cesium chloride is 1.29–1.30 g/ml for empty shells and 1.36–1.37 g/ml for complete particles.[41–43] The calf RV is stable, remaining viable and infectious at room temperature for seven months.[44] Morphologically intact human RV (HRV) particles were detected when stool samples were stored at −20°C for up to nine years.[45] In 1975, the Reoviridae working team was established under the sponsorship of the World Health Organization/Food and Agriculture Organization Comparative Virology Program. The generic name "rotavirus" was adopted for the reovirus-like agents associated with diarrhea in humans and animals, and the Nebraska calf diarrhea virus strain (NCDV) was selected as the reference strain.[46] Figure 7.2 shows RV particles as visualized by electron microscopy.

Antigenic Relationship of RVs

As stated earlier, RVs have been identified in a wide range of mammalian species. These RVs are not antigenically related to other known members of Reoviridae. They do, however, share a common antigen, as demonstrated by complement fixation, immunofluorescence, immunodiffusion, and IEM.[47] RVs of various species are distinguishable on the basis of virus neutralization and variation in RNA segments and structural proteins.[48,49]

RVs have a distinctive outer capsid with a more sharply defined edge than that of reoviruses or orbiviruses.[48] As determined by gel electrophoresis, RVs have an 11-segment genome, in contrast to the 10-segment genome of the known reoviruses and obviruses.[41,50–55] Gel electrophoresis of viral RNA can be used to distinguish members within the RV group.[52,53,55] HRV and bovine RV vary by as many as three to five RNA genome of the known reoviruses and obviruses.[41,50–55] Gel electropholamide gels.[52,53] Ovine RV differs in one segment from porcine RV,[51] while porcine and bovine RNA segments may be similar.[54] Strains of RV isolated from the same animal species also may show RNA segment variation. The molecular weights of RNA segments of an RV isolated

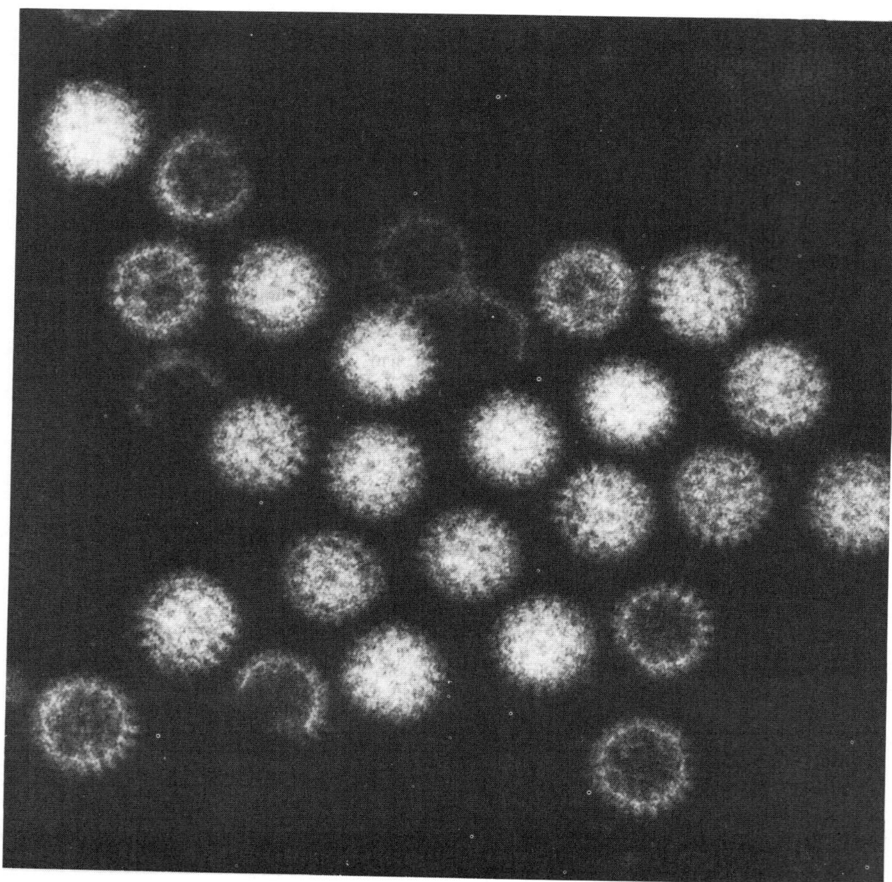

Figure 7.2. Electron micrograph of virus particles with partially removed capsids in a diarrheal stool specimen (phosphotungstic acid ×238,000). Prepared by J. J. Vollet, III, Ph.D.

from a calf with illness differed from the cell-cultured-adapted NCDV,[55] and small differences in electrophoretic mobility of RNA segments have been noted with HRV strains.[53]

Sera from infants and children who had recovered from illness contained immunofluorescent RV antibodies which failed to neutralize the calf virus.[30] Antisera to porcine RV did not neutralize bovine RV.[32,56] A lack of cross-neutralization also was noted between calf and lamb RV,[57] between human and simian RV,[58] and between human, porcine, and murine RV.[59]

RV Detection

Studies designed to determine the importance of RV in human illness have been limited because of an inability to efficiently grow the virus in cell culture systems. Identification of viral particles in stool specimens can be enhanced by incubation with serum containing antibody to the virus or by IEM, which encourages aggregation of the virions.[60] Due to the size of the RV (65–75 nm) and the high density of particles in diarrheal stools of children, direct visualization is possible without employing IEM (Figure 7.2). In adults, whose stool may contain a lower concentration of virus or by IEM, which encourages aggregation of the virions.[60] Due to been developed for detecting RV in stool specimens, including complement fixation,[62] counterimmunoelectroosmophoresis (CIEOP),[62–65] free viral immunofluorescence (IF) utilizing light microscopy,[66] a cell culture technique combined with IF,[67] solid-phase RIA,[68,69] a fluorescent virus precipitin test (FVPT),[70] ELISA,[71,72] and an enzyme-linked immunofluorescent assay (ELFA).[73] The procedures adaptable for efficient processing of large numbers of samples have been CIEOP, IF, FVPT, RIA, and ELISA. CIEOP may[65,74] or may not[62,64] be as sensitive as electron microscopy, while RIA appears to retain the sensitivity of electron microscopy.[69] The most important development to date in the area of RV detection has been ELISA. Here, alkaline phosphatase or other enzymes (not a radioisotope) is linked to anti-RV antibody. Antisera prepared against HRV or against the homologous virus probably should be used to assure optimal sensitivity.[75] Antibody is bound to the solid phase, a test solution containing antigen is added, and a second enzyme-labeled antibody is added. A substrate is then added, and enzyme activity is related to antigen concentration. A color change occurs which can be quantitated spectrophotometrically or read visually. ELISA is as sensitive as RIA and electron microscopy and as efficient as RIA.[72] ELISA can be used to differentiate RVs of the various animal species by employing a blocking technique[71] and to distinguish between the two major HRV types.[76] The procedure requires simple equipment and is adaptable to field conditions. Commercial colorimetric readers designed for ELISA plates are currently available. ELFA may prove to be more sensitive than the comparable ELISA due to sensitivity of detecting the fluorescent end product in a fluorocolorimeter.[73]

Pathogenesis of HRV Diarrhea

Although HRV was first identified in the duodenal mucosa of children with diarrhea,[13] much of the information on disease pathogenesis has been derived from animal studies in which similar intestinal changes following infection with the animal-adapted RV resulted.[77,78] Colostrum-deprived and gnotobiotic calves infected with NCDV (a calf RV) developed alterations of the upper small bowel during early infection: Villous epithelium was comprised of low columnar to cuboidal cells, denuded tips of many villi were visible, and there was an increase in the number of reticulum-like cells in the lamina propria. Transmission electron microscopy of villous epithelium revealed that a large number of viral particles were present in the cytoplasm and that epithelial cells contained a large quantity of viral antigen. In infants with infection, an indirect fluorescent antibody technique was used to localize RV in duodenal biopsy.[79] The virus was present only in the cytoplasm of villous epithelial cells and not in the lamina propria. The distribution of virus in epithelial cells was patchy, and virus rarely was identified in mucosal biopsies obtained more than four days after the onset of illness. Immunofluorescence testing revealed viral antigen in duodenal and upper jejunal epithelial cells but not in stomach, large bowel, or mesenteric lymph nodes.[80] Virus replication appeared to be confined to columnar epithelium of duodenum and upper jejunum.

Gnotobiotic calves have been infected successfully with HRV.[81] The sequence of events in small-intestinal infection included invasion of the absorptive villous epithelial cells, replacement of the tall columnar villous epithelial cells with cuboidal and squamous cells, shortening of villi, enlargement of reticular cells, and lymphocytic infiltration of the villous lamina propria.

It has been suggested that lactase in the brush border of intestinal epithelial cells may act as receptor site and uncoating enzyme for HRV.[82] This postulate was forwarded because of the ability of purified β-galactosidase to remove the outer capsid layer of virus *in vitro*, possibly explaining the tendency for HRV to infect only gut epithelial cells. However, lactase-deficient persons remain highly susceptible to HRV infection, casting doubt on this theory.[83]

Tallet *et al.*[84] found high fecal output with sodium and chloride loss during early illness, yet adenyl cyclase and cAMP levels were not increased. Decreased levels of mucosal disaccharidases were documented, as well as reduced Na^+, K^+, and ATPase activities reflected in sugar malabsorption and defective sodium absorption. A failure of glucose-stimulated sodium absorption was shown. Similar enzymatic and absorptive defects were noted in a piglet model used to study transmissible gastroenteritis virus.[85] In a study of 57 male infants and children in Bangladesh with RV diarrhea, 28 were given oral therapy with a sucrose electrolyte solution and 29 were given a glucose electrolyte preparation. A control group of 44 additional children received only intravenous hydration.[86] These groups did not differ clinically in the rate of rehydration or the rate of stooling, despite a documented defect of carbohydrate absorption.

Propagation of HRV

HRV has not grown efficiently in cell culture in studies carried out through 1979. A limited number of strains of NCDV have been propagated in cell culture, as well as SA11 (simian RV) and the "O" agent (which is found in sheep and cattle). Murine RV does not grow well in cell culture but has been grown in mouse embryonic intestinal organ cultures.[87] HRV was cultivated *in vitro* in human fetal intestinal organ cultures employing immunofluorescent staining techniques to detect viral antigens[88,89] and has been successfully passed in cultures of bovine,[90] human embryonic kidney,[91] and African green monkey (AGMK)[92] cell lines. Wyatt *et al.*[92] have reported in 1980 the efficient growth of HRV type 2 in primay AGMK cells. This finding should be of profound importance to our being able to characterize the agent further.

HRV was fed to germ-free and conventional piglets,[93] resulting in diarrhea in some of the animals. The virus was found in stool specimens and mucosal epithelial cells of the small intestine. Cross-infection between some of the conventional piglets was documented. HRV was transmitted successfully to gnotobiotic piglets after three serial passages.[94] Excretion of virus in stool was documented, and serum antibody development occurred. Colostrum-deprived one-day-old rhesus monkeys have been infected experimentally with HRV, while eight-day-old and juvenile monkeys were shown to resist clinical infection.[95]

Clinical, Epidemiologic, and Microbiologic Aspects of HRV Infection

The incubation period of HRV infection ranges from 48 hr to four days.[80,96,97] The most common symptoms are profuse watery diarrhea accompanied by low-grade fever and vomiting. A high frequency of vomiting (up to 80%) is the most characteristic clinical finding of HRV infection. Clinical illness generally lasts five to eight days but may rarely last as long as a month.[44] As with infection by Norwalk-like agents, transient disaccharidase deficiency and carbohydrate malabsorption may follow HRV infection.[13] While RV characteristically produces a transient diarrhea, it may cause a severely dehydrating illness necessitating hospitalization. Fatalities secondary to HRV infection have been documented.[80,96] HRV infection shows primarily a wintertime distribution in temperate climates, as determined by studies in Australia,[96] England,[68] Japan,[97,99] Canada,[80] and Washington, D.C.,[100] whereas there may be a less striking association with time of year in warmer climates.[101,102]

During the first several years of study, it was felt that HRV was a cause of diarrhea primarily among infants and children between the ages of six months and three years.[97,100] More recently, evidence has accumulated to suggest that persons of all ages are susceptible to infection. Although there is an increased resistance among infants less than six months of age,[98] newborns commonly become infected,[103,104] and parents of infected children often become infected secondarily or perhaps serve as primary sources of infection.[100,105,106] Infection by HRV among newborn infants is not usually associated with clinical symptoms and is more common in bottle-fed children than in those who are breast-fed.[107] Diarrhea among adults from the United States who travel to Mexico may occasionally be secondary to HRV infection,[61] and epidemics of RV diarrhea in adults have been described.[108] Undoubtedly, one reason that earlier studies failed to indicate the frequency of infection among adults relates to the insensitivity of the study techniques. Viral replication probably is limited in adults, and electron microscopic examination of stool may not document the low levels of viral excretion.

While most studies have shown that HRV is the most commonly discovered agent associated with endemic diarrhea among infants and children, epidemics of HRV infection also have been well documented in open pediatric populations,[97] in confined hospital pediatric populations,[44,109] in newborn nurseries,[103,104] and in populations of school children.[110] During hospital outbreaks, adult hospital personnel may become infected.[104]

Originally, it was thought that a single HRV was responsible for the illness, in view of seroconversion to a common complement-fixing antigen among infected children from various parts of the world. The notion was further supported by the finding that older children and adults had serum antibody and reduced susceptibility. However, multiple outbreaks of HRV diarrhea were reported among populations under study.[110] In the latter report, serologic differences were reported among the children with infection due to HRV. Zissis and Lambert[111] subsequently described two HRV serotypes. The same group of investigators[112] described two sequential outbreaks of diarrhea in a confined population. During the first epidemic, children were infected with HRV type 1 and during the second outbreak, which occured one year later, with HRV type 2. A separate report documented two attacks of HRV gastroenteritis with an 11-month separation in an infant.[113] HRV type 1 was identified during the first episode, when the infant was 12 weeks old, and seroconversion to HRV type 1 occurred; then, when the infant was 14 months old, a second illness was associated with intestinal excretion of HRV type 2. To determine the relative importance of the two known serotypes of HRV, an ELISA technique was employed to differentiate serotype-specific HRV antigen and antibody in pediatric diarrhea from various parts of the world.[76] HRV type 2 was implicated in 77% of 414 HRV isolations over a five-year period, while the remainder were due to type 1. Most children studied in the Washington, D.C., area had acquired antibody to both types of HRV by two years of age. Sequential illnesses usually indicated infection by the different serotypes where one agent did not produce immunity against the other. Recently, a third[114] and a fourth[115] HRV serotype have been identified.

Infected infants and children excrete the virus during the late incubation period and during the acute phase of the illness in densities of 10^7–10^{10} particles/g of stool. Virus excretion is greatest during the third and fourth days of illness and is rarely detectable after the eighth day,[96,97,116] although on occasion it may be found nearly a month after the onset of infection.[44] While HRV is occasionally identified along with other enteropathogens in stool of children,[100] there does not appear to be a relationship between HRV infection and infection by other agents in humans.[61,98,117,118]

Serology of HRV Infection

The most convincing evidence of the importance of the virus as a cause of illness in humans is the common development of humoral antibody during infection.[31,97,119,120] By complement-fixation testing, antibody has been detected as early as day 3 of illness, with peak antibody titers occurring during the second and third weeks of illness.[97] High titers of antibody are present 14 days after the onset of infection and persist without a fall for one to two years after infection.[120] The sequence of antibody acquisition may be similar to that seen with other viral agents,[121] with IgM antibody appearing rapidly and reaching maximum levels five to ten days after infection and IgG antibody becoming detectable later, reaching a peak two to three weeks after the onset of illness. The initial antibody in HRV infection, which develops two to three days after the onset of symptoms, is IgM,[79] while antibody resistant to 2-mercaptoethanol (probably IgG) is produced approximately ten days after the onset of disease.[97] Employing ELISA, it was verified that anti-HRV IgM antibody occurred early in the course of infection, while anti-HRV IgG antibodies were documented later in convalescence.[122] These findings, plus the observation that anti-HRV IgG occurred in 95% of adults without anti-HRV IgM, suggest that anti-IgM in the absence of anti-IgG signifies a recent infection with HRV. It appears that HRV has at least two antigenically unrelated capsid layers. The inner capsid layer may be common to all RVs, while the outer capsid layer may be type- or species-specific.[30,32] Antigen from the HRV outer capsid more accurately measures serum antibody during infection as compared to whole HRV employed as antigen.[100,118,119,123]

The ubiquity of HRV agents is suggested by the finding of an age-related antibody among children from six to 18 months of age, indicating that infection by HRV is common early in life.[123] This kind of age-related serotype response is characteristic of other ubiquitous viral agents.[124] Surveys among populations in Melbourne,[120] Washington, D.C.,[119] and Toronto[64] have shown that most children have experienced HRV infection by age three. Levels of antibody do not rise with age beyond this point.

A complement-fixation test was developed employing HRV antigen from stool specimens of infected children.[31] Because of the difficulty in collecting large quantities of diarrheal stools containing HRV, and because many stools possess anticomplementary activity, other serologic procedures have been developed. Table 7.2 lists many of the published studies on RV serology, detailing the viral antigens used and the specific serologic procedures. Morphologically related animal RVs have been shown to be antigenically similar to HRV, and infected children often have an increase in antibody to a common complement-fixing antigen.[125] SA11 virus, recovered from a verret monkey, O (offal) agent, originally recovered from intestinal washings of sheep and cattle, NCDV, and EDIM (epizootic diarrhea of infant mouse) virus have been used as substitutes for HRV. O agent was found to be the most efficient substitute antigen for HRV.[125] NCDV has been employed by many laboratories because of its cross-antigenicity with HRV and its availability.[30,119,123,126] Although NCDV is not as efficient as HRV as an antigen for viral detection, when a serologic procedure employing NCDV is coupled with direct examination of stools by electron microscopy, the diagnosis is usually made with accuracy. In addition to complement fixation, specific serologic procedures employed include IEM, indirect IF, ELISA, and hemagglutination inhibition (see Table 7.2 for references). Advantages of the ELISA technique are that it is easily performed, does not require tissue culture techniques or subjective readings, and can be performed with a single dilution of serum, using a volume as small as 3 μl.[122] In the indirect IF described by Davidson et al.,[79] human duodenal mucosal absorptive cells from infants infected with HRV were used as the antigen. Other sources of antigen have been human fetal intestinal organ

TABLE 7.2
Serologic Procedures Employed to Measure Humoral Immune Response to HRV

	Serologic procedure					
Antigen employed	Complement fixation	IEM	Indirect IF	ELISA	Hemagglutination inhibition	References
HRV	×					31, 97, 100, 106, 109, 120, 123
HRV		×				31, 97
HRV			×			79, 88
HRV				×		122
NCDV	×					100, 119, 123
NCDV			×			100, 119, 123, 132
NCDV					×	126
EDIM	×					31, 125
"O" agent	×					125
SA11	×					125

culture infected with HRV[88] and infant rhesus monkey intestine infected with HRV.[95]

In documenting HRV infection, serologic evidence of infection should be sought along with identification of viral agents in stool specimens.[100,120] There exists an 86% concordance between detection of HRV in stools and serum complement-fixing antibody response.[100] In children older than six months, serology is slightly more reliable than electron microscopic visualization, since viral replication in the gastrointestinal tract decreases with age. In contrast, infants younger than six months may have a poor antibody response to infection.[120]

New techniques by which HR may be propagated to high titers in cell culture[92] hold the potential for development of a standardized serologic procedure with wide-scale application.

Immunity in HRV Infection

Infants from six months to two years of age are the most susceptible to HRV infection. The lower incidence of infection among infants less than six months of age may relate to immunity acquired from the mother. The greatest resistance to infection appears to be among children above the age of two years and adults. Thus, it appears that natural immunization occurs, probably through repeated exposures to the virus or to an antigenically similar organism. The protective factor induced by infection has not been identified. It has been shown that there is no relationship between the level of serum antibody and susceptibility.[100,105] Immunity may be more related to resistance to clinical illness rather than resistance to infection, in view of the common finding of asymptomatic infection among adults and newborn infants.

Calves recovering from RV infection have been shown to be immune to reinoculation of virus from several days to four weeks after the initial infection.[77] The calf RV was attenuated by passing it approximately 140 times on bovine fetal kidney cells at 37°C and an additional 60 times on the same cell culture at 29–30°C. The strain was then employed as a vaccine. In a laboratory study it appeared to confer immunity to 6- to 7-hr-old calves, and in field studies carried out in 14 animal herds, it was shown further to protect calves when the animals were immunized within 24 hr of birth.[77,127] In view of the natural resistance of infants and because of possible limitations of active immunization,[128] passive immunization is being sought as a means of controlling infection. Two approaches have been taken in animals: immunization of the pregnant dam or artificial feeding of nonsuckling neonates with an antibody-containing preparation.[129] Antibody to RV is normally secreted in high concentrations in the colostrum of cattle and sheep during the first day postpartum but falls to negligible amounts three days later.[130,131] When high-titered (anti-RV antibody) colostrum was fed to calves, they were protected from infection by calf RV, as were lambs given sheep colostrum or human γ-globulin when exposed to lamb RV or HRV.[132,133] When fed daily to newborn animals, colostrum successfully prevented infection and clinical illness by RV. Use of antibody-containing colostrum may prove to be of value during the first few days to several weeks of life, when the newborn animals remain at high risk. Calves immunized *in utero* with NCDV were shown to resist challenge after birth by HRV type 2 or NCDV.[134] Similarity in the two viruses justifies further study of NCDV as a potential immunizing agent against human illness. Human colostrum and breast milk contain HRV-neutralizing antibody, and solid-phase RIA was employed to confirm that anti-HRV IgA antibody persisted in human milk for as long as nine months after delivery.[136] IgA antibody to HRV was found in colostral specimens from women living in Bangladesh, Guatemala, Costa Rica, and Washington, D.C.[76] Of the specimens, 88% had IgA antibody to HRV type 1 and 91% IgA antibody to HRV type 2. Infants who are breast-fed show a greater resistance to HRV infection than those who are bottle-fed, and when infection occurs, it generally produces no symptoms.[107]

Further studies are now needed to document the relative immunity of humans to HRV infection, considering that there are at least two important serotypes. The next step will be to compare antigenic similarities between HRVs identified in distinctly differing regions of the world. Finally, that efficient propagation of HRV to high titers in cell culture systems appears feasible, it should be possible to evaluate the possibility of controlling infection through immunophylaxis. The ubiquity of the virus and the profound magnitude of its impact on diarrhea, malnutrition, and death indicate the importance of pursuing the development and testing of immunizing agents.

REFERENCES

1. Cramblett, H. G., Moffet, H. L., Middleton, G. K., Jr., *et al.* ECHO 19 virus infections: Clinical and laboratory studies. *Arch. Intern. Med.* **110:**574–579, 1962.
2. Klein, J. O., Lerner, A. M., Finland, M. Acute gastroenteritis associated with ECHO virus, type 11 *Am. J. Med. Sci.* **240:**749–753, 1960.
3. Eichenwald, H. F., Ababio, A., Arky, A. M., *et al.* Epidemic diarrhea in premature and older infants caused by ECHO virus type 18. *J. Am. Med. Assoc.* **166:**1563–1566, 1958.
4. Scrimshaw, N. S., Salomon, J. B., Bruch, H. A., *et al.* Studies of diarrheal disease in Central America: VIII. Measles, diarrhea, and nutritional deficiency in rural Guatemala. *Am. J. Trop. Med.* **15:**625–631, 1966.
5. Salomon, J. E., Gordon, J. E., Scrimshaw, N. S. Studies of diarrheal disease in Central America: X. Associated chicken pox, diarrhea and kwashiorkor in a highland Guatemalan village. *Am. J. Trop. Med.* **15:**997–1002, 1966.
6. Sheehy, T. W., Artenstein, M. S., Green, R. W. Small intestinal mucosa in certain viral diseases. *J. Am. Med. Assoc.* **190:**1023–1028, 1964.
7. Gordon, J. E., Chicken pox: An epidemiological review. *Am. J. Med. Sci.* **244:**362–389, 1962.
8. Reimann, H. A., Price, A. H., Hodges, J. H. The cause of epidemic diarrhea nausea and vomiting (viral dysentery?) *Proc. Soc. Exp. Biol. Med.* **59:**8–9, 1945.
9. Gordon, I., Meneely, J. K., Jr., Currie, G. D., *et al.* Clinical laboratory studies in experimentally-induced epidemic nonbacterial gastroenteritis. *J. Lab. Clin. Med.* **41:**133–141, 1953.
10. Fukumi, H., Nakaya, R., Hatta, S., *et al.* An indication as to identity between the infectious diarrhea in Japan and the afebrile infectious nonbacterial gastroenteritis by human volunteer experiments. *Jpn. J. Med. Sci. Biol.* **10:**1–17, 1957.
11. Dolin, R., Blacklow, N. R., DuPont, H. L., *et al.* Transmission of acute infectious nonbacterial gastroenteritis to volunteers by oral administration of stool filtrates. *J. Infect. Dis.* **123:**307–312, 1971.
12. Kapikian, A. Z., Wyatt, R. G., Dolin, R., *et al.* Visualization by immune electron microscopy of a 27-nm particle associated with acute infectious non-bacterial gastroenteritis. *J. Virol.* **10:**1075–1081, 1972.
13. Bishop, R. F., Davidson, G. P., Holmes, I. H., *et al.* Virus particles in epithelial cells of

duodenal mucosa from children with acute non-bacterial gastroenteritis. *Lancet* **2:**1281–1283, 1973.

14. Wyatt, R. G., Dolin, R., Blacklow, N. R., *et al.* Comparison of three agents of acute infectious nonbacterial gastroenteritis by cross-challenge in volunteers. *J. Infect. Dis.* **129:**709–714, 1974.
15. Dolin, R., Blacklow, N. R., DuPont, H. L., *et al.* Biological properties of Norwalk agent of acute infectious nonbacterial gastroenteritis. *Proc. Soc. Exp. Biol. Med.* **140:**578–583, 1972.
16. Thornhill, T. S., Wyatt, R. G., Kalica, A. R., *et al.* Detection by immune electron microscopy of 26- to 27-nm viruslike particles associated with two family outbreaks of gastroenteritis. *J. Infect. Dis.* **135:**20–27, 1977.
17. Appleton, H., Buckley, M., Thom, B. T., *et al.* Virus-like particles in winter vomiting disease. *Lancet* **1:**409–411, 1977.
18. Clarke, S. K., Cook, G. T., Egglestone, S. I., *et al.* A virus from epidemic vomiting disease. *Br. Med. J.* **3:**86–89, 1972.
19. Appleton, H., Pereira, M. S. A possible virus aetiology in outbreaks of food-poisoning from cockles. *Lancet* **1:**780–781, 1977.
20. Greenberg, H. B., Kapikian, A. Z. Detection of Norwalk agent antibody and antigen by solid-phase radioimmunoassay and immune adherence hemagglutination assay. *J. Am. Vet. Med. Assoc.* **173:**620–623, 1978.
21. Wyatt, R. G., Greenberg, H. B., Dalgard, D. W., *et al.* Experimental infection of chimpanzees with the Norwalk agent of epidemic viral gastroenteritis. *J. Med. Virol.* **2:**89–96, 1978.
22. Thornhill, T. S., Kalica, A. R., Wyatt, R. G., *et al.* Pattern of shedding of the Norwalk particle in stools during experimentally induced gastroenteritis in volunteers as determined by immune electron microscopy. *J. Infect. Dis.* **132:**28–34, 1975.
23. Agus, S. G., Dolin, R., Wyatt, R. G., *et al.* Acute infectious nonbacterial gastroenteritis: Intestinal histopathology. Histologic and enzymatic alterations during illness produced by the Norwalk agent in man. *Ann. Intern. Med.* **79:**18–25, 1973.
24. Schreiber, D. S., Blacklow, N. R., Trier, J. S. The mucosal lesion of the proximal small intestine in acute infectious nonbacterial gastroenteritis. *N. Engl. J. Med.* **288:**1318–1323, 1973.
25. Schreiber, D. S., Blacklow, N. R., Trier, J. S. The small intestinal lesion induced by Hawaii agent acute infectious nonbacterial gastroenteritis. *J. Infect. Dis.* **129:**705–708, 1974.
26. Widerlite, L., Trier, J. S., Blacklow, N. R., *et al.* Structure of the gastric mucosa in acute infectious nonbacterial gastroenteritis. *Gastroenterology* **68:**425–430, 1975.
27. Dolin, R., Reichman, R. C., Fauci, A. S. Lymphocyte populations in acute viral gastroenteritis. *Infect. Immun.* **14:**422–428, 1976.
28. Parrino, T. A., Schreiber, D. S., Trier, J. S., *et al.* Clinical immunity in acute gastroenteritis caused by Norwalk agent. *N. Engl. J. Med.* **297:**86–89, 1977.
29. Agus, S. G., Falchuk, Z. M., Sessoms, C. S., *et al.* Increased jejunal IgA synthesis *in vitro* during acute infectious nonbacterial gastroenteritis. *Am. J. Dig. Dis.* **19:**127–131, 1974.
30. Flewett, T. H., Bryden, A. S., Davies, H., *et al.* Relation between viruses from acute gastroenteritis of children and newborn calves. *Lancet* **2:**61–63, 1974.
31. Kapikian, A. Z., Kim, H. W., Wyatt, R. G., *et al.* Reoviruslike agent in stools: Association with infantile diarrhea and development of serologic tests. *Science* **185:**1049–1053, 1974.
32. Woode, G. N., Bridger, J. C., Jones, J. M., *et al.* Morphological and antigenic relation-

ships between viruses (rotaviruses) from acute gastroenteritis of children, calves, piglets, mice and foals. *Infect. Immun.* **14**:804–810, 1976.

33. **Much, D.H., Zajac, I. Purification and characterization of epizootic diarrhea of infant mice virus. *Inject. Immun.* 6:1019–1924, 1972.**

34. Fernelius, A. L., Ritchie, A. E., Classick, L. G., *et al.* Cell culture adaptation and propagation of a reovirus-like agent of calf diarrhea from a field outbreak in Nebraska. *Arch. Gesamte Virusforsch.* **37**:114–130, 1972.

35. McNulty, M. S., Allan, G. M., Pearson, G. R., *et al.* Reovirus-like agent (rotavirus) from lambs. *Infect. Immun.* **14**:1332–1338, 1976.

36. Malherbe, H. H., Strickland-Cholmley, M. Simian virus SA11 and the related O agent. *Arch. Gesamte Virusforsch.* **22**:235–245, 1968.

37. Lecce, J. G., King, M. W., Mock, R. Reovirus-like agent associated with fatal diarrhea in neonatal pigs. *Infect. Immun.* **14**:816–825, 1976.

38. Flewett, T. H., Bryden, A. S., Davies, H. Virus diarrhoea in foals and other animals. *Vet. Rec.* **96**:477, 1975.

39. Bishop, R. F., Davidson, G. P., Holmes, I. H., *et al.* Detection of a new virus by electron microscopy of faecal extracts from children with acute gastroenteritis. *Lancet* **1**:149–151, 1974.

40. Holmes, I. H., Ruck, B. J., Bishop, R. F., *et al.* Infantile enteritis viruses: Morphogenesis and morphology. *J. Virol.* **16**:937–943, 1975.

41. Rodger, S. M., Schnagl, R. D., Holmes, I. H. Biochemical and biophysical characteristics of diarrhea viruses of human and calf origin. *J. Virol.* **16**:1229–1235, 1975.

42. Petric, M., Szymanski, M. T., Middleton, P. J. Purification and preliminary characterization of infantile gastroenteritis virus (orbivirus group). *Intervirology* **5**:233–238, 1975.

43. Kapikian, A. Z., Kalica, A. R., Shih, J. W., *et al.* Buoyant density in cesium chloride of the human reovirus-like agent of infantile gastroenteritis by ultracentrifugation, electron microscopy, and complement fixation. *Virology* **70**:564–569, 1976.

44. Flewett, T. H., Bryden, A. S., Davies, H., *et al.* Epidemic viral enteritis in a long-stay children's ward. *Lancet* **1**:4–5, 1975.

45. Albrey, M. B., Murphy, A. M. Rotaviruses and acute gastroenteritis of infants and children. *Med. J. Aust.* **1**:82–85, 1976.

46. Derbyshire, J B., Woode, G. N. Classification of rotaviruses: Report from the World Health Organization/Food and Agriculture Organization Comparative Virology Program. *J. Am. Vet. Med. Assoc.* **173**:519–521, 1978.

47. Flewett, T. H , Woode, G. N. The rotaviruses. *Arch. Virol.* **57**:1–23, 1978.

48. Kalica, A. R., Wyatt, R. G., Kapikian, A. Z. Detection of differences among human and animal rotaviruses, using analysis of viral RNA. *J. Am. Vet. Med. Assoc.* **173**:531–537, 1978.

49. Rodger, S. M., Schnagl, R. D., Holmes, I. H. Further biochemical characterization, including the detection of surface glycoproteins of human, calf, and simian rotaviruses. *J. Virol.* **24**:91–98, 1977.

50. Newman, J. F. E., Brown, F., Bridger, J. C., *et al.* Characterisation of a rotavirus. *Nature* **258**:631–633, 1975.

51. Todd, D., McNulty, M. S. Biochemical studies on a reovirus-like agent (rotavirus) from lambs. *J. Virol.* **21**:1215–1218, 1977.

52. Kalica, A. R., Garon, C. F., Wyatt, R. G., *et al.* Differentiation of human and calf reoviruslike agents associated with diarrhea using polyacrylamide gel electrophoresis of RNA. *Virology* **74**:86–92, 1976.

53. Schnagl, R. D., Holmes, I. H., Characteristics of the genome of human infantile enteritis virus (rotavirus). *J. Virol.* **19**:267–270, 1976.

54. Todd, D., McNulty, M. S. Characterization of pig rotavirus RNA. *J. Gen. Virol.* **33:** 147–150, 1976.
55. Verly, E., Cohen, J. Demonstration of size variation of RNA segments between different isolates of calf rotavirus. *J. Gen. Virol.* **35:**583–586, 1977.
56. Woode, G. N., Bridger, J. C., Hall, G. A., *et al.* The isolation of reovirus-like agents (rotaviruses) from acute gastroenteritis of piglets. *J. Med. Microbiol.* **9:**203–209, 1976.
57. Snodgrass, D. R., Herring, J. A., Gray, E. W., Experimental rotavirus infection in lambs. *J. Comp. Pathol.* **86:**637–642, 1976.
58. Schoub, B. D., Lecatsas, G., Prozesky, O. W. Antigenic relationship between human and simian rotaviruses. *J. Med. Microbiol.* **10:**1–6, 1977.
59. Thouless, M. E., Bryden, A. S., Flewett, T. H., *et al.* Serological relationships between rotaviruses from different species as studied by complement fixation and neutralization. *Arch. Virol.* **53:**287–294, 1977.
60. Almeida, J. D., Waterson, A. P. The morphology of virus–antibody interaction. *Adv. Virus Res.* **15:**307–338, 1969.
61. Bolivar, R., Conklin, R. H., Vollet, J. J., *et al.* Rotavirus in travelers' diarrhea: Study of an adult student population in Mexico. *J. Infect. Dis.* **137:**324–327, 1978.
62. Spence, L., Fauvel, M., Bouchard, S., *et al.* Test for reovirus-like agent. *Lancet* **2:**322, 1975.
63. Torres-Medina, A., Wyatt, R. G., Mebus, C. A., *et al.* Diarrhea caused in gnotobiotic piglets by the reovirus-like agent of human infantile gastroenteritis. *J. Infect. Dis.* **133:** 22–27, 1976.
64. Middleton, P. J., Petric, M., Hewitt, C. M., *et al.* Counter-immunoelectroosmophoresis for the detection of infantile gastroenteritis virus (orbigroup) antigen and antibody. *J. Clin. Pathol.* **29:**191–197, 1976.
65. Tufvesson, B., Johnsson, T. Immunoelectroosmophoresis for detection of reo-like virus: Methodology and comparison with electron microscopy. *Acta Pathol. Microbiol. Scand. Sect. B* **84:**225–228, 1976.
66. Yolken, R. H., Wyatt, R. G., Kalica, A. R., *et al.* Use of a free viral immunofluorescence assay to detect human reovirus-like agent in human stools. *Infect. Immun.* **16:**467–470, 1977.
67. Banatvala, J. E., Totterdell, B., Chrystie, I. L., *et al.* In-vitro detection of human rotaviruses. *Lancet* **2:**821, 1975.
68. Middleton, P. J., Holdaway, M. D., Petric, M., *et al.* Solid-phase radioimmunoassay for the detection of rotavirus. *Infect. Immun.* **16:**439–444, 1977.
69. Kalica, A. R., Purcell, R. H., Sereno, M. M., *et al.* A microtiter solid phase radioimmunoassay for detection of the human reovirus-like agent in stools. *J. Immunol.* **118:**1275–1279, 1977.
70. Peterson, M. W., Spendlove, R. S., Smart, R. A. Detection of neonatal calf diarrhea virus, infant reovirus-like diarrhea virus, and a coronarvirus using the fluorescent virus precipitin test. *J. Clin. Microbiol.* **3:**376–377, 1976.
71. Yolken, R. H., Barbour, B., Wyatt, R. G., *et al.* Enzyme-linked immunosorbent assay for identification of rotaviruses from different animal species. *Science* **201:**259–262, 1978.
72. Yolken, R. H., Kim, H. W., Clem, T., *et al.* Enzyme-linked immunosorbent assay (ELISA) for detection of human reovirus-like agent of infantile gastroenteritis. *Lancet* **2:**263–267, 1977.
73. Yolken, R. H., Stopa, P. J. Enzyme-linked immunofluorescence assay: Ultrasensitive solid-phase assay for detection of human rotavirus. *J. Clin. Microbiol.* **10:**317–321, 1979.
74. Spence, L. Fauvel, M., Petro, R., *et al.* Comparison of counterimmunoelectrophoresis

and electron microscopy for laboratory diagnosis of human reovirus-like agent-associated infantile gastroenteritis. *J. Clin. Microbiol.* **5:**248–249, 1977.

75. Yolken, R., Wyatt, R. G., Kapikian, A. Z. ELISA for rotavirus. *Lancet* **2:**819, 1977.

76. Yolken, R. H., Wyatt, R. G., Zissis, G., *et al.* Epidemiology of human rotavirus types 1 and 2 as studied by enzyme-linked immunosorbent assay. *N. Engl. J. Med.* **229:**1156–1161, 1978.

77. Mebus, C. A. Reovirus-like calf enteritis. *Am. J. Dig. Dis.* **21:**592–598, 1976.

78. Adams, W. R., Kraft, L. M. Electron-microscope study of the intestinal epithelium of mice infected with the agent of epizootic diarrhea of infant mice (EDIM virus). *Am. J. Pathol.* **51:**39–60, 1967.

79. Davidson, G. P., Goller, I., Bishop, R. F., *et al.* Immunofluorescence in duodenal mucosa of children with acute enteritis due to a new virus. *J. Clin. Pathol.* **28:**263–266, 1975.

80. Middleton, F. J., Szymanski, M. T., Abbott, G. D., *et al.* Orbivirus acute gastroenteritis of infancy. *Lancet* **1:**1241–1244, 1974.

81. Mebus, C. A., Wyatt, R. G., Kapikian, A. Z. Intestinal lesions induced in gnotobiotic calves by the virus of human infantile gastroenteritis. *Vet. Pathol.* **14:**273–282, 1977.

82. Holmes, I. H., Rodger, S. M., Schnagl, R. D., *et al.* Is lactase the receptor and uncoating enzyme for infantile enteritis (rota) viruses? *Lancet* **1:**1387–1389, 1976.

83. Schoub, B. D., Jenkins, T., Robins-Browne, R. M. Rotavirus infection in high-incidence lactase-deficiency population. *Lancet* **1:**328, 1978.

84. Tallett, S., Mackenzie, C., Middleton, P., *et al.* Clinical, laboratory, and epidemiological features of a viral gastroenteritis in infants and children. *Pediatrics* **60:**217–222, 1977.

85. Shepherd, R. W., Gall, D. G., Butler, D. G., *et al.* Determinants of diarrhea in viral enteritis: The role of ion transport and epithelial changes in the ileum in transmissible gastroenteritis in piglets. *Gastroenterology* **76:**20–24, 1979.

86. Sack, D.A., Chowdhury, A. M. A. K., Eusof, A. Oral hydration in rotavirus diarrhoea: A double-blind comparison of sucrose with glucose electrolyte solution. *Lancet* **2:**280–283, 1978.

87. Rubenstein, D., Milne, R. G., Buckland, R., *et al.* The growth of the virus of epidemic diarrhoea of infant mice (EDIM) in organ cultures of intestinal epithelium. *Br. J. Exp. Pathol.* **52:**442–445, 1971.

88. Wyatt, R. G., Kapikian, A. Z., Thronhill, T. S., *et al. In vitro* cultivation in human fetal intestinal organ culture of a reovirus-like agent associated with nonbacterial gastroenteritis in infants and children. *J. Infect. Dis.* **130:**523–528, 1974.

89. Wyatt, R. G., Kalica, A. R., Mebus, C. A., *et al.* Reovirus-like agents (rotaviruses) associated with diarrheal illness in animals and man. *Perspect. Virol.* **10:**121–145, 1978.

90. Albrey, M. B., Murphy, A. M. Rotavirus growth in bovine monolayers. *Lancet* **1:**753, 1976.

91. Wyatt, R. G., Gill, V. W., Sereno, M. M., *et al.* Probable *in vitro* cultivation of human reovirus-like agent of infantile diarrhoea *Lancet* **1:**98–99, 1976.

92. Wyatt, R. G, James, W. D., Bohl, E. H., *et al.* Human rotavirus type 2: Cultivation *in vitro. Science* **207:**187–191, 1980.

93. Middleton, P. J., Petric, M. Szymanski, M. T. Propagation of infantile gastroenteritis virus (orbigroup) in conventional and germfree piglets. *Infect. Immun.* **12:**1276–1280, 1975.

94. Bridger, J. C., Woode, G. N., Jones, J. M., *et al.* Transmission of human rotaviruses to gnotobiotic piglets. *J. Med. Microbiol.* **8:**565–569, 1975.

95. Wyatt, R. G., Sly, D. L., London, W. T., *et al.* Induction of diarrhea in colostrum-deprived newborn rhesus monkeys with the human reovirus-like agent of infantile gastroenteritis. *Arch. Virol.* **50:**17–27, 1976.

96. Davidson, G. P., Bishop, R. F., Townley, R. R. W., *et al.* Importance of a new virus in acute sporadic enteritis in children. *Lancet* **1**:242–246, 1975.

97. Konno, T., Suzuki, H., Imai, A., *et al.* Reovirus-like agent in acute epidemic gastroenteritis in Japanese infants: Fecal shedding and serologic response. *J. Infect. Dis.* **135**:259–266, 1977.

98. Bryden, A. S., Davies, H. A., Hadley, R. E., *et al.* Rotavirus enteritis in the West Midlands during 1974. *Lancet* **2**:241–243, 1975.

99. Konno, T., Suzuki, H., Imai, A., *et al.* A long-term survey of rotovirus infection in Japanese children with acute gastroenteritis. *J. Infect. Dis.* **138**:569–576, 1978.

100. Kapikian, A. Z., Kim, H. W., Wyatt, R. G., *et al.* Human reovirus-like agent as the major pathogen associated with "winter" gastroenteritis in hospitalized infants and young children. *N. Eng. J. Med.* **294**:965–972, 1976.

101. Pickering, L. K., Evans, D. J., Jr., Muñoz, O., *et al.* Prospective study of enteropathogens in children with diarrhea in Houston and Mexico. *J. Pediatr.* **93**:383–388, 1978.

102. Hieber, J. P., Shelton, S., Nelson, J. D., *et al.* Comparison of human rotavirus disease in tropical and temperate settings. *Am. J. Dis. Child.* **132**:853–858, 1978.

103. Murphy, A. M., Albrey, M. B., Crewe, E. B. Rotavirus infections of neonates. *Lancet* **2**:1149–1150, 1977.

104. Chrystie, I. L., Totterdell, B. M., Banatvala, J. E. Asymptomatic endemic rotavirus infections in the newborn. *Lancet* **1**:1176–1178, 1978.

105. Kim, H. W., Brandt, C. D., Kapikian, A. Z., *et al.* Human reovirus-like agent infection: Occurrence in adult contacts of pediatric patients with gastroenteritis. *J. Am. Med. Assoc.* **238**:404–407, 1977.

106. Gomez-Barreto, J., Palmer, E., Nahmias, A. J., *et al.* Acute enteritis associated with reovirus-like agents. *J. Am. Med. Assoc.* **235**:1857–1860, 1976.

107. Banatvala, J. E., Chrystie, I. L., Totterdell, B. M. Rotaviral infections in human neonates. *J. Am. Vet. Med. Assoc.* **173**:527–530, 1978.

108. Lycke, E., Blomberg, J., Berg, G., *et al.* Epidemic acute diarrhoea in adults associated with infantile gastroenteritis virus. *Lancet* **2**:1056–1057, 1978.

109. Ryder, R. W., McGowan, J. E., Jr., Hatch, M. H., *et al.* Reovirus-like agent as a cause of nosocomial diarrhea in infants. *J. Pediatr.* **90**:698–702, 1977.

110. Hara, M., Mukoyama, J., Tsuruhara, T., *et al.* Acute gastroenteritis among school children associated with reovirus-like agent. *Am. J. Epidemiol* **107**:161–169, 1978.

111. Zissis, G., Lambert, J. P. Different serotypes of human rotaviruses. *Lancet* **1**:38–39, 1978.

112. Fonteyne, J., Zissis, G., Lambert, J. P. Recurrent rotavirus gastroenteritis. *Lancet* **1**:983, 1978.

113. Rodriguez, W. J., Kim, H. W., Brandt, C. D., *et al.* Sequential enteric illnesses associated with different rotavirus serotypes. *Lancet* **2**:37, 1978.

114. Thouless, M. E., Bryden, A. S., Flewett, T. H. Serotypes of human rotavirus. *Lancet* **1**:39, 1978.

115. Flewett, T. H., Thouless, M. E., Pilfold, J. N., *et al.* More serotypes of human rotavirus (letter). *Lancet* **2**:632, 1978.

116. Flewett, T. H., Davies, H., Bryden, A. S., *et al.* Diagnostic electron microscopy of faeces: II. Acute gastroenteritis associated with reovirus-like particles. *J. Clin. Pathol.* **27**:608–614, 1974.

117. Echeverria, P., Blacklow, N. R., Smith, D. H. Role of heat-labile toxigenic *Escherichia coli* and reovirus-like agent in diarrhea in Boston children. *Lancet* **2**:1113–1116, 1975.

118. Ryder, R. W., Sack, D. A., Kapikian, A. Z., *et al.* Enterotoxigenic *Escherichia coli* and reovirus-like agent in rural Bangladesh. *Lancet* **1**:659–663, 1976.

119. Kapikian, A. Z., Cline, W. L., Mebus, C. A., *et al.* New complement-fixation test for the human reovirus-like agent of infantile gastroenteritis. *Lancet* **1:**1056–1061, 1975.

120. Gust, I. D., Pringle, R. C., Barnes, G. L., *et al.* Complement-fixing antibody response to rotavirus infection. *J. Clin. Microbiol.* **5:**125–130, 1977.

121. Cowan, K. M. Antibody response to viral antigens. *Adv. Immunol.* **17:**195–2563, 1973.

122. Yolken, R. H., Wyatt, R. G., Kim, H. W., *et al.* Immunological response to infection with human recvirus-like agent: Measurement of anti-human reovirus-like agent immunoglobulin G and M levels by the method of enzyme-linked immunosorbent assay. *Infect. Immun.* **19:**540–546, 1978.

123. Blacklow, N. R., Echeverria, P., Smith, D. H. Serological studies with reovirus-like enteritis agent. *Infect. Immun.* **13:**1563–1566, 1976.

124. Merigan, T. C. Host defenses against viral disease. *N. Engl. J. Med.* **290:**323–329, 1974.

125. Kapikian, A. Z., Cline, W. L., Kim, H. W., *et al.* Antigenic relationships among five reovirus-like (RVL) agents by complement fixation (CF) and development of new substitute CF antigens for the human RVL agent of infantile gastroenteritis. *Proc. Soc. Exp. Biol. Med.* **152:**535–539, 1976.

126. Shinozaki, T., Fujii, R., Sato, K., *et al.* Haemagglutinin from human reovirus-like agent (letter). *Lancet* **1:**877–878, 1978.

127. Mebus, C. A., White, R. G., Bass, E. P., *et al.* Immunity to neonatal calf diarrhea virus. *J. Am. Vet. Med. Assoc.* **163:**880–883, 1973.

128. Acres, S. D., Radostits, O. M. The efficacy of a modified live reo-like virus vaccine and an *E. coli* bacterin for prevention of acute undifferentiated neonatal diarrhea of beef calves. *Can. Vet. J.* **17:**197–212, 1976.

129. Snodgrass, D. R., Wells, P. W. Passive immunity in rotaviral infections. *J. Am. Vet. Med. Assoc.* **173:**565–568, 1978.

130. Wells, P. W., Snodgrass, D. R., Herring, J. A., *et al.* Antibody titers to lamb rotavirus in colostrum and milk of suckled ewes. *Vet. Rec.* **103:**46–48, 1978.

131. Woode, G. N., Jones, J., Bridger, J. Levels of colostral antibodies against neonatal calf diarrhoea virus. *Vet. Rec.* **97:**148–149, 1975.

132. Snodgrass, D. R., Madeley, C. R., Wells, P. W., *et al.* Human rotavirus in lambs: Infection and passive protection. *Infect. Immun.* **16:**268–270, 1977.

133. Snodgrass, D. R., Wells, P. W. Rotavirus infection in lambs: Studies on passive protection. *Arch. Virol.* **52:**201–205, 1976.

134. Wyatt, R. G., Mebus, C. A., Yolken, R. H., *et al.* Rotaviral immunity in gnotobiotic calves: Heterologous resistance to human virus induced by bovine virus. *Science* **203:**548–550, 1979.

135. Thouless, M. E., Bryden, A. S., Flewett, T. H. Rotavirus neutralisation by human milk. *Br. Med. J.* **2:**1390, 1977.

136. Cukor, G., Blacklow, N., Capozza, F., *et al.* Secretory IgA antibody to rotavirus in human milk 6–9 months postpartum (letter). *Lancet* **2:**631–632, 1978.

137. Blacklow, N. R., Dolin, R., Fedson, D. S., *et al.* Acute infectious nonbacterial gastroenteritis: Etiology and pathogenesis. *Ann. Intern. Med.* **76:**993–1008, 1972.

8

Relative Importance of Enteropathogens in Acute Endemic Diarrhea and Food-Borne Diarrheal Illness

INTRODUCTION

Establishing the etiology of acute diarrhea is complex because of the many variables influencing its cause and/or detection, including age, geographic location, season, and availability of laboratory procedures necessary to fully identify the various agents. Regardless of the part of the world in which it occurs, acute infectious diarrhea cannot be attributed to any one enteropathogen. The presence of rotavirus (RV) in stool specimens of a substantial proportion of children with diarrhea is evidence of the importance of this agent in endemic illness. A correlation exists between identification of RV in stool specimens and serologic response to infection. Enterotoxigenic *E. coli.* (ETEC) is an important cause of diarrhea in persons from industrialized countries during travel to developing regions, but it does not account for a large number of endemic cases of diarrhea in children in the United States. Serotype-determined enteropathogenic *E. coli* (EPEC) is an important cause of infantile diarrhea, yet the relative frequency of occurrence and mechanisms of pathogenesis are unknown. Intestinal infections due to *Shigella* and *Salmonella* generally occur in the summer months in children over 3 months of age and in adults. *G. lamblia* is a cause of acute, chronic, and recurrent diarrhea in all age groups. Other agents which require specialized laboratory techniques for identification have been shown to cause diarrhea on occasion.

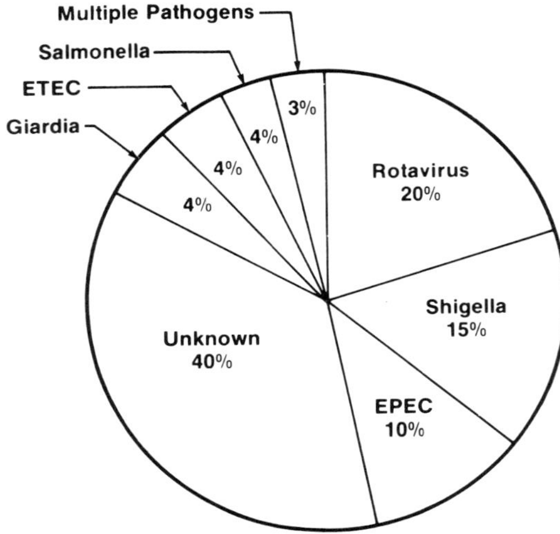

Figure 8.1. Approximate relative importance of infectious agents in endemic pediatric diarrhea.

Up to this point, the text has dealt with specific etiologic classifications of enteric infection. This chapter will serve to review their relative importance in patients with acute diarrheal disease. The percentages given are speculations based on noncoordinated studies, with an emphasis on prospective, longitudinal investigations including controls. Figure 8.1 gives the causes of acute infectious diarrhea of children in the United States and their estimated relative frequency of occurrence. Figure 8.2 compares the relative importance of causative agents of food-borne illness in this country.

ACUTE ENDEMIC DIARRHEA

Rotavirus (RV)

The human rotavirus (HRV) has been established as a major cause of acute gastroenteritis among infants and children in many parts of the world. In several investigations from diverse geographic locations, HRV has accounted for 10–50% of the cases of diarrhea in children and has been present in stool specimens of up to 70% of children with diarrhea acquired during the winter months in colder climates. Viral particles are uncommon among healthy children, a finding which confirms the low incidence of carriage of this agent, even in areas of poor sanitation. Although HRV gastroenteritis has been reported to occur primarily dur-

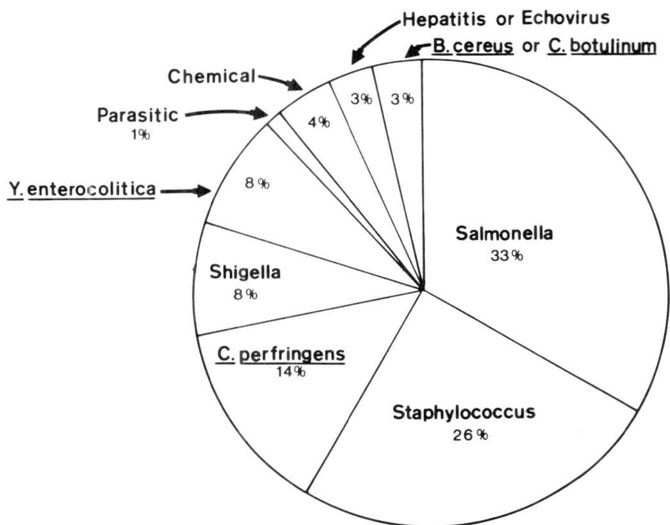

Figure 8.2. Confirmed cases of food-borne disease by etiology, 1976. Reported in *Food-Borne and Waterborne Disease Outbreaks: Annual Summary, 1976, 1977.* United States Department of Health, Education and Welfare, Center for Disease Control, Atlanta, 1977.

ing winter months in temperate climates, a less significant seasonal occurrence has been reported in studies conducted in tropical or semitropical climates. The majority of patients with HRV infections are between six and 24 months of age, although HRV has been reported to be a cause of gastroenteritis in newborn infants and adults and has been detected in stool specimens of asymptomatic infants. Reinfection with HRV has been reported and probably reflects the differing serotypes which exist.

A large prospective study of gastroenteritis in Canada[1] revealed that the overall incidence of HRV infection among children with gastroenteritis was 11%, while the rate was 25% during the winter months. In our survey,[2] HRV was related to 10% of diarrhea episodes in children living in Houston, Texas, 17% of children living in Mexico. In comparing the various published studies, it is reasonable to assume that at least 20% of cases of pediatric diarrhea worldwide are due to this agent and its related serotypes.

Norwalk-Like Agents

Distinct epidemics have been shown to be caused by infection with Norwalk-like agents. Agents responsible for the outbreaks have been named after the place of occurrence: the Norwalk, Hawaii, and Montgomery County agents. Although Norwalk-like agents are important causes of epidemic diarrhea, their role in the cause of endemic diarrhea is unknown. A major reason that so little is known about the importance of these agents relates to the difficulty in detecting the small particles in stool. Immune electron microscopy (IEM) is the only recognized technique for determining infection by Norwalk-like agents, and this procedure is not applicable for routine screening of stool specimens by laboratories other than those with special equipment, reagents, and interest in this area. Greenberg and associates[3] have developed a solid-phase microtiter radioimmunoassay (RIA) for detecting the Norwalk agent and specific humoral antibodies. Such techniques will be important to allow the efficient study of Norwalk infection and may let us determine the importance of this group of agents.

Enterotoxigenic *E. coli* (ETEC)

(ETEC) has been shown to be of major importance to adults from the United States who travel to Mexico and to the animal industry as a cause of scours among the newborns of swine and cattle. (See Chapter 9 for a discussion of the role of ETEC in travelers' diarrhea). Only three of the many studies from North America have shown high rates of identification of these organisms in children with diarrhea. In one of the first such studies from Chicago, Illinois, ETEC was found in 24 of 29 infants with diarrhea.[4] In a later report from Dallas, Texas, *E. coli* that produced heat-stable enterotoxin (ST) was found in 86% and invasive *E. coli* in 30% of children with diarrhea.[5] However, ST-producing organisms were found in 41% and invasive *E. coli* in 12% of controls in the same study. Sack and associates[6] isolated ETEC strains from 16% of Apache children with diarrhea. Other published reports of diarrhea in North America and Hawaii showed a low prevalence of toxin-producing or invasive *E. coli*.[1,2,7–10] Longitudinal, prospective studies of diarrhea in children in Canada and the United States have established that ETEC and invasive *E. coli* are not commonly associated with endemic diarrhea of children in North America.[1,2] Toxin-producing *E. coli* were isolated from stool of 1% and 4%, respectively, of children with diarrhea in Canada and the United States,[1,2] and invasive *E. coli* were not found in one study[1] and identified in only one of 255 children with gastroenteritis in the other.[2]

Studies evaluating the importance of ETEC as a cause of endemic diarrhea in children in Mexico have produced varying results. In two studies evaluating hospitalized children from an indigent population over a short period of time, ETEC strains were detected in 47% and 16%

respectively, of Mexican children with diarrhea.[11,12] In a 21-month study of outpatient children from a middle socioeconomic class, ETEC were detected in stool from 7% of Mexican children with diarrhea and 3% of controls.[2] Differences in socioeconomic class or severity of illness may have accounted for this disparity. Evidence has been put forth that asymptomatic ETEC infection in childhood may be common, in view of an increase in serum antibody to the heat-labile toxin (LT) with age.[2,13] This age-related acquisition of antibody was particularly common among Mexican children, indicating the ubiquity of the agent in that part of the world.

Serotype-Identified Enteropathogenic *E. coli* (EPEC)

The significance of EPEC as a cause of diarrhea in infants and children has been questioned, particularly since these bacteria apparently do not produce enterotoxins and are not invasive by conventional testing. The findings that these bacteria are associated with a distinct clinical illness,[14] cause diarrhea in adult volunteers,[15] and produce toxins which are nonreactive in the standard suckling mouse and tissue culture assays[16] stress the importance of reevaluating their role as a cause of gastroenteritis. The incidence of EPEC in stool specimens of children with diarrhea varies from 7 to 20%.[1,6,12,17] In a prospective study of diarrhea, Gurwith and Williams[1] reported that EPEC were found in stool of 10% of children with diarrhea, a finding which is in agreement with the many other published reports.

Shigella

Children between the ages of one and four are at highest risk of developing shigellosis. *Shigella* strains often produce outbreaks involving persons in close contact with one another, as is seen in institutions for the mentally retarded, prisons, day-care centers, and family units. This reflects the unique communicability of this enteropathogen.

In a two-year prospective study of diarrhea among children in Houston, Texas, *Shigella* was the major enteropathogen associated with endemic infectious gastroenteritis, accounting for 25% of the episodes.[2] In another prospective study of gastroenteritis among children in Canada,[1] *Shigella* accounted for 12% of diarrhea cases. Diarrhea due to this organism most commonly occurs in summer, although cases are seen throughout the year.

Salmonella

Salmonellosis has a well-established seasonal pattern, with the disease occurring most commonly during the summer months and during the November and December holidays when turkey consumption increases. It is primarily a disease of children, with over half of the cases being children less than five years of age. The attack rate among infants under one year of age has become progressively greater in recent years. Outbreaks of disease due to *Salmonella* often occur because of mishandling of food. Poultry, meat, eggs, and dairy products have been the most important vehicles of transmission, but person-to-person spread also occurs, particularly among the young, the elderly, and those confined to institutions. Gastroenteritis associated with *Salmonella* accounts for approximately 2–4% of the episodes of endemic diarrhea in children in North America.[1,2] Large outbreaks occur on occasion when a contaminated food is served to persons at restaurants and other social gatherings. These outbreaks explain the disparity between low endemic rates and apparently higher numbers of reported isolates each year (Fig. 8.1 vs. Fig. 8.2).

Multiple Enteropathogens

The finding of multiple enteropathogens in stool occurs in 2–3% of children with diarrhea in North America. The occurrence of multiple enteropathogens also has been noted in stool of children with diarrhea from Brazil (13%)[18] and the Philippines (10%)[19] and of children[2,11,12] and adults[20] from Mexico (10–25%). These combinations reflect the prevalent enteropathogens in each location and make it difficult to define the relative roles of each pathogen in episodes of gastroenteritis. Associations of multiple agents, particularly virus–bacteria interactions, have been shown in veterinary diarrhea, but there is no evidence that such a relationship exists in humans.

The Remaining Forty Percent

The various studies carried out with tissue culture assays, serologic procedures, and electron microscopic techniques still have failed to ascribe an etiologic agent in approximately 40% of diarrhea cases. Some of this diarrhea is undoubtedly caused by recently described agents such as *Campylobacter, Y. enterocolitica,* and Norwalk-like agents. Other non-*E. coli* gram-negative enteric bacteria possessing virulence properties ordinarily identified with *E. coli* and as yet undetectable viral agents will prove to also play roles in human illness. A percentage will be noninfectious in origin.

Other Toxin Producers

Enterotoxin production by gram-negative bacilli other than *V. cholerae* and *E. coli* has been recognized although not thoroughly evaluated. *Klebsiella, Aeromonas, Proteus,* and *Shigella* strains have been incriminated on occasion as toxin-producing organisms.[1,18,19,21] The significance of these strains and the nature of the substances produced are unknown. There has been no systematic search for toxin-producing Enterobacteriaceae other than *E. coli* in children with gastroenteritis, so that their relative importance is unknown.

Since we have not focused previously on *Campylobacter, noncholera vibrios, V. parahemolyticus,* and *Y. enterocolitica,* some detail will be given here.

Campylobacter

In 1957, King[22] described a group of vibrios which were similar to but not the same as *Vibrio fetus.* She suspected them of being causative agents of enteritis in infants and children. They provisionally were called "related vibrios." The term "campylobacter," meaning curved rod, was coined by Sebald and Véron when they distinguished these organisms from the true vibrios such as *V. cholerae* and *V. parahemolyticus.*[23] Véron and Chatelain considered them to be represented by two species, *Campylobacter jejuni* and *C. coli.* Smibert[24] classified them in *Bergey's Manual* as *C. fetus* ssp. *jejuni.*

Infections caused by *Campylobacter* species are common in animals and well known to veterinarians. Table 8.1 reviews important differences in these species. *C. fetus* ssp. *fetus* infects cattle and produces abortion and sterility but is not a cause of human disease. Other members of the genus have been associated with disease of domestic animals, including enteritis of calves and pigs. *C. fetus* ssp. *intestinalis* causes perinatal infections of human mothers and infants similar to those seen in cattle and sheep. *C. fetus* ssp. *jejuni* is a frequent commensal in swine and has been isolated from asymptomatic cattle, monkeys, cats, and birds.[25,26]

These organisms appear to produce disease in humans after oral ingestion,[26] although the number of organisms required to produce disease is unknown. Both common-source outbreaks and person-to-person spread have been documented.[26] In Vermont, a large outbreak of gas-

TABLE 8.1
Species of *Campylobacter fetus*

Species	Hosts	Disease states	Routes of transmission
ssp. *fetus (Vibrio fetus* ssp. *venerealis)*	Cattle	Abortion and sterility in cattle	Venereal
ssp. *intestinalis (Vibrio fetus* ssp. *intestinalis)*	Humans, cattle, chickens, goats, sheep, turkeys, other birds and mammals	Septic abortion in humans, sheep, goats, and cattle; systemic disease in humans	Contaminated food and water; direct contact with animals
ssp. *jejuni* (Related vibrio) *(Vibrio jejuni)*	Humans, cattle, chickens, dogs, goats, monkeys, sheep, swine, turkeys	Diarrhea in humans, other mammals, and birds; rarely a cause of systemic diseases in humans	Raw milk; contaminated food and water; contact with infected animals or humans

troenteritis due to *C. fetus* ssp. *jejuni* was associated with consumption of contaminated water from a public supply.[27] Some consider animal reservoirs as a likely source of *Campylobacter* infection in humans,[22] since many species such as poultry, pigs, sheep, and cattle harbor *Campylobacter*. Human infections have been traced to contact with poultry and dogs with diarrhea.[28–31] Unpasteurized milk has been suggested as a vehicle for infection by *Campylobacter*.[32–34] We do not yet know the extent to which animals contribute to human infection, either directly or indirectly.

The site of infection in affected patients appears to be the jejunum, ileum, and probably colon. *Campylobacter* has been isolated from ileal, jejunal, and gastric aspirates,[28,35,36] and acute inflammation of the jejunum has been seen at laparotomy. Karmali and Fleming[37] reported the occurrence of bloody diarrhea characteristically appearing two to four days after the onset of symptoms, suggesting the occurrence of colitis.

Clinical manifestations of infections due to *Campylobacter* include (1) perinatal infections of mothers and infants similar to those seen in cattle[38,39]; (2) gastroenteritis; and (3) bacteremia. *Campylobacter* infection usually constitutes an acute diarrheal illness, with *C. fetus* ssp. *jejuni* as the most common cause. It persists for several days with or without fever.[28] Diarrhea is the most significant feature and may be mild or profuse. The occurrence of mucus and blood in stool has varied in reports from a low of 15%[40] to 50–90% of patients with diarrhea. Most investigators feel that a bloody, mucoid stool (dysentery) is the only characteristic finding of infection. Apart from diarrhea and dysentery, outstanding symptoms include abdominal pain, fever, malaise, and occasionally headache, nausea, and vomiting.[37,40] A small number of patients (8%) may have persistent or recurrent diarrhea[40] or, less commonly, relapsing fever.[22,41] *Campylobacter* organisms may enter the bloodstream, producing septicemia during an episode of gastroenteritis. The latter is more commonly seen in patients with immunologic deficiency,[36,42] chronic alcoholism,[41] or cardiovascular disorders.[41]

A method for isolating *Campylobacter* from stool was first reported by Dekeyser and associates[43] in 1972. Using this method, which consisted of filtering stool suspensions through a 0.65-μm Millipore membrane filter, Butzler and associates[44] demonstrated that *C. fetus* commonly was associated with gastroenteritis. Subsequently, Skirrow[28] devised a selective antibiotic-containing medium for isolating the organism from stool. Specific complement-fixing antibodies to the strain of *C. fetus* ssp. *jejuni* isolated from their stool have been demonstrated in children with diarrhea.[45] Specific agglutinating antibodies appear in most patients during illness,[28,37,45] reflecting the invasive character of the organism.

The role of this organism as a cause of gastoenteritis in humans has been investigated. Studies of patients with diarrhea in Europe,[28,29,35,44] Africa,[45,46] and North America[22,27,30,32,37,47] have shown that *Campylobacter* agents can be identified in stool specimens of 3–8% of patients with diarrhea and 0–2% of healthy persons.[28,35,37,46,48] The incidence of gastroenteritis due to *Campylobacter* appears to be greatest in young children, but people of all ages may be affected.[28] Day-care nursery outbreaks of *Campylobacter* enteritis have been reported.[35] The relative importance of *Campylobacter* as a cause of gastroenteritis may be underestimated due to the special techniques required for culture and isolation of this organism. It has been estimated that the additional cost to a community hospital to culture for *Campylobacter* is $2.50/specimen.[49]

Several studies have evaluated the sensitivity of *Campylobacter* species to antimicrobial agents.[50–52] Furazolidine, the aminoglycosides, tetracycline, erythromycin, and chloramphenicol were active against most strains tested, while penicillin, ampicillin, and the cephalosporins were relatively inactive. Clindamycin, metronidazole, ticarcillin, and carbenicillin also may show activity against *Campylobacter* isolates.[52] Isolation of *Campylobacter* from stool does not imply the need for antibotics. The decision should be made on clinical grounds; however, therapy may reduce fecal losses.[37] In patients with *Campylobacter* enteritis, either erythromycin or tetracyline probably represents the agent of choice when a decision has been made to initiate therapy. The treatment of choice for patients with septicemia appears to be an aminoglycoside, although chloramphenicol, tetracycline, and erythromycin have been effective.

Noncholera Vibrios and *V. parahemolyticus*

V. cholerae is classified by biochemical reaction. To be further differentiated into the causative agent of cholera, the strain must agglutinate in vibrio O group 1 antiserum.[53] Noncholera vibrios (NCVs), also referred to as nonagglutinable vibrios (NAGs), biochemically are identical to *V. cholerae* (and they are so classed), but they are not agglutinable. The NCV strains generally share common proteases, alkaline phosphatases, and H antigen with the cholera bacillus,[54] and a similar enterotoxin may be elaborated.[55,56] NCV strains cause an illness similar to cholera, and although severe dehydration requiring hospitalization and intravenous therapy may occur, lower case fatalities than those produced by cholera have been reported.[57,58] NCV infections may occur during cholera epidemics,[57,58] although they also occur in areas where cholera is not endemic, including the United States.[59] The usual mode of transmission is ingestion of contaminated seafood, especially shellfish, although water may be a source in developing regions. NCVs can also cause septicemia, biliary tract infection, and wound infection.[59] When wound infection occurs, it usually follows exposure to salt water.[60]

V. parahemolyticus, a motile halophilic vibrio, is part of the normal flora of estuarine waters during warm months.[61,62] It has been known to be the major cause of food poisoning in Japan for more than two decades.[63] Food-borne illness in the western hemisphere was first reported to have occurred in 1971.[64] Nearly all strains associated with human illness produce hemolysis on Watatsuma blood agar. These strains are said to be Kanagawa-positive. Most strains isolated from fish and water are Kanagawa-negative, or "nonhemolytic."[65] In all probability, these strains differ quantitatively in hemolysin production.[66] Strains of *V. parahemolyticus*, especially those found to be Kanagawa-positive, produce fluid distention of the ligated rabbit ileal loop,[63–67] although false-positive reactions due to high salt concentrations of the filtrates may be a factor.[68] *V. parahemolyticus* infection results when seafood contaminated with the organism is ingested. In Japan, the problem is so prevalent because of the common consumption of raw or poorly cooked seafood. In the United States, seafood that is recontaminated after cooking may be the most common setting for disease occurrence.[64,69] The disease is associated with abdominal cramps, nausea, vomiting, and diarrhea. A dysenteric form of the disease occurs.[70] The incubation period is between 4 and 96 hr and typically occurs after 15 hr.[69]

The importance of noncholera vibrios and *V. parahemolyticus* as causes of enteric infection is unknown. A major problem in most regions where cholera is not seen is failure to use proper media to isolate the agents. The preferred medium is thiosulfate–citrate bile salts–sucrose (TCBS) agar.[71] We will not consider the other vibrios for which little information exists regarding pathogenicity and role in human illness: *Vibrio alginolyticus*, "unnamed" marine vibrios, and the miscellaneous halophilic vibrios.

Yersinia enterocolitica

Yersinia enterocolitica is a member of the Enterobacteriaceae family and belongs to the genus that includes *Y. pestis* and *Y. pseudotuberculosis*. It is a gram-negative, coccobacillary organism first reported as pathogenic for humans in New York State in 1933.[72] It appears to be a common cause of gastroenteritis among children in Europe and Canada[73–77] only rarely being recognized in the United States. Since the identification of *Y. enterocolitica* in stool is difficult when using conventional culture methods, the specific frequency of occurrence of this agent as a cause of gastroenteritis in the United States is unknown.

While most reported cases of disease due to *Y. enterocolitica* have been reported from Europe, particularly the Scandinavian countries, the organism is prevalent worldwide.[78] The incidence of gastroenteritis due to this organism has been reported to be lower in summer months, but this pattern has not been consistent.[73,76,79,80] *Y. enterocolitica* has been recovered from wild and domestic animals,[81–83] raw and pasteurized milk,[84,85] water,[86,87] and oysters.[83] Infection in humans has been associated with exposure to contaminated milk,[85] water,[88] and animals,[83,89–91] although the overall significance of environmental exposure remains obscure. Person-to-person transmission has been documented.[74,75,79,88,92,93]

Clinical manifestations (Table 8.2) produced by *Y. enterocolitica* vary with age and state of health. The illness associated with this organism that occurs most commonly in children less than five years of age is a self-limiting gastroenteritis. The stools may contain blood and mucus,[75,94,95] indicating the presence of a colitis, or profuse watery diarrhea, thought to be due to toxin production, may occur.[96] Associated symptoms consisting of fever, vomiting, or abdominal pain are reported in up to 60–80% of these patients.[75,76,85,93,94] Duration of illness is generally two weeks; however, chronic diarrhea, intestinal ulceration, or perforation and peritonitis may occur.[93,94,97] Children over five years of age present with abdominal pain that mimics acute appendicitis[76,85,91] and is often associated with colitis and aphthous ulcers of the gastrointestinal

Table 8.2
Clinical Characteristics of Patients with *Yersinia enterocolitica* Infection

Patients	Clinical manifestations
Infants and young children (<5 yr)	Gastroenteritis with fever
Older children	Pseudoappendicitis, diarrhea
Adults	Arthralgia, polyarthritis, erythema nodosum, diarrhea and abdominal pain (less often)
Immunocompromised	Bacteremia, abscesses of liver and spleen

tract.[98] Adults develop diarrhea and abdominal pain less often than do children but may present with polyarthritis, arthralgia, or erythema nodosum.[79,80,91,99–101] Septicemia has been reported in otherwise healthy children and adults[88,94,102] but generally occurs in immunocompromised patients.[73,93,103–105]

The isolation of *Y. enterocolitica* from blood or other normally sterile body fluids is not difficult; however, its isolation from stool specimens by conventional methods is difficult due to overgrowth by other bacteria. The ability of *Yersinia* to grow at 4 and 25°C offers a means of isolating it from stool that contains other gram-negative bacilli.[106] There is evidence that *Y. enterocolitica* is both invasive to the intestinal tract and enterotoxigenic. Undoubtedly, the dysenteric form reflects the invasive character of the organism, and certain isolates have been shown to invade He La cells[107] and produce keratoconjunctivitis in the guinea pig eye model.[108] The syndrome of profuse diarrhea probably reflects active small-intestinal secretion, perhaps secondary to elaboration of a heat-stable enterotoxin.[108,109]

The efficacy of antibiotic therapy in eradicating clinical symptoms and fecal shedding of the organism in patients with gastroenteritis is unknown.[75,78,85] In patients with chronic or fulminating infection, success has been achieved with chloramphenicol, gentamicin, or colistin[73,88,104]; however, the results have been variable, and the drug of choice has not been established. There is little information at present to indicate that antibiotics shorten the course of gastroenteritis.

FOOD-BORNE DIARRHEAL ILLNESS

Food serves as an excellent culture medium for microbial agents and probably is a more important vehicle of disease transmission than is usually considered. Development of symptomatic disease following ingestion of food contaminated with microorganisms generally correlates with one of three factors: (1) the number of viable organisms per gram of food; (2) the presence of a highly virulent or aggressive agent which is able to either produce a toxin or invade the intestinal lining; and (3) the presence of a host factor such as achlorhydria, prior gastric surgery, agammaglobulinemia, protein–calorie malnutrition, or extremes of age.

Almost any bacterial species is capable of producing intestinal symptoms if swallowed in sufficient numbers. If the organism is not a high-grade (virulent) pathogen, only one to several loose bowel movements develop when a large inoculum of bacteria is ingested. On the other hand, a far lower number of bacteria produces striking diarrhea when the agent possesses inherent virulence properties (*Shigella, Salmonella*, ETEC, *Giardia* or *E. histolytica* cysts, etc.). Finally, recurrent diarrhea occurs in persons lacking local intestinal immune factors such as high gastric acidity, normal intestinal motility patterns, or local antibody production (see Chapter 1, which deals with intestinal immune factors) when contaminated food is ingested.

TABLE 8.3
The Important Causes of Food-Borne Diarrheal Illness

| Agent | Epidemiology | | Clinical features | | |
	Incubation period (hr)	Secondary spread	Fever	Vomiting	Diagnosis
Staphylococcus aureus	1–5	None	Absent	Profuse	Characteristic epidemiologic and clinical picture
Clostridium perfringens	8–22	Unusual	Absent	Minimal	Characteristic epidemiologic and clinical picture
Enterotoxigenic Esherichia coli	8–96	Unknown	Absent or low-grade	Occasional	Detection of agent in stool specimens or rise in humoral antibody to toxin
Bacillus cereus	2–20	Unusual	Absent	Occasional	Isolation of organism from food and/or stool
Salmonella	8–24	Occasional	Common	Common	Isolation of organism from food and/or stool
Shigella	7–120	Common	Common	Occasional	Isolation of organism from food and/or stool
Vibrio parahemolyticus	12–24	Unusual	Occasional	Occasional	Isolation of organism from food and/or stool

Figure 8.2 illustrates the relative importance of the common causes of food-borne diarrhea in the United States. Listed are percentages of the total number of cases of diarrhea confirmed by etiology. Infection by certain agents such as *C. perfringens* and *Salmonella* species produces large outbreaks, so that the number of cases is large but the number of outbreaks is rather small. This is in sharp contrast to agents which usually produce only a few cases per outbreak, such as *Clostridium botulinum.*

Table 8.3 demonstrates the clinical features of food-borne diarrhea which separate the various agents. By determining the number of associated cases, the incubation period, and the degree of vomiting and fever, the etiologic diagnosis should be suspected before the laboratory is able to offer confirmation.

Food-borne diarrhea is suggested when two or more persons experience a similar illness after ingestion of a common meal. It is important to attempt to establish an etiology of food-borne disease, since it will allow the development of an optimal plan for treating affected patients and for instituting appropriate measures to limit secondary spread or prevent further cases in an epidemic. Also, knowledge of the specific agent may help suggest the food that is responsible, implicate a food handler, or identify faulty food-handling practices.

REFERENCES

1. Gurwith, M. J., Williams, T. W. Gastroenteritis in children: A two-year review in Manitobia: I. Etiology. *J. Infect. Dis.* **136**:239–247, 1977.
2. Pickering, L. K., Evans, D. J., Jr., Mũnoz, O., et al. Prospective study of enteropathogens in children with diarrhea in Houston and Mexico. *J. Pediatr.* **93**:383–388, 1978.
3. Greenberg, H. B., Wyatt, R. G., Valdesuso, J., et al. Solid-phase microtiter radioimmunoassay for detection of the Norwalk strain of acute nonbacterial, epidemic gastroenteritis virus and its antibody. *J. Med. Virol.* **2**:97–108, 1978.
4. Gorbach, S. L., Khurana, C. M. Toxigenic *Escherichia coli*: A cause of infantile diarrhea in Chicago. *N. Engl. J. Med.* **287**:791–795, 1972.
5. Rudoy, R. C., Nelson, J. D. Enteroinvasive and enterotoxigenic *Escherichia coli*: Occurrence in acute diarrhea of infants and children. *Am. J. Dis. Child.* **129**:668–672, 1975.
6. Sack, R. B., Hirschhorn, N., Brownlee, I., et al. Enterotoxigenic *Escherichia coli*-associated diarrheal disease in Apache children. *N. Engl. J. Med.* **292**:1041–1045, 1975.
7. Kapikian, A. Z., Kim, H. W., Wyatt, R. G., et al. Human reovirus-like agent as the major pathogen associated with "winter" gastroenteritis in hospitalized infants and young children. *N. Engl. J. Med.* **294**:965–972, 1976.
8. Echeverria, P., Ho, M. T., Blacklow, N. R., et al. Relative importance of viruses and bacteria in the etiology of pediatric diarrhea in Taiwan. *J. Infect. Dis.* **136**:383–390, 1977.
9. Echeverria, P., Blacklow, N. R., Smith, D. H., Role of heat-labile toxigenic *Escherichia coli* and reovirus-like agent in diarrhoea in Boston children. *Lancet* **2**:1113–1116, 1975.
10. Dean, A. G., Ching, Y. C., Williams, R. G., et al. Test for *Escherichia coli* enterotoxin using infant mice: Application in a study of diarrhea in children in Honolulu. *J. Infect. Dis.* **125**:407–411, 1972.

11. Evans, D. G., Olarte, J., DuPont, H. L., *et al.* Enteropathogens associated with pediatric diarrhea in Mexico City. *J. Pediatr.* **91**:65–68, 1977.

12. Donta, S. T., Wallace, R. B., Whipp, S. C., *et al.* Enterotoxigenic *Escherichia coli* and diarrheal disease in Mexican children. *J. Infect. Dis.* **135**:482–485, 1977.

13. Ruiz-Palacios, G., Evans, D. G., Evans, D. J., Jr., *et al.* Age-related acquisition of IgG and IgM antibodies to heat-labile enterotoxin of *Escherichia coli* (abstract). In *Abstracts of the Annual Meeting of the American Society for Microbiology,* Las Vegas, Nev., May 17, 1978.

14. Gurwith, M. J., Wiseman, D. A., Chow, P. Clinical and laboratory assessment of the pathogenicity of serotyped enteropathogenic *Escherichia coli. J. Infect. Dis.* **135**:735–743, 1977.

15. Levine, M. M., Berggwist, E. J., Nalin, D. R., *et al. Escherichia coli* strains that cause diarrhoea but do not produce heat-labile or heat-stable enterotoxins and are non-invasive. *Lancet* **2**:1119–1122, 1978.

16. Klipstein F. A., Rowe, B., Engert, R. F., *et al.* Enterotoxigenicity of enteropathogenic serotypes of *Escherichia coli* isolated from infants with epidemic diarrhea. *Infect. Immun.* **21**:171–178, 1978.

17. Rodriguez, W. J., Kim, H. W., Arrobio, J. O., *et al.* Clinical features of acute gastroenteritis associated with human reovirus-like agent in infants and young children. *J. Pediatr.* **91**:188–193, 1977.

18. Guerrant, R. L., Moore, R. A., Kirshenfeld, P. M., *et al.* Role of toxigenic and invasive bacteria in acute diarrhea of childhood. *N. Engl. J. Med.* **293**:567–572, 1975.

19. Echeverria, P., Blacklow, N. R., Vollet, J. L., III, *et al.* Reovirus-like agent and enterotoxigenic *Escherichia coli* infections in pediatric diarrhea in the Philippines. *J. Infect. Dis.* **138**:326–332, 1978.

20. DuPont, H. L., Olarte, J., Evans, D. G., *et al.* Comparative susceptibility of Latin American and United States students to enteric pathogens. *N. Engl. J. Med.* **295**:1520–1521, 1976.

21. Wadstrom, T., Aust-Kettis, A., Habte, D., *et al.* Enterotoxin-producing bacteria and parasites in stools of Ethiopian children with diarrheal disease. *Arch. Dis. Child.* **51**:865–870, 1976.

22. King, E. O. Human infections with *Vibrio fetus* and a closely related vibrio. *J. Infect. Dis.* **101**:119–128, 1957.

23. Véron, M., Chatelain, R. Taxonomic study of the genus *Campylobacter* Sebald and Véron and designation of the neotype strain for the type species, *Campylobacter fetus* (Smith and Taylor) Sebald and Veron. *Int. J. Syst. Bacteriol.* **23**:122–134, 1973.

24. Smibert, R. M. In R. E. Buchanan & N.E. Gibbons (eds.), *Bergey's Manual of Determinative Bacteriology,* 8th ed. Williams & Wilkins, Baltimore, 1974, pp. 207–212.

25. Bryner, J. H., O'Berry, P. A., Estes, P. C., *et al.* Studies of vibrios from gallbladder of market sheep and cattle. *Am. J. Vet. Res.* **33**:1439–1444, 1972.

26. Butzler, J. P., Dekegel, D., Hubrechts, J. M., *et al.* Mode of transmission of human campylobacteriosis. In W. Siegenthaler & R. Luthy (eds.), *Current Chemotherapy: Proceedings of the 10th International Congress of Chemotherapy,* Vol. 1. American Society for Microbiology, Washington, D. C., 1978, pp. 174–175.

27. United States Department of Health, Education and Welfare, Public Health Service, Center for Disease Control. Waterborne *Campylobacter* gastroenteritis—Vermont. *Morbid. Mortal. Week. Rep.* **27**:207, 1978.

28. Skirrow, M. B. *Campylobacter* enteritis: A "new" disease. *Br. Med. J.* **2**:9–11, 1977.

29. Lindquist, B., Kjellander, J., Kosunen, T. *Campylobacter* enteritis in Sweden. *Br. Med. J.* **1**:303, 1978.

30. Wheeler, W. E., Borchers, J. Vibrionic enteritis in infants. *Am. J. Dis. Child.* **101**:60–66, 1961.

31. Blaser, M., Carvens, J., Powers, B. W., *et al. Campylobacter* enteritis associated with canine infection. *Lancet* **2**:979–981, 1978.
32. United States Department of Health, Education and Welfare, Public Health Service, Center for Disease Control. *Campylobacter* enteritis—Colorado. *Morbid. Mortal. Week. Rep.* **27**:226, 231, 1978.
33. Levy, A. J. A gastro-enteritis outbreak probably due to a bovine strain of vibrio. *Yale J. Biol. Med.* **18**:243–258, 1946.
34. Communicable Disease Surveillance Centre. Outbreaks of campylobacter infection. *Commun. Dis. Rep.* **78**:20, 1978.
35. Lauwers, S., DeBoeck, M., Butzler, J. P. *Campylobacter* enteritis in Brussels. *Lancet* **1**:604–605, 1978.
36. Cadranel, S., Rodesch, P., Butzler, J. P., *et al.* Enteritis due to "related vibrio" in children. *Am. J. Dis. Child.* **126**:152–155, 1973.
37. Karmali, M. A., Fleming, P. C. *Campylobacter* enteritis in children. *J. Pediatr.* **94**:527–533, 1979.
38. Vinzent, R., Dumas, J., Picard, N. Septicémie grave au cours de la grossesse, due à un vibrion: Avortement consécutif. *Bull. Acad. Natl. Méd. Paris* **131**:90–92, 1947.
39. Eden, A. N. Perinatal mortality caused by *Vibrio fetus. J. Pediatr.* **68**:297–304, 1966.
40. Communicable Disease Surveillance Centre. Reports of campylobacter isolates in 1977. *Commun. Dis. Rep.* **78**:13, 1978.
41. Bokkenheuser, V. *Vibrio fetus* infection in man: I. Ten new cases and some epidemiologic observations. *Am. J. Epidemiol.* **91**:400–409, 1970.
42. Wyatt, R. A., Younoszai, K., Anuras, S., *et al. Campylobacter fetus* septicemia and hepatitis in a child with agammaglobulinemia. *J. Pediatr.* **91**:441–442, 1977.
43. Dekeyser, P., Gossuin-Detrain, M., Butzler, J. P., *et al.* Acute enteritis due to related vibrio: First positive stool cultures. *J. Infect. Dis.* **125**:390–392, 1972.
44. Butzler, J. P., Dekeyser, P., Detrain, M., *et al.* Related vibrio in stool. *J. Pediatr.* **82**:493–495, 1973.
45. Butzler, J. P. Related vibrios in Africa. *Lancet* **2**:858, 1973.
46. DeMol, P., Bosmans, E. *Campylobacter* enteritis in central Africa. *Lancet* **1**:604, 1978.
47. Laboratory Centre for Disease Control. *Campylobacter* enteritis—Ontario. *Can. Dis. Week. Rep.* **4**:57–58, 1978.
48. Butzler, J. P., Dereume, J. P., Barbier, P., *et al.* L'origine digestive des septicèmies à campylobacter. *Nouv. Presse. Méd.* **6**:1033–1035, 1977.
49. United States Department of Health, Education and Welfare, Public Health Service, Center for Disease Control. *Campylobacter* enteritis—Iowa. *Morbid. Mortal. Week. Rep.* **28**:565–566, 1979.
50. Butzler, J. P., Dekeyser, P., Lafontaine, T. Susceptibility of related vibrios and *Vibrio fetus* to twelve antibiotics. *Antimicrob. Agents Chemother.* **5**:86–89, 1974.
51. Vanhoof, R., Vanderlinden, M. P., Dierickx, R., *et al.* Susceptibility of *Campylobacter fetus* subsp. *jejuni* to twenty-nine antimicrobial agents. *Antimicrob. Agents Chemother.* **14**:553–556, 1978.
52. Chow, A. W., Patten, V., Bednorz, D. Susceptibility of *Campylobacter fetus* to twenty-two antimicrobial agents. *Antimicrob. Agents Chemother.* **13**:416–418, 1978.
53. Gardner, A. D., Venkatraman, K. V. The antigens of the cholera group of vibrios. *J. Hyg. (London)* **35**:262–282, 1935.
54. Hsi-Chia, H., Liu, P. V. Serological identities of proteases and alkaline phosphatases of the so-called nonagglutinable (NAG) vibrios and those of *Vibrio cholerae. J. Infect. Dis.* **121**:251–259, 1970.
55. Zinnaka, Y., Carpenter, C. C., J., Jr. An enterotoxin produced by noncholera vibrios. *Johns Hopkins Med. J.* **131**:403–411, 1972.
56. Ohashi, M., Shimada, T., Fukumi, H. *In vitro* production of enterotoxin and hemorrhagic principle by *Vibrio cholerae*, NAG. *Jpn. J. Med. Sci. Biol.* **25**:179–194, 1972.

57. McIntyre, O. R., Feeley, J. C., Greenough, W. B., III, *et al.* Diarrhea caused by noncholera vibrios. *Am. J. Trop. Med.* **14**:412–418, 1965.

58. El-Shawi, N., Thewaini, A. J. Nonagglutinable vibrios isolated in the 1966 epidemic of cholera in Iraq. *Bull. W. H. O.* **40**:163–166, 1969.

59. Hughes, J. M., Hollis, D. G., Gangarosa, E. J., *et al.* Noncholera vibrio infections in the United States. Clinical, epidemiologic and laboratory features. *Ann. Intern. Med.* **88**:602–606, 1978.

60. Back, E., Ljunggren, A., Smith, H., Jr. Noncholera vibrios in Sweden. Lancet **1**:723–724, 1974.

61. Miyamoto, Y., Nakamura, K., Takizawa, K. Seasonal distribution of *Oceanomonas* spp., halophilic bacteria, in the coastal sea: Its significance in epidemiology and marine industry. *Jap. J. Microbiol.* **6**:141–158, 1962.

62. Kaneko, T., Colwell, R. R. Distribution of *Vibrio parahaemolyticus* and related organisms in the Atlantic Ocean off South Carolina and Georgia. *Appl. Microbiol* **28**:1009–1017, 1974.

63. Sakazaki, R., Iwanami, S., Fukumi, H. Studies on the enteropathogenic, facultatively halophilic bacteria, *Vibrio parahaemolyticus:* I. Morphological, cultural, and biochemical properties and its taxonomical position. *Jpn. J. Med. Sci. Biol.* **16**:161–188, 1963.

64. Dadisman, T. A., Jr., Nelson, R., Molenda, J. R., *et al. Vibrio parahaemolyticus* gastroenteritis in Maryland: I. Clinical and epidemiologic aspects. *Am. J. Epidemiol.* **96**:414–426, 1972.

65. Sakazaki, R., Tamura, K., Kato, T., *et al.* Studies on the enteropathogenic, facultatively halophilic bacteria, *Vibrio parahaemolyticus:* III. Enteropathogenicity. *Jpn. J. Med. Sci. Biol.* **21**:325–331, 1968.

66. Chun, D., Chung, J. K., Tak, R., *et al.* Nature of the Kanagawa phenomenon of *Vibrio parahaemolyticus. Infect. Immun.* **12**:81–87, 1975.

67. Zen-Yoji, H., Sakai, S., Terayama, T.,*et al.* Epidemiology, enteropathogenicity, and classification of *Vibrio parahaemolyticus. J. Infect. Dis.* **115**:436–444, 1965.

68. Johnson, D. E., Calia, F. M., False-positive rabbit ileal loop reactions attributed to *Vibrio parahaemolyticus* broth filtrates. *J. Infect. Dis.* **133**:436–440, 1976.

69. Lawrence, D. N., Blake, R. A., Yashuk, J. C., *et al. Vibrio parahaemolyticus* gastroenteritis outbreaks aboard two cruise ships. *Am. J. Epidemiol.* **109**:71–80, 1979.

70. Hughes, J. M., Boyce, J. M., Aleem, A. R. M. A., *et al. Vibrio parahaemolyticus* gastroenteritis in Bangladesh: Report of an outbreak. *Am. J. Trop. Med. Hyg.* **27**:106–112, 1978.

71. Gangarosa, E. J., Dewitt, W. E., Hug, I., *et al.* Laboratory methods in cholera: Isolation of *Vibrio cholerae* (El Tor and classical) on TCBS medium in minimally equipped laboratories. *Trans. R. Soc. Trop. Med. Hyg.* **62**:693–699, 1968.

72. Gilbert, R. Interesting cases and unusual specimens. *N.Y. State Dep. Health Annu. Rep. Div. Lab. Res.* **1933**:57.

73. Mollaret, H. H. L'infection humaine à "*Yersinia enterocolitica*" en 1970, à la lumière de 642 cas recents: Aspects cliniques et perspectives epidemiologiques. *Pathol. Biol.* **19**:189–205, 1971.

74. Lafleur, L., Marineau, B., Chicoine, L. *Yersinia enterocolitica:* Aspects biologiques, épidémiologiques et cliniques de 67 cas observés à l'Hôpital Sainte-Justine (Montreal, Canada). *Union Méd. Can.* **101**:2407–2413, 1972.

75. Bergstrand, C. G., Winblad, S. Clinical manifestations of infection with *Yersinia enterocolitica* in children. *Acta Paediatr. Scand.* **63**:875–877, 1974.

76. Delorme, J., Laverdiere, M., Martineau, B., *et al.* Yersiniosis in children. *Can. Med. Assoc. J.* **110**:281–284, 1974.

77. Schieven, B. C., Randall, C. Enteritis due to *Yersinia enterocolitica. J. Pediatr.* **84**:402–404, 1974.

78. Bottone, E. J. *Yersinia enterocolitica:* A panoramic view of a charismatic microorganism. *CRC Crit. Rev. Microbiol.* **52:**211–241, 1977.
79. Arvastson, B., Damgaard, K., Winblad, S. Clinical symptoms of infection with *Yersinia enterocolitica. Scand. J. Infect. Dis.* **3:**37–40,1971.
80. Leino, R., Kalliomaki, J. L. Yersiniosis as an internal disease. *Ann. Intern. Med.* **81:**458–461, 1974.
81. Hubbert, W. T. Yersiniosis in mammals and birds in the United States: Case reports and review. *Am. J. Trop. Med. Hyg.* **21:**458–463, 1972.
82. Mair, N. S. Yersiniosis in wildlife and its public health implications. *J. Wildl. Dis.* **9:**64–71, 1973.
83. Toma, S. Survey on the incidence of *Yersinia enterocolitica* in the province of Ontario. *Can. J. Public Health* **64:**477–487, 1973.
84. Schieman, D. A., Toma, S. Isolation of *Yersinia enterocolitica* from raw milk. *Appl. Environ. Microbiol.* **35:**54–58, 1978.
85. Black, R. E., Jackson, R. J., Tsai, T., *et al.* Epidemic *Yersinia enterocolitica* infection due to contaminated chocolate milk. *N. Engl. J. Med.* **289:**76–79, 1978.
86. Highsmith, A. K., Feeley, J. C., Skaliy, P., *et al.* Isolation of *Yersinia enterocolitica* from well water and growth in distilled water. *Appl. Environ. Microbiol.* **34:**745–750, 1977.
87. Lassen, J. *Yersinia enterocolitica* in drinking water. *Scand. J. Infect. Dis.* **4:**125–127, 1972.
88. Keet, E. E. *Yersinia enterocolitica* septicemia—source of infection and incubation period identified. *N. Y. State J. Med.* **74:**2226–2230, 1974.
89. Tsubokura, M., Otsuki, K., Itagaki, K. Studies on *Yersinia enterocolitica:* I. Isolation of *Y. enterocolitica* from swine. *Jpn. J. Vet. Sci.* **35:**419–424, 1973.
90. Rabson, A. R., Koornhof, H. J., Notman, J., *et al.* Hepatosplenic abscesses due to *Yersinia enterocolitica. Br. Med. J.* **4:**341, 1972.
91. Ahvonen, P. Human yersiniosis in Finland: II. Clinical features. *Ann. Clin. Res.* **4:**39–48, 1972.
92. Toivanen, P., Toivanen, A., Olkkonen, L., *et al.* Hospital outbreak of *Yersinia enterocolitica* infection. *Lancet* **1:**801–803, 1973.
93. Kohl, S., Jacobson, J. A., Nahmias, A. *Yersinia enterocolitica* infections in children. *J. Pediatr.* **89:**77–79, 1976.
94. Gutman, L. T., Ottesen, E. A., Quan, T. J., *et al.* An inter-familial outbreak of *Yersinia enterocolitica* enteritis. *N. Engl. J. Med.* **288:**1372–1377, 1973.
95. Maki, M., Gronroos, P., Vesikari, T. *In vitro* Invasiveness of *Yersinia enterocolitica* isolated from children with diarrhea. *J. Infect. Dis.* **138:**677–680, 1978.
96. Pai, C. H., Mors, V., Toma, S. Prevalence of enterotoxigenicity in human and nonhuman isolates of *Yersinia enterocolitica. Infect. Immun.* **22:**334–338, 1978.
97. Bradford, W. D., Noce, P. S., Gutman, L. T. Pathologic features of enteric infection with *Yersinia enterocolitica. Arch. Pathol.* **98:**17–22, 1974.
98. Vantrappen, G., Agg, H. O., Ponette, E., *et al. Yersinia* enteritis and enterocolitis: Gastroenterological aspects. *Gastroenterology* **72:**220–227, 1977.
99. Ahvonen, P., Rossi, T. Familial occurrence of *Yersinia enterocolitica* infection and acute arthritis. *Acta Paediatr. Scand. Suppl.* **206:**121–122, 1970.
100. Laitinen, O., Tuuhea, J., Ahvonen, P. Polyarthritis associated with *Yersinia enterocolitica* infection: Clinical features and laboratory findings in nine cases with severe joint symptoms. *Ann. Rheum. Dis.* **31:**34–39, 1972.
101. Winblad, S. Erythema nodosum associated with infection with *Yersinia enterocolitica. Scand. J. Infect. Dis.* **1:**11–16, 1969.

102. Bissett, M. L. *Yersinia enterocolitica* isolates from humans in California, 1968–1975. *J. Clin. Microbiol.* **4**:137–144, 1976.
103. Abramovitch, H., Butas, C. A. Septicemia due to *Yersinia enterocolitica. Can. Med. Assoc. J.* **109**:1112–1115, 1973.
104. Rabson, A. R., Hallett, A. F., Koornhof, H. J. Generalized *Yersinia enterocolitica* infection. *J. Infect. Dis.* **131**:447–451, 1975.
105. Spira, T. J., Kabins, S. A. *Yersinia enterocolitica* septicemia with septic arthritis. *Arch. Intern. Med.* **136**:1305–1308, 1976.
106. Nilehn, B. Studies on *Yersinia enterocolitica* with special reference to bacterial diagnosis and occurrence in human enteric disease. *Acta Pathol. Microbiol. Scand. Suppl.* **206**:1–48, 1969.
107. Lee. W. H., McGrath, P. P., Carter, P. H., *et al.* The ability of some *Yersinia enterocolitica* strains to invade HeLa cells. *Can. J. Microbiol.* **23**:1714–1722, 1977.
108. Boyce, J. M., Evans, D. J., Jr., Evans, D. G., *et al.* Production of heat-stable, methanol-soluble enterotoxin by *Yersinia enterocolitica. Infect. Immun.* **25**:532–537, 1979.
109. Pai, C. H., Mors, V., Toma, S. Prevalence of enterotoxigenicity in human and nonhuman isolates of *Yersinia enterocolitica. Infect. Immun.* **22**:234–338, 1978.

9

Diarrhea of Travelers (Emporiatric Enteritis)

INTRODUCTION

Travelers from certain industrialized countries who visit less well-developed areas, particularly areas with reduced levels of food hygiene and water sanitation, run a special risk of developing diarrhea. Thoughts of how to prevent the common problem or how best to treat it occupy the minds of nearly all travelers. The economic aspects of travelers' diarrhea are profound. Considering that $45 billion per year is spent by persons crossing national boundaries, that a high percentage of travelers develop troublesome diarrhea which often modifies the travel itinerary, and that nearly everyone purchases drugs to prevent or treat the disorder, the overall cost to the traveler is great. The economic implications to developing countries are of even greater importance. It has been projected that by the early 1980s, persons from various regions will spend $100 billion in foreign travel.[1] If the current travel trends continue, 80% of these dollars will be spent in travel to Canada, Japan, and western Europe, while only 20% will be spent in the developing areas where economic support is needed the most. If the threat of diarrhea could be lessened, greater travel to Latin America, Africa, and Asia undoubtedly would be stimulated. A great deal of new information recently has become available in this area, and many researchers in the field are encouraged about the future.

MAGNITUDE OF THE PROBLEM AND POPULATIONS AT RISK

Travelers from the United States to Mexico commonly experience diarrhea, usually within the first two weeks after arrival. The frequency of troublesome illness among travelers ranges from 30 to 80% in published studies and generally occurs in about half. The problem is most profound for persons from industrialized countries who travel to developing areas with decreased levels of food and personal hygiene. Diarrhea is most important for persons from the United States, Canada, northern Europe, and Australia who travel to Latin America or Asia; illness is less important for those from Italy, Spain, Portugal, the Far East, Africa, and Latin America when traveling to the same countries.[2,3] High rates of illness among foreign travelers to a country appear to parallel high rates of diarrhea endemicity among the indigenous population, as has been observed in Latin America,[2,4-7] Iran,[3] and Egypt.[8] Younger-aged travelers seem to be more susceptible to developing enteric symptoms.[5,9] In studies of British troops stationed in Egypt during 1939–1945, it was observed that high rates of illness were characteristic during the first months after arrival and dramatically fell during the second year in Egypt.[10] Similar observations were made among United States students in Mexico, where diarrhea rates were 40% per month for those newly arrived from the United States and half that, or 20%, for others who had been attending classes at the school for a year or longer.[7] In this same study, the diarrhea rates and severity of illness among Latin American students were the lowest (see Table 9.1). Serum antibody titers to heat-labile *E. coli* enterotoxin (LT) among the students correlated with susceptibility to infection (see Figure 9.1). Among those developing illness, there was a rise in the geometric mean serum LT antibody titer during convalescence. It was of interest that the lowest baseline antibody titers were seen in the newly arrived United States students and in the Latin American students who developed illness. The highest baseline titers were seen in the Latin American students who failed to develop illness.

Kean and Smillie found that the incidence of diarrhea among United States students visiting northern Europe during the summer of 1953 was half that of students visiting Mediterranean countries.[11] Others have commented upon the common occurrence of illness among travelers to Mediterranean countries as compared to England and Scandinavia.[9] These various studies have identified high-risk areas—Latin America, Mediterranean European countries, Far East, and Africa (with the exception of the developed cities of South Africa)—and low-risk areas—United States, Canada, northern Europe, and Australia. The risk of acquiring

TABLE 9.1
Incidence of Acute Diarrhea among Students in Mexico during a One-Month Period of Study

Prior geographic location	Number studied	Diarrhea[a,b]
United States		
Newly arrived students	55	22 (40)
Full-time students	142	28 (20)
Latin America	95	11 (12)

[a]Defined as twice the normal daily frequency of unformed stools together with abdominal cramps, pain, fever, nausea, or vomiting.
[b]Numbers in parentheses represent percentages.

illness in the remaining countries is unknown (see Figure 9.2). There is epidemiologic information that persons traveling from one high-risk area to a different high-risk area experience fewer problems,[2,3,7] indicating the ubiquity of the common enteropathogens in each of these areas. There is evidence that persons from high-risk areas such as Mexico or Asia may experience diarrhea when traveling to an area of low risk such as the United States[12–14] and that persons from low-risk areas may commonly experience diarrhea when traveling to another low-risk country.[14] However, this concept has been overemphasized. Diarrhea occurred in only three of 147 foreign study participants at a conference held in Miami, Florida.[15] A prospective study of Mexican students traveling to California suggested that diarrhea was common among those newly arrived but that it was mild and clinically unimportant.[13] A mild to moderate change in bowel habits probably is common among travelers regardless of country of origin and place of travel, possibly due to altered dietary and alcohol consumption patterns, exposure to normally nonpathogenic bacteria in higher than usual concentrations (as, for example, in food), or psychic or emotional factors. It is likely that the severe and disabling form of illness is common, however, only to travelers from low to high risk areas. Figure 9.3 demonstrates a relationship between the number of diarrheal stools passed during a 48-hr period of observation and the identification of an enteropathogen in a United States student population newly arrived in Mexico for study. An agent was identified in stool in slightly more than one-third of cases when the illness consisted of passing fewer than ten unformed stools during a 48-hr period. In more intense disease (ten or more unformed stools during the time of observation), an enteropathogen was confirmed in diarrheal stool of 85% of students. These data support our hypotheses that diarrhea is common among travelers and that it may not always reflect intestinal infection, particularly

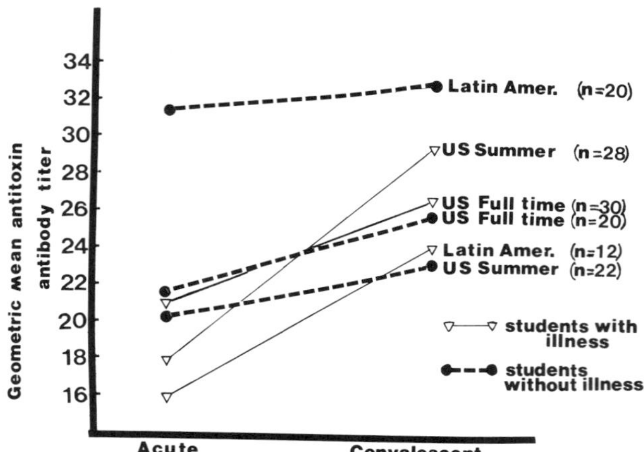

Figure 9.1. Acute and convalescent serum antibody titers to heat-labile *Escherichia coli* enterotoxin (LT) by passive immune hemolysis technique. Subjects studied are students who did or did not develop diarrhea while attending classes in Mexico. Adapted from Evans *et al.*[45]

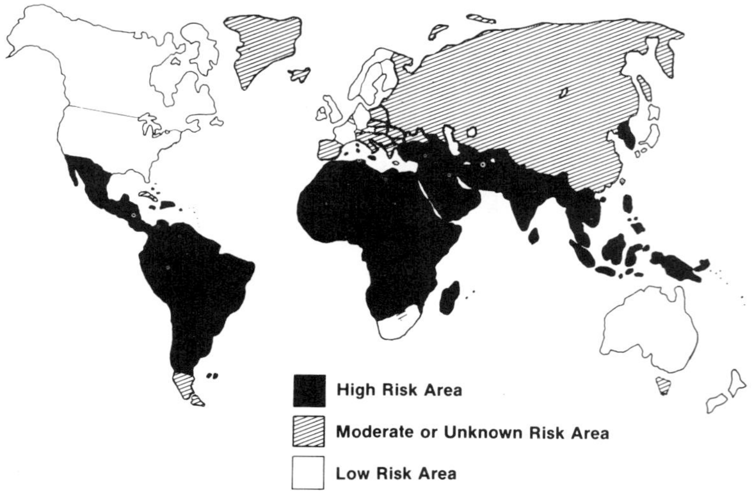

Figure 9.2. Division of regions of the world into low, moderate (or unknown), or high risk for developing diarrhea. From DuPont, H.L., and DuPont, M.W.[44]

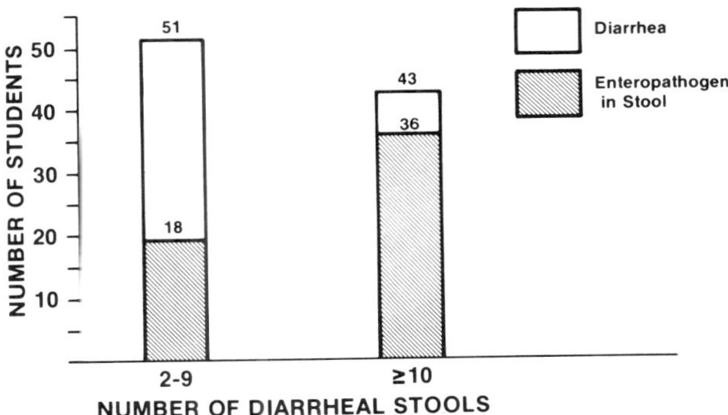

Figure 9.3. Relationship between identification of an enteropathogen in stool and number of diarrheal stools passed during a 48-hr period by United States summer students in Mexico.

when symptoms are not severe. On the other hand, when a striking illness occurs which is likely to temporarily incapacitate a person, infection with a high-grade pathogen is more likely.

CLINICAL ASPECTS

Characteristically, the problem occurs within the first two weeks of arrival in the foreign country. The clinical illness is highly variable, probably reflecting the diversity of etiologic agents responsible and the variation in host response to enteric infection. Approximately one-third of affected persons are incapacitated by the illness or find that their activities must be significantly altered.[6,7] The average number of stools passed over a five-day period is 12.[7] The problem may occur after the traveler has returned home.

ETIOLOGY

Until the early 1970s, there was little information about the common cause of the illness. In 1970, Rowe *et al.*[16] described an outbreak of diarrhea among British soldiers who had traveled to Aden. An *E. coli* serotyped as O148:K?:H28 was isolated from 54% of the soldiers, and the strain later produced illness in a technician working with it in the laboratory. Subsequent to the initial publication, this strain also was shown to produce an enterotoxin. In a separate report, 11 of 28 student travelers (39%) to Asia, Africa, or Latin America developed illness while under surveillance, and in four of 11 cases of illness (36%), an enterotoxigenic

E. coli (ETEC) was demonstrated in diarrheal stools by the use of a suckling mouse assay.[17] Gorbach *et al.*[18] next studied diarrheal disease in a group of 133 United States students attending classes during the summer of 1973 at Universidad de las Américas in Cholula, Puebla, Mexico. They were able to identify LT-producing *E. coli* in stool specimens of 72% of students with illness and 15% of those without symptoms. In a separate investigation carried out in Kenya, 27 of 39 Peace Corps volunteers from the United States developed diarrhea during their first five weeks in the African country, and in 17 (62%) there was evidence of infection by ETEC.[19] A study done by the Center for Disease Control,[6] appropriately at an international conference of gastroenterologists in Mexico City, confirmed that LT-producing *E. coli* was a common cause of illness (seen in 45% of cases). They also found other enteropathogens to be associated with illness, including *Salmonella* and *Shigella* strains. Studies subsequently carried out among students studying in Mexico[20,21] also demonstrated that LT-producing *E. coli* was an important cause of illness yet offered evidence that *Shigella* and *Salmonella* strains, rotaviruses, and *G. lamblia* also were important causes of disease. Figure 9.4 indicates the relative importance of the various enteropathogens as causative agents of diarrhea among United States students in Mexico. The percentages are averages obtained by us over a three-year period of study in multiple areas of Mexico. The single most important cause of illness

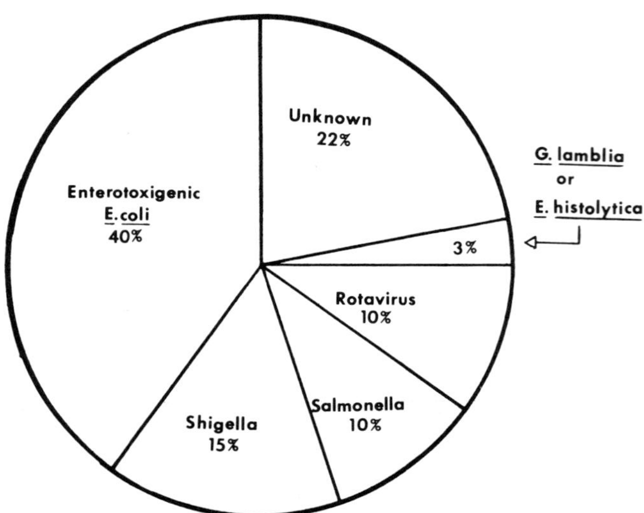

Figure 9.4. Approximate relative importance of enteropathogens in diarrhea of newly arrived United States students in Mexico. Results of several years of experience in three areas of Mexico (Cholula, Puebla; Guadalajara, Jalisco; Xalapa, Vera Cruz).

was ETEC, accounting for 40% of cases. There can no longer be doubt that this is the most important cause of diarrhea when a person travels from a low-risk to a high-risk area of the world. It is an error, however, to assume that this agent produces all of the illness. *Shigella, Salmonella,* and RV were all shown by us to be common causes of diarrhea. Although *Giardia* was not a common cause of acute diarrhea, it was identified in 3% of cases. Giardiasis should always be suspected in a traveler to the Soviet Union (particularly to Leningrad)[22,23] or to the Rocky Mountain area of the United States.[24,25] It should be considered in a person traveling to any region of the world when diarrhea is protracted or recurrent. In our studies carried out in Mexico, none of these enteropathogens was found to be an important cause of diarrhea among Latin American students, suggesting the development of natural immunity following prior exposure to the agents. The resistance to infection among Latin American students was most pronounced for ETEC.

PREVENTION OF TRAVELERS' DIARRHEA AND THE SOURCE OF THE PROBLEM

Table 9.2 lists the important placebo-controlled trials in which agents have been employed chemoprophylactically in the prevention of travelers' diarrhea. There is little doubt that many antimicrobial agents favorably reduce the rates of diarrhea, presumably because of their effect on the relatively antibiotic susceptible ETEC.[26] Drugs favorably reducing the rates of diarrhea include phthalylsulfathiazole, neomycin, trisulfonamides plus streptomycin (Streptotriad), and doxycycline. Enterovioform has been used with mixed success. Subacute myelo-optic neuropathy has been reported to develop among persons taking this drug,[27] and its use has been discouraged.[28] Although Enterovioform is no longer licensed in the United States, it is readily available in other countries. Some feel that general use of antimicrobials among travelers will not select antibiotic-resistant pathogens.[29] We feel that the problems of drug toxicity, potential enhancement of susceptibility to infection by *Salmonella* strains,[30] and possible encouragement of the development of antibiotic resistance among a variety of enteropathogens justify caution among those of us working in the field before recommending widespread employment of antibiotic chemoprophylaxis. One published study already has demonstrated that antibiotics used to prevent travelers' diarrhea can lead to an increase in salmonellosis.[31] Recent studies demonstrated that plasmids controlling enterotoxigenicity were transferred to susceptible bacteria along with R (antibiotic resistance) factors during bacterial conjugation.[32] It is therefore theoretically possible to increase the reservoir of ETEC

TABLE 9.2
Placebo-Controlled Trials Employing Chemoprophylactic Agents in the Prevention of Travelers' Diarrhea

Population	Foreign country	Chemoprophylactic agent	Results of study	References
North American	Mexico	Phthalylsulfathiazole 1 g b.i.d.	Effective	5, 38
North American	Mexico	Neomycin sulfate 500 mg b.i.d.	Effective	4, 5, 38
North American	Mexico	Furazolidone 100 mg b.i.d.	Ineffective	5
North American	Mexico	Enterovioform 375 mg b.i.d.	Ineffective	4
North American	Mexico	Bismuth subsalicylate 60 ml q.i.d.	Effective	33
North American	Mexico	*Lactobacillus acidophilus,* *L. bulgaricus* 4 tablets t.i.d.	Ineffective	39
North American	Kenya	Doxycycline 100 mg/day	Effective	29
North American	Mexico	TMP 160 mg + SMX 800 mg b.i.d.	Effective	43
British	Various countries	Enterovioform 250 mg t.i.d. or q.i.d.	Effective	40
British	Various countries	Streptotriad[a] 1 tablet b.i.d. for 2 weeks, then 1 tablet daily for third week	Effective	41
British	East of Suez	Furazolidone 100 mg/day or 100 mg b.i.d.	Effective	42

[a]Trisulfonamides plus streptomycin.

strains by routinely employing antibiotics to prevent the problem. We routinely advise chemoprophylaxis for two types of travelers: (1) those whose occupations necessitate productive interaction with business associates for a brief but important meeting and (2) those who have experienced the disease before demonstrating susceptibility. It is of interest that bismuth subsalicylate (Pepto-Bismol), a popular over-the-counter antidiarrheal, protected United States students in Mexico from developing diarrhea.[33] It therefore may be possible to utilize a chemoprophylactic agent which might be effective through nonspecific mechanisms.

The major area for the prevention of illness is the prevention of exposure to the infectious agents. Evidence is mounting that contaminated food is the single most important vehicle of disease transmission in Mexico.[6,34,35] This is particularly the case for ETEC diarrhea, shigellosis, and salmonellosis. Many public restaurants and cafeterias often fail to meet adequate food hygienic standards, and food served may be contaminated with fecal coliforms, including *Shigella* and *Salmonella*.[34] A series of errors in food preparation and preservation are commonly made. Vegetables may be grown in soil containing human excreta, they may be improperly washed, foods may be put back into their original contaminated containers after adequate processing or cooking, adequate and timely refrigeration may be lacking, and, finally, food preparers are not encouraged to wash their hands thoroughly nor are they prevented from working while convalescing from a bout of diarrhea (which is so common in these areas). In all probability, the single most important thing that can be done to minimize the potential for eating contaminated food is to select a restaurant for eating meals where local experienced persons can verify a record of safety for those patronizing the establishment. Such persons may be friends or associates living in the area, tour guides, or a hotel manager. We have been unable to predict the degree of bacterial contamination of food encountered by examining the appearance and outward cleanliness of public eating establishments, making advice from local persons extremely important. Cooked foods are safest, and they should be brought to the table steaming hot. Cooked foods (such as cooked hamburgers) tend to become recontaminated if not served immediately, making terminal heating necessary. Bottled drinks generally are safe, although they should be carbonated and the top of the bottle carefully cleaned by wiping it with a napkin before drinking. Peeled fruits are safe. Leafy vegetables should be considered contaminated unless adequately cleansed at home, and the hot sauces in public restaurants are often contaminated. The very hot spices in these preparations do not appear to have any antibacterial activity. Milk should be considered unsafe. Eating at street vendors or very small restaurants is not wise due to predictable contamination at these establishments. Acquisition of diarrhea among travelers taking a chemoprophylactic agent is still influenced by eating habits.[35]

Contaminated water may be important in diarrhea among travelers to many areas of the world, particularly in more remote areas with inadequate water sanitation standards and treatment facilities. In larger cities with adequate water treatment centers, water may become contaminated in homes due to inadequate standards of care of water reservoirs and cisterns. RV-associated gastroenteritis among United States travelers, in contrast to bacterial-agent-induced diarrhea, is not associated with place of food consumption.[36] Future study will probably reveal water to be the source of this important viral pathogen. In areas where water standards are unknown, tap water and ice probably should be avoided. In areas where water contamination is likely, bottled water should be used for drinking and for brushing teeth. It is likely that water from a faucet dispensing heated water is safer than the cold water and may be used for brushing teeth when bottled water is unavailable.[37]

Since a high percentage of persons traveling from a low-risk to a high-risk area are susceptible to infection by strains of ETEC, and because local populations who are chronically exposed to this agent show increased resistance, attempts are actively being made to develop an immunizing agent to prevent the disease. Antibody preparations are being evaluated which may offer short-term passive immunity during short visits to high-risk areas, while other groups are pursuing the development of purified antigen preparations [either a toxoid preparation or one composed of colonization factor antigen (CFA)] which will be administered as an active immunizing agent. See Chapter 6 for a discussion of *E. coli* vaccine development.

REFERENCES

1. International conference on the diarrhea of travelers—new directions in research: A summary. *J. Infect. Dis.* **137**:355–369, 1978.
2. Loewenstein, M. S., Balows, A., Gangarosa, E. J. Turista at an international congress in Mexico. *Lancet* **1**:529–531, 1973.
3. Kean, B. H. Turista in Teheran: Travellers' diarrhoea at the Eighth International Congresses of Tropical Medicine and Malaria. *Lancet* **2**:583–584, 1969.
4. Kean, B. H., Waters, S. The diarrhea of travelers: III. Drug prophylaxis in Mexico. *N. Engl. J. Med.* **261**:71–74, 1959.
5. Kean, B. H. The diarrhea of travelers to Mexico: Summary of five-year study. *Ann. Intern. Med.* **59**:605–614, 1963.
6. Merson, M. H., Morris, G. K., Sack, D. A., et al. Travelers' diarrhea in Mexico: A prospective study of physicians and family members attending a congress. *N. Engl. J. Med.* **294**:1299–1305, 1976.
7. DuPont, H. L., Haynes, G. A., Pickering, L. K., et al. Diarrhea of travelers to Mexico: Relative susceptibility of United States and Latin American students attending a Mexican university. *Am. J. Epidemiol.* **105**:37–41, 1977.
8. Higgins, A. R. Observations on health of United States personnel living in Cairo, Egypt. *Am. J. Trop. Med.* **4**:970–979, 1955.
9. Kean, B. H., Waters, S. The diarrhea of travelers: 1. Incidence in travelers returning to the United States from Mexico. *Arch. Ind. Health* **18**:148–150, 1958.
10. Bulmer, E. A survey of tropical diseases as seen in the Middle East. *Trans. R. Soc. Trop. Med. Hyg.* **37**:225–242, 1944.
11. Kean, B. H., Smillie, W. G. Intestinal protozoa of American travelers returning from Europe. *N. Engl. J. Med.* **251**:471–475, 1954.
12. Travellers' diarrhoea (annotations). *Lancet* **2**:85–86, 1962.
13. Dandoy, S. The diarrhea of travelers: Incidence in foreign students in the United States. *Calif. Med.* **104**:458–462, 1966.
14. Macdonald, I., Kean, B. H. Diarrhea of travelers (letters). *J. Am. Med. Assoc.* **181**:804, 1962.
15. Ryder, R. W., Wells, J. G., Gangarosa, E. J. A study of travelers' diarrhea in foreign visitors to the United States. *J. Infect. Dis.* **136**:605–607, 1977.
16. Rowe, B., Taylor, J., Bettelheim, K. A. An investigation of travellers' diarrhoea. *Lancet* **1**:1–5, 1970.
17. Shore, E. G., Dean, A. G., Holik, K. J., et al. Enterotoxin-producing *Escherichia coli* and diarrheal disease in adult travelers: A prospective study. *J. Infect. Dis.* **129**:577–582, 1974.
18. Gorbach, S. L., Kean, B. H., Evans, D. G., et al. Travelers' diarrhea and toxigenic *Escherichia coli*. *N. Engl. J. Med.* **292**:933–936, 1975.

19. Sack, D. A., Kaminsky, D. C., Sack, R. B., *et al.* Enterotoxigenic *Escherichia coli* diarrhea of travelers: A prospective study of American Peace Corps volunteers. *Johns Hopkins Med. J.* **141**:63–70, 1977.
20. DuPont, H. L., Olarte, J., Evans, D. G., *et al.* Comparative susceptibility of Latin American and United States students to enteric pathogens. *N. Engl. J. Med.* **295**:1520–1521, 1976.
21. Bolivar, R., Conklin, R. H., Vollet, J. J., *et al.* Rotavirus in travelers' diarrhea: Study of an adult student population in Mexico. *J. Infect. Dis.* **137**:324–327, 1978.
22. Brodsky, R. E., Spencer, H. C., Jr., Schultz, M. G. Giardiasis in American travelers to the Soviet Union. *J. Infect. Dis.* **130**:319–323, 1974.
23. Jokipii, L., Jokipii, A. M. Giardiasis in travelers: A prospective study. *J. Infect. Dis.* **130**:295–299, 1974.
24. Schultz, M. G. Giardiasis (editorial). *J. Am. Med. Assoc.* **233**:1383–1384, 1975.
25. Wanner, R. G., Atchley, F. O., Wasley, M. A. Association of diarrhea with *Giardia lamblia* in families observed weekly for occurrence of enteric infections. *Am. J. Trop. Med. Hyg.* **12**:851–853, 1963.
26. DuPont, H. L., West, H., Evans, D. G., *et al.* Antimicrobial susceptibility of enterotoxigenic *Escherichia coli*. *J. Antimicrob. Chemother.* **4**:100–102, 1978.
27. Kono, R. Subacute myelo-optic-neuropathy, a new neurological disease prevailing in Japan. *Jpn. J. Med. Sci. Biol.* **24**:195–216, 1971.
28. Oakley, G. P., Jr. The neurotoxicity of the halogenated hydroxyquinolines: A commentary. *J. Am. Med. Assoc.* **225**:395–397, 1973.
29. Sack, D. A., Kaminsky, D. C., Sack, R. B., *et al.* Prophylactic doxycycline for travelers' diarrhea: Results of a prospective double-blind study of Peace Corps volunteers in Kenya. *N. Engl. J. Med.* **298**:758–763, 1978.
30. Aserkoff, B., Bennett, J. V. Effect of antibiotic therapy in acute salmonellosis on the fecal excretion of salmonellae. *N. Engl. J. Med.* **281**:636–640, 1969.
31. Mentzing, L. O. Salmonella infection in tourists: 2. Prophylaxis against salmonellosis. *Acta Pathol. Microbiol. Scand.* **74**:405–413, 1968.
32. Echeverria, P., Verhaert, L., Ulyangco, C. V., *et al.* Antimicrobial resistance and enterotoxin production among isolates of *Escherichia coli* in the Far East. *Lancet* **2**:589–592, 1978.
33. DuPont, H. L., Sullivan, P., Evans, D. G., *et al.* Prevention of travelers' diarrhea (emporiatric enteritis): Prophylactic administration of subsalicylate bismuth. *J. Am. Med. Assoc.* **243**:237–241, 1980.
34. Tjoa, W., DuPont, H. L., Sullivan, P., *et al.* Location of food consumption and travelers' diarrhea. *Am. J. Epidemiol.* **106**:61–66, 1977.
35. Ericsson, C. D., Pickering, L. K., Sullivan, P., *et al.* The role of location of food consumption in the prevention of travelers' diarrhea in Mexico. *Gastroenterology* (in press).
36. Vollet, J. J., III, Ericsson, C. D., Gibson, G., *et al.* Human rotavirus in an adult population traveler's diarrhea and its relationship to the location of food consumption. *J. Med. Virol.* **4**:81–87, 1979.
37. Neumann, H. H. Travellers' diarrhoea. *Lancet* **1**:420, 1970.
38. Kean, B. H., Schaffner, W., Brennan, R. W., *et al.* The diarrhea of travelers: V. Prophylaxis with phthalylsulfathiazole and neomycin sulphate. *J. Am. Med. Assoc.* **180**:367–371, 1962.
39. Pozo-Olano, J., Warram, J. H., Jr., Gómez, R. G., *et al.* Effect of a lactobacilli preparation on traveler's diarrhea: A randomized, double-blind clinical trial. *Gastroenterology* **74**:829–830, 1978.
40. Richards, D. A. A controlled trial in travellers' diarrhoea. *Practitioner* **204**:822–824, 1970.

41. Turner, A. C. Travellers' diarrhoea: A survey of symptoms, occurrence and possible prophylaxis. *Br. Med. J.* **4:**653–654, 1967.
42. Nelson, S. R. C., Jones, H. L., Ross, J. B. Trial of furazolidone as a prophylactic in travellers' diarrhoea. *Practitioner* **188:**654–655, 1962.
43. DuPont, H. L., Evans, D. G., Vollet, J. J., III, *et al.* Prevention of traveler's diarrhea with trimethoprim/sulfamethoxazole. *Rev. Inf. Dis.* (in press).
44. DuPont, H. L., DuPont, M. W. *Travel with Health.* Appleton-Century-Crofts, New York, 1980.
45. Evans, D. J., Jr., Ruiz-Palacios, G., Evans, D. G., *et al.* Humoral immune response to the heat-labile enterotoxin of *Escherichia coli* in naturally acquired diarrhea and antitoxin determination by passive immune hemolysis. *Infect. Immun.* **16:**781–788, 1977.

10

Diagnosis and Treatment of Acute Diarrhea

INTRODUCTION

A patient has diarrhea if unformed bowel movements occur at a daily rate twice that of the usual rate. Diarrhea of infectious origin generally is associated with one or more symptoms of intestinal infection: fever, nausea, vomiting, abdominal pain or cramps, or dysentery (bloody and mucoid stools). The number of persons exposed to enteropathogens who develop illness depends upon the inoculum size. Host factors and virulence properties of the organism affect the clinical response.

Enteric infection generally is a self-limiting condition; however, in some cases, nonspecific therapy can provide relief, and specific therapy can shorten the duration of the illness and eradicate fecal shedding of the organism. When a patient complains of diarrhea, a decision should be made as to whether the patient should be admitted to the hospital or treated as an outpatient. Once this decision is made, appropriate therapy can be instituted. In the past, physicians have treated all patients with acute diarrhea in a similar fashion since the specific cause rarely was determined.[1] Most diarrheal illness can now be classified into one of several categories based upon the causative agent, its pathophysiologic mechanism, and the clinical response. This new information allows us to approach both nonspecific and specific therapy in a more rational manner. This chapter will deal with the methods of pathogen detection and nonfluid therapy of infectious agents that cause acute diarrhea. Fluid treatment and dietary management are discussed in Chapter 11.

DIAGNOSTIC PROCEDURES

Fecal Leukocytes

The examination of diarrheal stools for fecal leukocytes provides information concerning the cause of diarrhea in addition to the anatomical location and extent of mucosal inflammation.[2,3] Fecal leukocytes are produced in response to bacteria that diffusely invade the colonic mucosa and are an indication that the patient has colitis. Other disorders associated with colonic mucosal inflammation and destruction, such as ulcerative colitis and antibiotic-associated colitis, often are associated with a fecal exudate containing leukocytes. Fecal leukocytes generally are not present in stools of patients with diarrhea secondary to enterotoxigenic bacteria, viruses, and parasites (Table 10.1). The fecal leukocyte examination is performed by placing a small fleck of stool (mucus, if present) on a clean glass slide and mixing it thoroughly with two drops of Loeffler's methylene blue. A coverslip is placed over the specimen which is then examined microscopically (see Figure 4.2, Chapter 4). While the presence of fecal leukocytes is not pathognomonic of disease due to a specific microorganism, this finding in a patient with acute diarrhea and bloody stools generally indicates bacillary dysentery (shigellosis), and the patient can be treated empirically with an antimicrobial agent. Confirmatory stool culture results usually require an additional 48 hr.

TABLE 10.1
Occurrence of Fecal Leukocytes in Enteric Disease

Absent	Present
Toxigenic bacteria	*Shigella*
Escherichia coli	
Staphylococcus aureus	*Salmonella*
Clostridium perfringens	
Vibrio cholerae	*Yersinia enterocolitica*
	Invasive *Escherchia coli*
Viruses	
Rotavirus	*Campylobacter*
Norwalk-like agents	
	Vibrio parahemolyticus
Parasites	*Ulcerative colitis*
Giardia lamblia	
Strongyloides stercoralis	*Allergic and antibiotic-associated colitis*
Entamoeba histolytica[a]	

[a]Leukocytes may be present in low numbers (especially lymphocytes, eosinophils).

Serotyping of *E. coli*

During the 1940s and 1950s, outbreaks of acute diarrhea occurred in hospital nurseries, and strains of *E. coli* identified by serotype were isolated from stool and occasionally from blood of affected infants. At present, there are 11 distinct antigenic serotypes of *E. coli* which are referred to as the classic enteropathogenic serotypes (see Table 6.5 Chapter 6). It generally is agreed that the classic serotypes of EPEC possess virulence properties other than conventional LT or ST production or invasiveness for colonic mucosa.[4] At the present time, the major value of serotyping *E. coli* using the pools of commercial antisera currently available in the United States is in evaluating epidemic situations, particularly in newborn nurseries. Serotyping, like phage typing of staphylococci, can help to ascertain whether an epidemic is in progress. It is likely that prevalent serotypes of EPEC will have to be reevaluated on a prospective basis to allow laboratories to keep abreast of shifts in serotype which undoubtedly must occur with *E. coli* as it does with other microbial agents. Chapter 6 details the methods of serotyping *E. coli*.

Stool Culture

Routine Diagnostic Culture

From a cost/benefit standpoint, laboratory studies of stool specimens for etiologic agents cannot be justified in all patients with acute diarrhea. Patients with mild, self-limiting illness may not need to have stool cultured; however, they should receive symptomatic fluid and electrolyte treatment and diet modification. The finding of numerous white cells in stool of a patient with acute diarrhea usually is associated with invasive colonic pathogens such as *Shigella* or *Salmonella* (Table 10.1). These organisms are enteropathogens which routinely are detected by most microbiology laboratories and are found in stool of about 10–20% of patients with acute diarrhea. Other infectious agents which cause colitis producing leukocytes in stool require modified laboratory procedures for their identification. If *Vibrio, Yersinia,* or *Campylobacter* organisms are suspected, the laboratory should be notified so that appropriate culture methods can be used.

Special Diagnostic Cultures

Y. enterocolitica can be identified by most hospital laboratories if they are specifically alerted. Recovering the organism from blood, joint fluid, or other normally sterile fluid can be accomplished without difficulty; however, isolation of the organism from feces can be difficult due to overgrowth by normal flora. Media should be incubated at 22°C and 25°C as well as 37°C, since *Yersinia* will grow at low temperatures.[5,6] Optimal recovery from fecal material may be further achieved by suspending a sample in 0.067 M phosphate buffered saline, pH 7.6, and incubating at 4°C for four weeks.

Selective techniques are required to culture *Campylobacter*.[7] The culture medium should be made selective by the addition of vancomycin (10 mg/liter), polymyxin B (2.5 IU/ml), and trimethoprim (5 mg/liter). *Campylobacter* organisms have a growth requirement of an atmosphere in which the oxygen tension is reduced and the carbon dioxide tension increased. Plates should be incubated at 43°C in an atmosphere of 5% oxygen, 10% carbon dioxide, and 85% hydrogen. *Campylobacter* colonies can be recognized after an 18–hr incubation. Gram staining of the colonies reveals small spiral or S-shaped gram-negative bacilli. Cholera and noncholera vibrios are best recovered on TCBS agar.

Invasion of Intestinal Mucosa

Strains of *E. coli* have been identified that invade intestinal mucosa and produce typical bacillary dysentery similar to that produced by *Shigella*.[8] To detect an invasive strain (either *E. coli* or *Shigella*), the most reliable laboratory evaluation is the guinea pig eye model referred to as the Serény test.[9] Heavy suspensions of the freshly isolated strain are dropped into the conjunctival sac of a guinea pig. Invasive organisms will produce purulent keratoconjunctivitis within one to seven days after inoculation (Figure 4.3, Chapter 4).

Toxin Detection Assays

Bacteria may produce diarrhea secondary to toxin production, causing watery diarrhea without intestinal inflammation or fecal leukocytic exudate. Although microbiology laboratories can isolate *E. coli* specialized laboratory facilities are necessary to identify enterotoxigenic bacteria. The standard tests for the detection of LT are the Y1 adrenal cell (Figures 6.2 and 6.3, Chapter 6), CHO cell, and ligated rabbit loop (Figure 6.4, Chapter 6) models.[8,10,11] ST is best detected by the suckling mouse assay (Figure 6.5, Chapter 6).[12,13] Most ETEC that currently cause diarrhea worldwide are of relatively few serotypes, different from those that previously were incriminated in outbreaks of diarrheal disease,[14] indicating the need to determine the relationships between ETEC strains, EPEC strains, and serotype of *E. coli*. Chapter 6 describes the available toxin assay systems.

Ova and Parasites

Parasites that cause diarrhea usually do not produce numerous fecal leukocytes. Patients that have fecal-leukocyte-positive stools need not normally have these stools examined for ova and parasites unless (1) there is a history of recent travel to high-risk areas, (2) stool cultures are repeatedly negative for other enteropathogens, and (3) diarrhea persists for longer than one week.

Giardiasis should be considered in the diagnosis of any patient with diarrhea that lasts one week or longer. *G. lamblia* trophozoites or cysts in stool specimens may be detected by examination of fecal smears. Due to the intermittent passage of parasites, at least three stools should be examined. The sensitivity of stool examination can be improved by the use of a concentration technique such as the zinc sulfate concentration method. Negative stool findings for *G. lamblia* may necessitate sampling of duodenal contents either by intubation and aspiration or by duodenal biopsy. Many antibiotics and antidiarrheal compounds can cause a temporary disappearance of parasites from the stool or can interfere with recognition of parasites.

A diagnosis of *E. histolytica* can be made by examination of stool specimens or bowel-wall scrapings for cysts or trophozoites. Trophozoites generally are found in liquid stool, while cysts are detected in formed specimens. A concentration technique may be helpful in the demonstration of amebic cysts. Examination of several stool samples by an experienced technician may be necessary, since excretion of cysts often is intermittent and interpretation difficult. Confusion in differentiating *E. histolytica* from fecal leukocytes is common.[15] Serology for amebiasis is helpful in the diagnosis of acute amebic dysentery and hepatic amebiasis.[16]

Virus Detection

RV does not grow efficiently in tissue culture systems. Attempts at *in vitro* propagation of the Norwalk agent by routine techniques have been unsuccessful, and no readily available animal model has been developed for the study of Norwalk-like agents. This has made it difficult to study these agents by conventional neutralization test methods. RV can be detected by examination of stools for typical particles by electron microscopy.[17] IEM has proved useful in the study of volunteers with experimental Norwalk agent gastroenteritis[18]; however, the usefulness of IEM in the diagnosis of naturally occurring gastroenteritis caused by Norwalk-like agents remains to be established. These techniques are time-consuming and require trained personnel and specialized equipment. The ELISA for the detection of antibody against the HRV[19,20] and the RIA to measure Norwalk agent antibodies[21] are not readily available but are used to assist in the diagnosis of infection caused by these viruses.

NONSPECIFIC THERAPY—ANTIDIARRHEAL COMPOUNDS

Many compounds are available for the symptomatic treatment of patients with diarrhea.[22, 23] These over-the-counter and ethical (prescription) preparations have different mechanisms of action on the gastrointestinal tract. Table 10.2 lists some of the important drugs, offers statements about major value and toxicity, and identifies published studies employing the agents. In the United States, compounds are prescribed by physicians or administered by parents or patients eagerly focusing on relief of symptoms of acute diarrheal disease with little thought as to the specific cause.

Enteropathogens produce diarrhea by several different known virulence mechanisms: (1) invasion of intestinal mucosa with disruption of the villous architecture, (2) enterotoxin production with fluid and electrolyte accumulation in the lumen of the gastrointestinal tract, and (3) colonization or adherence of enteropathogens in the intestine with variable degrees of local destruction. In nearly all forms of acute infectious diarrhea, the abnormally formed stools reflect small-bowel hypersecretion of fluid and electrolytes and do not represent increased intestinal motility. Drugs that act strictly through effects on intestinal motility may not be useful in these instances and may on rare occasion worsen the symptoms by inhibiting intestinal transit and allowing the enteropathogen to be in contact with the intestinal mucosa for a longer period of time.

Drugs that Alter Intestinal Motility

Drugs that alter intestinal motility can be classified into three groups: (1) antimuscarinics, (2) opium alkaloids, and (3) synthetic opium alkaloids. Drugs that act through effects on intestinal motility patterns usually

TABLE 10.2
Antidiarrheal Compounds Used as Nonspecific Therapy for Patients with Acute
Diarrhea

Mechanism of action	Classification	Value	Comment	References
Alteration of intestinal motility	Antimuscarinics (belladonna alkaloids) Atropine Homatropine Mepenzolate (Cantil)[a] Scopolamine Thiphenamil Opium alkaloids Codeine (methylmorphine) Morphine Paregoric (camphorated opium tincture) Synthetic opium alkaloids Diphenoxylate Meperidine (Demerol) Loperamide	Decreased diarrhea Decreased cramps	Not recommended for infants or young children May rarely potentiate *Shigella* or *Salmonella* infections Convenient to transport and rapid onset of action	22, 23, 25–27, 30, 32, 34
Adsorption	Aluminum hydroxide Kaolin Pectin Kaolin + pectin (Kaopectate) Cholestyramine Activated charcoal	Increased stool form	Safe Minimally effective in increasing form of stool	32–34
Alteration of intestinal flora	*Lactobacillus acidophilus* *Lactobacillus bulgaricus* *Lactulose*	Unproven	Safe	35, 36
Inhibition of intestinal secretion	Bismuth subsalicylate Indomethacin (possible)	Decreased diarrhea Decreased cramps	Delayed onset (4 hr) Bulky and difficult to carry on trips	41

[a]We have shown recently that this preparation is without beneficial effect in the symptomatic treatment of acute diarrhea.

have a rapid onset of action. They decrease diarrhea and relieve abdominal cramps and pain, probably by producing segmental contractions of the intestine which serve to retard movement of intestinal contents responsible for diarrhea and by restricting the intestinal distention which is normally responsible for abdominal pain. These agents may also directly inhibit intestinal secretion.[24] Disadvantages of such drugs include overdose toxicity, lack of proven efficacy in infants and young children, and rarely, accentuation or prolongation of bacterial diarrhea in which the pathogen invades the bowel wall, such as in shigellosis or salmonellosis. Two to four doses of these compounds over a 24-hr period may be used by adults to treat severe cramps, but prolonged therapy is not advised.

Antimuscarinics

The naturally occurring antimuscarinic drugs are the alkaloids of the belladonna plant. The most important of these are atropine and scopolamine. These drugs antagonize the muscarinic actions of acetylcholine. Actions on the gastrointestinal tract include reduction in volume of both salivary and gastric secretion and decrease in tone, amplitude, and frequency of peristaltic contractions. Side effects that invariably occur when therapeutic doses of these drugs are given include dry mouth and blurred vision; less commonly, dry, flushed skin, photophobia, confusion, difficulty in urination, and psychosis; and, rarely, death. Infants and young children are especially susceptible to side effects of this class of drugs, and, therefore, antidiarrheal compounds containing belladonna alkaloids should not be used by children. A recently completed study carried out by our research team failed to identify beneficial effects when Cantil (mepenzolate bromide) was used to treat acute diarrhea. Side effects of the drug were common.

Opium Alkaloids

The term "opioid" refers to any natural or synthetic drug that has morphine-like pharmacologic actions. Morphine, the alkaloid that gives opium its analgesic actions, produces its major effects on the central nervous system and bowel. The use of opium for relief of diarrhea and dysentery preceded for many centuries its use for analgesia. These compounds cause an enhancement in amplitude of the nonpropulsive type of rhythmic contractions, but propulsive contractions are decreased markedly in both the small and large intestine. There is an increase in tone of the first part of the duodenum, ileocecal valve, and anal sphincter. The opioids are useful in treating exhausting diarrhea due to a number of causes. Side effects include dependency in adults and overdose in children. The dose of these drugs needed to affect the gastrointestinal tract is less than the analgesic dose.

Opium preparations such as opium tincture and camphorated opium tincture (paregoric) are more widely used as antidiarrheals than are morphine and codeine.

Synthetic Opium Alkaloids

Meperidine (Demerol) is a synthetic analgesic drug. It acts directly on the smooth muscle of the gastrointestinal tract to increase tone and decrease motility. Diphenoxylate is a meperidine congener that has the treatment of diarrhea as its only recognized use.[25-27] Lomotil is the combination of diphenoxylate and atropine. The atropine is present in subtherapeutic levels and is contained only to prevent the taking of excessive dosage where objectionable atropine symptoms theoretically would result before toxic levels of diphenoxylate are reached. Toxicity has, however, been reported in children who have ingested this drug.[28,29] It is currently contraindicated in children under two years of age and has been shown to rarely worsen clinical shigellosis[30] and possibly salmonellosis[31] in adults. Its side effects and lack of proven efficacy make it unacceptable for use in children. Its use in adults should be limited, as outlined above, with avoidance in patients with high fever or systemic toxicity and in those with bloody, mucoid stools.

Adsorbents

A number of chemically inert powders are used internally as adsorbents.[32-34] When these substances are given by mouth, they can adsorb not only bacteria and toxins but also drugs, nutrients, and enzymes. Aluminum hydroxide is an adsorbent, but it neutralizes hydrochloric acid so efficiently that it also serves as an antacid. Kaolin is a native, hydrated aluminum silicate. Pectin is a purified carbohydrate which consists chiefly of polygalacturonic acid. The mechanism of action of pectin in the treatment of diarrhea is unknown. It is often used in combination with an adsorbent such as kaolin. Cholestyramine is a nonabsorbable anion-exchange resin that binds bile acids and other substances in the intestine. There are no controlled studies showing the effectiveness of adsorbents in reducing the duration of diarrheal disease or diminishing the loss of fluid and electrolytes in diarrheal stool. The use of adsorbents results in the production of stools of increased form. Theoretical disadvantages include the nonspecific adsorption of nutrients, enzymes, and antibiotics, particularly if used for a prolonged period of time. This group of agents probably is the safest to use for the brief treatments of acute diarrhea.

Agents That Influence Intestinal Flora

Lactobacillus preparations are given to recolonize the intestine with saccharolytic flora and to alter the intestinal pH so as to deter potential pathogens. Lactulose, lactobacilli, and yogurt acidify the intestinal fluid and may inhibit the growth of enteropathogens. Lactulose is a synthetic derivative of lactose, containing one molecule of galactose and one of fructose. It is neither absorbed nor hydrolyzed by the human intestine but passes intact into the human colon, where it is actively metabolized by the normal gut flora, resulting in an increased production of short-chain fatty acids, a decrease in pH, and softening of stool consistency. Since short-chain fatty acids inhibit the growth of *Salmonella* and *Shigella,* it has been postulated that lactulose therapy may be an effective nonabsorbable therapy for persons with bacterial diarrhea, although its effectiveness may be limited since the changes in flora and resultant metabolites are restricted to the colon. There is no evidence of the effectiveness of these compounds in the symptomatic treatment of diarrhea.[35,36]

Agents That Inhibit Intestinal Secretion

Bismuth subsalicylate, indomethacin, and acetylsalicylic acid (aspirin) inhibit intestinal secretion of fluid and electrolytes.[37-40] Indomethacin and aspirin act as prostaglandin inhibitors. It is known that prostaglandin increases mucosal adenyl cyclase, thereby increasing the concentration of cAMP and stimulating small-bowel water and electrolyte secretion. Although prostaglandins may be shown to play a part in some diarrheal states such as carcinoid syndrome and medullary carcinoma of the thyroid, they may not be of importance in the pathogenesis of the small-bowel fluid loss of cholera or ETEC diarrhea. The specific mechanism of action of bismuth subsalicylate is unknown. Laboratory studies have shown that bismuth subsalicylate inhibits intestinal secretion secondary to *E. coli* and cholera enterotoxins.[37] It also has been shown to be effective in improving diarrhea acquired by adult students in Mexico[41] and as a prophylactic agent in the prevention of diarrhea among United States students traveling to Mexico.[42]

SPECIFIC ANTIMICROBIAL THERAPY

General

Antimicrobial therapy is administered to patients with gastroenteritis to abbreviate the clinical course and/or to decrease excretion of the causative organisms. A stool culture should be obtained and antibiotic sensitivity of the suspected pathogen determined to insure optimal therapy for complicated cases. Changing sensitivity patterns often make the initial selection of antimicrobial agents difficult. Antimicrobial agents should not be used routinely or liberally for gastroenteritis of unknown etiology.

Shigella

Patients with *Shigella* isolated from stool may present with three clinical patterns: (1) transient excretion, (2) enterotoxin-like diarrhea, and (3) bacillary dysentery. The finding of *Shigella* or other enteropathogens in the stool of asymptomatic persons indicates that the presence of these organisms need not be associated with disease. Healthy, transient carriers may be an important reservoir for, and mode of spread of, these organisms.[43] Treatment may be necessary to prevent spread of the disease in day-care centers or among family members. Persons with involvement of only the small intestine, which occurs during the early stages of illness, may present with fever and pass large volumes of liquid stool which do not contain blood, mucus, or leukocytes. Patients may complain of abdominal cramps, nausea, or vomiting. Patients with dysentery (bloody, mucoid stool) usually have been ill for several days with fever, urgency and tenesmus. They excrete smaller volumes of stool (fractional stools) but with greater frequency.

Several antibiotics have been used successfully in eradicating clinical symptoms and fecal shedding of *Shigella*.[44-48] Approximately half of the *S. sonnei* strains are resistant to ampicillin, whereas *S. flexneri* strains generally have remained relatively susceptible to ampicillin. Table 10.3 outlines suggested antimicrobial therapy for children and adults who have *Shigella* isolated from stool. In children infected with known ampicillin-sensitive strains, ampicillin is the treatment of choice and can be given orally or parenterally. Single-dose tetracycline therapy is effective in the treatment of *Shigella* infection in adults, regardless of clinical expression of illness.[44] Therapy decreases the excretion of the organism in stool and abbreviates the clinical course of both mild and severe disease. Treatment

TABLE 10.3
Antimicrobial Therapy of Shigellosis

	Infection due to *Shigella* strains of		
	Unknown sensitivity		Known ampicillin sensitivity
	Antimicrobial agent	Alternative	
Children	TMP 10 mg/kg/day plus SMX 50 mg/kg/day (p.o.) in 2 equally divided doses for 5 days	Ampicillin 50–75 mg/kg/ day (p.o. or i.v.) in 4 equally divided doses for 5 days	Ampicillin 50–75 mg/kg/ day (p.o. or i.v.) in 4 equally divided doses for 5 days
Adults	Tetracycline 2.5 g (p.o.) in a single dose or TMP 160 mg plus SMX 800 mg (p.o.) b.i.d. for 5 days	Oxolinic acid 750 mg (p.o.) b.i.d. for 5 days	Ampicillin 500 mg (p.o.) q.i.d. for 5 days

with tetracycline should be limited to adults because of side effects, including discoloration of teeth in children younger than eight years of age. Patients who are transient asymptomatic carriers may be managed without antimicrobial therapy if they understand and employ excellent standards of personal hygiene and if regular contact with children can be avoided.[48] Treatment of these patients, however, should reduce fecal shedding of the organism and prevent spread of infection. TMP plus SMX or oxolinic acid may become the treatment of choice in shigellosis due to the increasing frequency of ampicillin resistance among *Shigella* isolates.[45,46] At present, TMP plus SMX is recommended for use in patients with shigellosis of unknown sensitivity.

Sulfonamides are as effective as ampicillin if the organism is susceptible, but most *Shigella* strains are resistant. Nonabsorbable antibiotics such as neomycin, kanamycin, and gentamicin will not alter the course of the disease or fecal excretion of *Shigella*. Amoxicillin is not effective in shigellosis,[49] probably because the infecting strains are less susceptible to amoxicillin than ampicillin (higher minimal inhibitory concentration). Also, the profoundly greater intestinal absorption of amoxicillin may be a liability in the treatment of shigellosis.

Salmonella

More than 1400 serotypes have been identified within the genus *Salmonella;* however, the majority of cases of illness are caused by fewer than 20 serotypic variations. There are four clinical *Salmonella* syndromes: (1) carrier state, (2) acute gastroenteritis, (3) bacteremia and/or enteric fever, and (4) dissemination with localized suppuration (abscesses, osteomyelitis, etc.).[50]

Table 10.4 outlines the various clinical manifestations and antimicrobial therapy of patients infected with a *Salmonella* strain. Antibiotics should not be used in the treatment of persons who are nontyphoid *Salmonella* carriers or in patients with mild gastroenteritis. Antimicrobial therapy may on occasion convert an intestinal carriage into systemic disease with bacteremia,[51] prolong excretion of *Salmonella*,[52] or encourage the development or selection of resistant strains. Antibiotic treatment of patients with *Salmonella* infection is restricted to those with (1) typhoid fever, (2) bacteremia due to nontyphoidal strains, and (3) dissemination with localized suppuration. Since chloramphenicol-resistant strains of *Salmonella* have emerged in all parts of the world, ampicillin is

TABLE 10.4
Clinical Manifestations and Antimicrobial Therapy of *Salmonella* Infections in Children and Adults

Clinical manifestation	Antimicrobial therapy	
	Children	Adults
Carrier state	None	None
Acute gastroenteritis	Probably none[a]	Probably none[a]
Bacteremia and/ or enteric fever	Ampicillin 200 mg/kg/day (i.v.) in 6 equally divided doses for 2 weeks or Chloramphenicol 75 mg/kg/day (p.o. or i.v.) in 4 equally divided doses for 2 weeks or TMP 10 mg/kg/day plus SMX 50 mg/kg/day in 2 equally divided doses for 2 weeks	Ampicillin 6 g/day (i.v.) in 6 equally divided doses for 2 weeks or Chloramphenicol 3 g/day (p.o. or i.v.) in 3 equally divided doses (every 8 hr) for 2 weeks or TMP 160 mg plus SMX 800 mg (p.o.) b.i.d. for 2 weeks
Dissemination with localized suppuration (osteomyelitis)	Ampicillin, chloramphenicol, or TMP–SMX in same dosage as above; administer for 4–6 weeks for osteomyelitis or other infection showing slow response to treatment	Ampicillin, chloramphenicol, or TMP–SMX in same dosage as above; administer for 4–6 weeks for osteomyelitis or other infection showing slow response to treatment

[a]Patients with hyperpyrexia and systemic toxicity should be treated as if they have bacteremia; 7-to 10-day course of therapy is probably sufficient.

probably the current drug of choice when testing for organism susceptibility has not been performed.

Miscellaneous Bacterial Agents

Antimicrobial agents improve the diarrhea associated with cholera, reduce the volume of fluid loss, decrease the fluid replacement requirement, and eradicate the vibrios from the gastrointestinal tract.[53-55] Antimicrobial agents may be given orally or intravenously. Generally, cholera in adults is treated with tetracycline in a dosage schedule of 500 mg (p.o.) q.i.d. for two days (total of eight doses). Children with cholera who live in endemic areas are usually treated with tetracycline 50 mg/kg/day in four divided doses. Alternatives that do not have the dental staining problem of tetracycline are furazolidone 5 mg/kg/day in four divided doses and chloramphenicol 75 mg/kg/day in four divided doses. Each preparation is given for 72 hr. Studies to establish the value of antimicrobial therapy in the treatment of diarrhea due to ETEC are needed. It is reasonable to assume that antimicrobial agents would decrease diarrhea and fluid replacement, in view of the clinical similarity of this disease with cholera. A preliminary report suggested that antimicrobials may have some value in the treatment of ETEC diarrhea.[56]

Antimicrobial agents have been employed frequently in attempting to treat infantile gastroenteritis due to EPEC strains and as a means of controlling their spread in hospital nurseries. Although there are no definitive studies of the effectiveness of these drugs, they may be of use in certain situations, particularly when life-threatening infection occurs or when epidemic spread of the strains continues despite the institution of strict aseptic techniques and appropriate isolation and cohorting of active cases. Antimicrobial agents used in the treatment of EPEC diarrhea include neomycin, colymycin, and gentamicin, generally given orally.[57-61] Problems with antibiotic usage in EPEC infection are development of resistance to the drug used[62] and failure to adequately control epidemic spread of disease.[63]

Y. enterocolitica causes mild to moderately severe diarrhea, acute mesenteric adenitis clinically resembling acute appendicitis,[64] and other syndromes, including gastroenteritis with fever, arthritis, and sepsis. Treatment of patients with mild gastroenteritis is generally not necessary. Patients with severe gastroenteritis or systemic infections present a management problem, since they often respond poorly to antimicrobial agents, including those considered the drugs of choice in *Yersinia* bacteremia: chloramphenicol, the aminoglycosides (gentamicin, kanamycin, tobramycin, or amikacin), or tetracycline. Some have suggested the use of

TMP plus SMX. One of these agents should be employed in the septicemic form of illness or in any patient with life-threatening illness. Erythromycin given orally has been advocated for the therapy of *Campylobacter* diarrhea. There are no data supporting the use of antimicrobial agents in diarrheal disease due to noncholera vibrios, or *V. parahemolyticus.*

Protozoal Agents

A clear relationship between infection by parasitic agents and occurence of acute diarrhea exists only for *G. lamblia* and *E. histolytica.* They should be considered as the cause of diarrhea that persists longer than one to two weeks. In chronic diarrhea, *G. lamblia* is often underestimated as the causative agent, while *E. histolytica* is often overestimated, particularly in areas of the world where these agents are prevalent.

G. lamblia

G. lamblia is a flagellate protozoan that resides in the upper small intestine of humans.[65] It occurs in all parts of the world and has been the cause of numerous epidemics of diarrhea. *Giardia* is a particular problem to travelers to developing parts of the world, the Soviet Union, or mountain ski resorts.[66-69] The parasite exists in two forms: (1) trophozoites, which are usually seen in duodenal aspirates and in loose stools, and (2) cysts, which may remain viable and infectious in water for longer than three months. Infection is spread either by direct fecal–oral contamination or by transmission of cysts in food or water. Individuals vary in their response to *G. lamblia,* with the following clinical manifestations: (1) asymptomatic; (2) acute illness with sudden onset of explosive, watery, foul-smelling stools without blood or mucus, flatulence, distention, nausea, and anorexia; and (3) chronic diarrhea and malabsorption with flatulence, distention, and abdominal pain often lasting for months.

Quinacrine hydrochloride and metronidazole are effective in treating patients with giardiasis.[65,70] Metronidazole may be better tolerated than quinacrine, but it is far more expensive and no more effective. Neither of the drugs is available in liquid form and therefore must be specially prepared for children. The dosage schedule of quinacrine for treatment of children is 7 mg/kg/day in equally divided doses t.i.d. (maximum daily dose 300 mg) for seven days. For adults, the proper dosage is 100 mg t.i.d. for seven days. Metronidazole is given to children in a dosage of 20 mg/kg/day in equally divided doses q.i.d. (maximum daily dose 750 mg), and adults receive 250 mg t.i.d.; both receive the drug for ten days. Furazolidone is available in liquid form and, like quinacrine, is lower in cost than metronidazole. The dosage of furazolidone is 5 mg/kg/day (p.o.) in four divided doses for children and 100 mg (p.o.) q.i.d. for adults, both for seven days.

E. histolytica

E. histolytica is a parasitic protozoan that is more prevalent in tropical climates. The trophozoites of *E. histolytica* live and multiply in the large intestine, especially the cecum. As the contents of the lumen advance and become less fluid, the trophozoites change into cysts. Amebiasis spreads by ingestion of cysts which contaminate food and drink. Clinical patterns seen with amebiasis consist of (1) intestinal amebiasis with gradual onset of colicky abdominal pain, frequent bowel movements, tenesmus, and little or no constitutional disturbance; (2) amebic dysentery characterized by profuse diarrhea containing blood and mucus and the presence of constitutional signs such as fever, dehydration, and electrolyte alterations; and (3) hepatic amebiasis, which usually presents as abscess formation with or without gastrointestinal symptoms; patients may have tender hepatomegaly, jaundice, weight loss, fever, and anorexia.

In treating patients with amebiasis, diiodohydroxyquin is the best lumenal amebicide presently available. This drug is effective against both cysts and trophozoites in the lumen of the gut but is ineffective against tissue forms of the disease. Invasive amebiasis of the intestine, liver, or other organs necessitates the additional use of a tissue amebicide such as metronidazole.

The treatment of choice for the asymptomatic cyst excretor is diloxanide furoate (20 mg/kg/day for children and 500 mg t.i.d. for adults) given orally for ten days. For intestinal amebiasis, metronidazole is given orally (50 mg/kg/day for children and 750 mg t.i.d. for adults) for ten days, followed by a course of oral diiodohydroxyquin (40 mg/kg/day for children and 650 mg t.i.d. for adults) for 21 days. Liver abscess or other extraintestinal form of disease should be treated with metronidazole in the dosage recommended for intestinal disease. A single drug probably is satisfactory, although some would also administer chloroquine. Table 2.4, Chapter 2 lists alternative choices for therapy of amebiasis.

REFERENCES

1. Cramblett, H. G., Siewers, C. M. The etiology of gastroenteritis in infants and children, with emphasis on the occurrence of simultaneous mixed viral–bacterial infections. *Pediatrics* **35**:885–898, 1965.
2. Harris, J. C., DuPont, H. L., Hornick, R. B. Fecal leukocytes in diarrheal illness. *Ann. Intern. Med.* **76**:697–703, 1972.

3. Pickering, L K., DuPont, H. L., Olarte, J., *et al.* Fecal leukocytes in enteric infections. *Am. J. Clin. Pathol.* **68**:562–565, 1977.

4. Goldschmidt, M. C., DuPont, H. L. Enteropathogenic *Escherichia coli:* Lack of correlation of serotype with pathogenicity. *J. Infect. Dis.* **133**:153–156, 1976.

5. Bottone, E. J. *Yersinia enterocolitica:* A panoramic view of a charismatic microorganism. *CRC Crit. Rev. Microbiol.* **5**:211–241, 1977.

6. Kohl, S. *Yersinia enterocolitica* infection. *Pediatr. Clin. North Am.* **26**:433–444, 1979.

7. Skirrow, M. B. *Campylobacter* enteritis: A "new" disease. *Br. Med. J.* **2**:9–11, 1977.

8. DuPont, H. L., Formal, S. B., Hornick, R. B., *et al.* Pathogenesis of *Escherichia coli* diarrhea. *N. Engl. J. Med.* **285**:1–9, 1971.

9. Serény, B. Experimental shigella keratoconjunctivitis: A preliminary report. *Acta Microbiol. Acad. Sci. Hung.* **2**:293–296, 1955.

10. Donta, S. T., Moon, H. W., Whipp, S. C. Detection of heat-labile *Escherichia coli* enterotoxin with the use of adrenal cells in tissue culture. *Science* **183**:334–336, 1974.

11. Donta, S. T., Smith, D. M. Stimulation of steroidogenesis in tissue culture by enterotoxigenic *Escherichia coli* and the neutralization by specific antiserum. *Infect. Immun.* **9**:500–505, 1974.

12. Dean, A. G., Ching, Y. C., Williams, R. G., *et al.* Test for *Escherichia coli* enterotoxin using infant mice: Application in a study of diarrhea in children in Honolulu. *J. Infect. Dis.* **125**:407–411, 1972.

13. Byers, P. A., DuPont, H. L., Evans, D. J., Jr. Pooling method for screening large numbers of *Escherichia coli* for production of heat-stable enterotoxin, and its application in field studies. *J. Clin. Microbiol.* **9**:541–543, 1979.

14. Ørskov, F., Ørskov, I., Evans, D. J., Jr., *et al.* Special *Escherichia coli* serotypes among enterotoxigenic strains from diarrhoea in adults and children. *Med. Microbiol. Immunol.* **162**:73–80, 1976.

15. Krogstad, D. J., Spencer, H. C., Jr., Healy, G. R., *et al.* Amebiasis: Epidemiologic studies in the United States, 1971–1974. *Ann. Intern. Med.* **88**:89–97, 1978.

16. Mahmoud, A. A. F., Warren, K. S. Algorithms in the diagnosis and management of exotic diseases: XVII. Amebiasis. *J. Infect. Dis.* **134**:639–643, 1976.

17. Bishop, R. F., Davidson, G. P., Holmes, I. H., *et al.* Detection of a new virus by electron microscopy of faecal extracts from children with acute gastroenteritis. *Lancet* **1**: 149–151, 1974.

18. Kapikian, A. Z., Wyatt, R. G., Dolin, R., *et al.* Visualization by immune electron microscopy of a 27-nm particle associated with acute infectious non-bacterial gastroenteritis. *J. Virol.* **10**:1075–1081, 1972.

19. Yolken, R. H., Kim, H. W., Clem, T., *et al.* Enzyme-linked immunosorbent assay (ELISA) for detection of human reovirus-like agent of infantile gastroenteritis. *Lancet* **2**:263–267, 1977.

20. Yolken, R. H., Barbour, B., Wyatt, R. G., *et al.* Enzyme-linked immunosorbent assay for identification of rotaviruses from different animal species. *Science* **201**:259–262, 1978.

21. Greenberg, H. B., Kapikian, A. Z. Detection of Norwalk agent antibody and antigen by solid-phase radioimmunoassay and immune adherence hemagglutination assay. *J. Am. Vet. Med. Assoc.* **173**:620–623, 1978.

22. Murphy, J. E. A comparison of antidiarrhoeal preparations in acute diarrhoea in general practice. *Practitioner* **200**:570–574, 1968.

23. Adams, L. A., Clark-Wilson, L. J., Giwelb, H. J., *et al.* Anti-diarrhoeal agents compared. *Practitioner* **202**:569–571, 1969.

24. Higgins, J. A., Code, C. F., Orvis, A. L. The influence of motility on the rate of absorption of sodium and water from the small intestine of healthy persons. *Gastroenterology* **31**:708–716, 1956.

25. Barowsky, H., Schwartz, S. A. Method for evaluating diphenoxylate hydrochloride: Comparison of its antidiarrheal effect with that of camphorated tincture of opium. *J. Am. Med. Assoc.* **180**:1058–1061, 1962.

26. Harris, M. J., Beveridge, J. Diphenoxylate in the treatment of acute gastro-enteritis in children. *Med. J. Aust.* **2**:921–922, 1965.

27. Cornett, J. W. D., Aspeling, R. L., Mallegol, D. A double-blind comparative evaluation of loperamide versus diphenoxylate with atropine in acute diarrhea. *Curr. Ther. Res. Clin. Exp.* **21**:629–637, 1977.

28. Ginsburg, C. M. Lomotil (diphenoxylate and atropine) intoxication. *Am. J. Dis. Child.* **125**:241–242, 1973.

29. Rumack, B. H., Temple, A. R. Lomotil poisoning. *Pediatrics* **53**:495–500, 1974.

30. DuPont, H. L., Hornick, R. B. Adverse effect of Lomotil therapy in shigellosis. *J. Am. Med. Assoc.* **226**:1525–1528, 1973.

31. Sprinz, H. Pathogenesis of intestinal infections. *Arch. Pathol.* **87**:556–562, 1969.

32. Portnoy, B. L., DuPont, H. L., Pruitt, D., *et al.* Antidiarrheal agents in the treatment of acute diarrhea in children. *J. Am. Med. Assoc.* **236**:844–846, 1976.

33. McCloy, R. M., Hofmann, A. F. Tropical diarrhea in Vietnam—a controlled study of cholestyramine therapy. *N. Engl. J. Med.* **284**:139–140, 1971.

34. Dubow, E. "Nonspecific" diarrhea in infants and young children: Observations on pathogenesis and therapy. *Clin. Pediatr. (Philadelphia)* **3**:168–170, 1964.

35. Pearce, J. L., Hamilton, J. R. Controlled trial of orally administered lactobacilli in acute infantile diarrhea. *J. Pediatr.* **84**:261–262, 1974.

36. Levine, M. M., Hornick, R. B. Lactulose therapy in *Shigella* carrier state and acute dysentery. *Antimicrob. Agents Chemother.* **8**:581–584, 1975.

37. Ericsson, C. D., Evans, D. G., DuPont, H. L., *et al.* Bismuth subsalicylate inhibits activity of crude toxins of *Escherichia coli* and *Vibrio cholerae. J. Infect. Dis.* **136**:693–696, 1977.

38. Gots, R. E., Formal, S. B., Giannella, R. A. Indomethacin inhibition of *Salmonella typhimurium, Shigella flexneri,* and cholera-mediated rabbit ileal secretion. *J. Infect. Dis.* **130**:280–284, 1974.

39. Giannella, R. A., Rout, W. R., Formal, S. B. Effect of indomethacin on intestinal water transport in salmonella-infected rhesus monkeys. *Infect. Immun.* **17**:136–139, 1977.

40. Mennie, A. T., Dalley, V. M., Dinneen, L. C., *et al.* Treatment of radiation-induced gastrointestinal distress with acetylsalicylate. *Lancet* **2**:942–943, 1975.

41. DuPont, H. L., Sullivan, P., Pickering, L. K., *et al.* Symptomatic treatment of diarrhea with bismuth subsalicylate among students attending a Mexican university. *Gastroenterology* **73**:715–718, 1977.

42. DuPont, H. L., Sullivan, P., Evans, D. G., *et al.* Prevention of traveler's diarrhea (emporiatric enteritis): Prophylactic administration of subsalicylate bismuth. *J. Am. Med. Assoc.* **243**:237–241, 1980.

43. Pickering, L. K, DuPont, H. L., Evans, D. G., *et al.* Isolation of enteric pathogens from asymptomatic students from the United States and Latin America. *J. Infect. Dis.* **135**:1003–1005, 1977.

44. Pickering, L. K., DuPont, H. L., Olarte, J. Single-dose tetracycline therapy for shigellosis in adults. *J. Am. Med. Assoc.* **239**:853–854, 1978.

45. Nelson, J. D., Kusmiesz, H., Jackson, L. H., *et al.* Trimethoprim–sulfamethoxazole therapy for shigellosis. *J. Am. Med. Assoc.* **235**:1239–1243, 1976.

46. Haltalin, K. C., Nelson, J. D., Kusmiesz, H. T. Comparative efficacy of nalidixic acid and ampicillin for severe shigellosis. *Arch. Dis. Child.* **48**:305–312, 1973.

47. Weissman, J. B., Gangarosa, E. J., DuPont, H. L. Changing needs in the antimicrobial therapy of shigellosis. *J. Infect. Dis.* **127**:611–613, 1973.

48. Weissman, J. B., Gangarosa, E. J., DuPont, H. L., *et al.* Shigellosis: To treat or not to treat? *J. Am. Med. Assoc.* **229**:1215–1216, 1974.

49. Nelson, J. D., Haltalin, K. C. Amoxicillin less effective than ampicillin against *Shigella in vitro* and *in vivo:* Relationship of efficacy to activity in serum. *J. Infect. Dis. Suppl.* **129:**S222–S227, 1974.

50. Cohen, M. L., Gangarosa, E. J. Nontyphoid salmonellosis. *South. Med. J.* **71:**1540–1545, 1978.

51. Rosenthal, S. L. Exacerbation of salmonella enteritis due to ampicillin. *N. Engl. J. Med.* **280:**147–148, 1969.

52. Aserkoff, B., Bennett, J. V. Effect of antibiotic therapy in acute salmonellosis on the fecal excretion of salmonellae. *N. Engl. J. Med.* **281:**636–640, 1969.

53. Kobari, K., Uylangco, C., Vasco, J. *et al.* Observations on cholera treated orally and intravenously with antibiotics: With particular reference to the number of vibrios excreted in the stool. *Bull. W.H.O.* **37:**751–762, 1967.

54. Wallace, C. K., Anderson, P. N., Brown, T. C., *et al.* Optimal antibiotic therapy in cholera. *Bull. W.H.O.* **39:**239–245, 1968.

55. Rahaman, M. M., Majid, M. A., Alam, A. K. M., *et al.* Effects of doxycycline in actively purging cholera patients: A double-blind clinical trial. *Antimicrob. Agents Chemother.* **10:**610–612, 1976.

56. Merson, M. H., Sack, R. B., Islam, S., *et al.* Enterotoxigenic *Escherichia coli* (ETEC) disease in Bangladesh: Clinical, therapeutic and laboratory aspects. In *Proceedings of XIII Joint Conference on Cholera, the U.S.–Japan Cooperative Medical Science Program*, Atlanta, September, 1977, pp. 343–359.

57. Wheeler, W. E. Spread and control of *Escherichia coli* diarrheal disease. *Ann. N.Y. Acad. Sci.* **66:**112–117, 1956.

58. Rogers, K. B., Benson, R. P., Foster, W. P., *et al.* Phthalylsulphacetamide and neomycin in the treatment of infantile gastro-enteritis. *Lancet* **2:**599–604, 1956.

59. Neter, E. Enteritis due to enteropathogenic *Escherichia coli.* Present-day status and unsolved problems. *J. Pediatr.* **55:**223–239, 1959.

60. South, M. A., Yow, M. D., Robinson, N. M., *et al.* Antibiotic sensitivity patterns of strains of enteropathogenic *Escherichia coli* isolated in various areas of the United States and Mexico. In J. C. Sylvester, (ed.), *Antimicrobial Agents and Chemotherapy— 1963 (Proceedings of the Third Interscience Conference on Antimicrobial Agents and Chemotherapy*, Washington, D.C., October 28–30, 1963). American Society for Microbiology, Ann Arbor, 1963, pp. 402–405.

61. Riley, H. D., Jr. Antibiotic therapy in neonatal enteric disease. *Ann. N.Y. Acad. Sci.* **176:**360–370, 1971.

62. Kessner, D. M., Shaughnessy, H. J., Googins, J., *et al.* An extensive community outbreak of diarrhea due to enteropathogenic *Escherichia coli* O111:B4: I. Epidemiologic studies. *Am. J. Hyg.* **76:**27–43, 1962.

63. Ryder, R. W., Wachsmuth, I. K., Buxton, A. E., *et al.* Infantile diarrhea produced by heat-stable enterotoxigenic *Escherichia coli. N. Engl. J. Med.* **295:**849–853, 1976.

64. Kohl, S., Jacobson, J. A., Nahmias, A. *Yersinia enterocolitica* infections in children. *J. Pediatr.* **89:**77–79, 1976.

65. Wolfe, M. S. Giardiasis. *J. Am. Med. Assoc.* **233:**1362–1365, 1975.

66. Wright, R. A., Spencer, H. C., Brodsky, R. E., *et al.* Giardiasis in Colorado: Epidemiologic study. *Am. J. Epidemiol.* **105:**330–336, 1977.

67. Babb, R. R., Peck. O. C., Vescia, F. G. Giardiasis: A cause of travelers' diarrhea. *J. Am. Med. Assoc.* **217:**1359–1361, 1971.

68. Brodsky, R. E., Spencer, H. C., Jr., Schultz, M. G. Giardiasis in American travelers to the Soviet Union. *J. Infect. Dis.* **130:**319–323, 1974.

69. Jokipii, L., Jokipii, A. M. Giardiasis in travelers: A prospective study. *J. Infect. Dis.* **130:**295–299, 1974.

70. Mahmoud, A. A., Warren, K. S. Algorithms in the diagnosis and management of exotic diseases: II. Giardiasis. *J. Infect. Dis.* **131:**621–624, 1975.

11

Fluid and Dietary Management of Acute Diarrhea

INTRODUCTION

Patients who develop diarrhea generally experience an excess loss of fluid and electrolytes via the gastrointestinal tract. If vomiting complicates the illness, this loss is compounded. Continued loss of fluid and/or electrolytes leads to dehydration, which is the most severe complication of diarrheal disease. Children and especially infants are more susceptible to dehydration because of the greater rate of water turnover in relation to their total body weight.[1,2] Elderly patients and patients of any age with an underlying disorder such as cardiovascular disease are more susceptible to dehydration and its sequelae. Maintaining optimal hydration and electrolyte balance is critical in any patient with diarrhea. This chapter will deal with fluid and electrolyte and dietary management of patients with diarrhea.

MECHANISMS OF FLUID AND ELECTROLYTE LOSS BY CAUSATIVE AGENT

Recent studies of the etiology of acute diarrhea have focused attention on RV and enterotoxin-producing strains of *E. coli*. RV is a major cause of acute diarrhea in children under two years of age, with worldwide distribution, while ETEC infection appears to be an uncommon cause of endemic diarrhea in children and adults in developed countries. It is useful to determine the relative incidence of different causative agents in acute diarrhea in children since appropriate rehydration measures may depend upon the mechanism of diarrheal fluid loss. ETEC causes fluid loss through a mechanism similar to that of *V. cholerae.* Attachment of enterotoxin to membrane receptors in the intestinal lumen activates adenyl cyclase, which leads to increased levels of cAMP and altered cellular function, resulting in loss of fluid and electrolytes from the mucosa into the lumen of the small intestine (see Figure 6.1, Chapter 6). While chloride may be the primary ion moved by the toxin, stools contain a high concentration of sodium and potassium. Glucose-mediated sodium absorption is intact, which explains the success of oral glucose-electrolyte solution in the treatment of cholera and related diarrhea. There is evidence that the mechanism of fluid loss in viral diarrhea may be quite different.

Studies in gnotobiotic piglets infected with transmissible gastroenteritis virus[3] have demonstrated an intact adenyl cyclase system and a defect in the jejunal glucose-mediated sodium transport. Davidson and coworkers[4] established a model of RV infection in piglets. Their studies have served to identify histologic and pathophysiologic responses associated with altered glucose transport and diminished disaccharidase activity. These findings suggest that the pathophysiology of RV diarrhea differs markedly from the secretory enterotoxigenic diarrhea of cholera and *E. coli.* In viral gastroenteritis, which is not primarily a secretory type of diarrhea, the sodium and potassium content of stool is significantly less (approximately 26 mEq/liter) than that seen in stool of patients with diarrhea due to organisms that produce an enterotoxin (100 mEq/liter). If solutions with a high sodium concentration are used without supervision to rehydrate infants with RV gastroenteritis, the extracellular volume and renal function tolerance of the infected infants could be exceeded, with

TABLE 11.1
Sodium and Potassium Content (mEq/liter) of Stool Characterized by Organism
Causing Diarrhea

Type of stool	Na	K	References
Normal	18	45	5, 6, 14
Diarrhea			
Mixed or unknown cause	48	37	5–12, 15
Cholera	100	27	13
RV	26	44	16, 38

development of hypernatremia. Table 11.1 lists fecal sodium and potassium content with regard to the cause of gastroenteritis.[5-16]

FLUID AND ELECTROLYTE THERAPY

There are four important factors to be considered in evaluating patients with diarrhea and possible dehydration: (1) an estimation of deficiency, (2) ongoing daily requirements, (3) the occurrence of continued losses and their replacement, and (4) correction of the underlying cause. Clinical signs and symptoms which may help in estimating deficiencies and determining the severity of dehydration are listed in Table 11.2. These signs and symptoms may be misleading in patients who are malnourished or in those with hypertonic dehydration. Although a person may not be dehydrated upon the initial visit to a physician, the risk of impending dehydration must be considered if continued losses occur from a large number of stools or if vomiting is present, impeding oral alimentation. Young children and the elderly with diarrhea must have someone caring for them who can follow instructions, look for signs and symptoms of dehydration, and understand the need for medical intervention if the disease persists or worsens.

Fluids should not be withheld in the outpatient treatment of patients, particularly children, with diarrheal disease. Oral therapy generally consists of two stages: (1) rehydration and maintenance for a 12- to 48-hr period with a glucose–electrolyte solution, followed by (2) initiation of a modified diet.

TABLE 11.2
Signs and Symptoms of Dehydration

Percentage rapid weight loss	Clinical finding
<3	Thirst
3–10	Dryness of mucous membranes and skin; slight tachycardia; oliguria
> 10	Marked tachycardia; extreme dryness of mucous membranes; lack of tears; oliguria approaching anuria; fontanel, if open, palpably depressed; eyeballs sunken; loss of skin elasticity and turgor; skin mottling; extremities cool to touch; apathy and mild somnolence
>15	Complete circulatory collapse

Oral Rehydration

Mild Dehydration

Patients with mild diarrhea without clinical dehydration (less than 3% weight loss) can be managed at home initially with oral hypotonic electrolyte solutions containing glucose. The glucose in these solutions is necessary to promote intestinal absorption of sodium and water in the small intestine.[17–19] Kinetic studies suggest that sodium binds to a carrier along with glucose but at a different binding site.[17] Glucose is released inside the cell wall, and the sodium moves down a concentration gradient into the cell to subsequently be pumped out at the lateral membrane of the cell by an active process.

Commercial preparations of ready-to-feed glucose–electrolyte solutions are available and should be utilized. The sodium and potassium contents of various commercially available preparations are outlined in Table 11.3.[20–22] Pedialyte, Lytren, and Gatorade are the best available solutions; however, they may not supply an adequate quantity of electrolytes necessary to replace continued stool losses if severe diarrhea occurs. The preparation of sugar-and-salt solutions at home is no longer recommended because of the frequent errors in preparing the solutions which may result in hypertonic dehydration if used in infants.[23–25] The controversy which exists in the literature about the optimal oral rehydration solution relates to the different populations treated and the causes of diarrhea in these populations. Most studies that have advocated solutions with high sodium content[26,27] have centered about rehydration of malnourished and dehydrated children over two years of age with cholera or other severe diarrhea, often in developing parts of the world. The appro-

TABLE 11.3
Sodium and Potassium Content (mEq/liter) of
Solutions Used for Oral Rehydration

	Na	K
Pedialyte	30	20
Lytren	30	25
Gatorade	23	3
Pepsi-Cola	6.5	0.8
7-Up	4.6	0.1
Coca-Cola	0.4	1–13
Root beer	3.5	0.1
Ginger ale	3.5	0.2
Apple juice, canned	1.7	26
Kool-Aid	3	0.1
Tea	1	6.8

priate caution put forth by others[28] relates to concern about the use of such solutions in younger well-nourished children and infants with mild or absent dehydration in the United States. It is unlikely that a single electrolyte solution will answer the needs for all clinical situations.

Other commercially available preparations which may be used at home include decarbonated soda beverages or fruit juices, which contain small amounts of sodium and potassium. These solutions may not be useful if rehydration requires more than two or three feedings. Kool-Aid and tea are not useful, since they are low in both sodium and potassium and have no advantage over water.[20] Children who have diarrhea accompanied by vomiting are initially given small volumes—0.5–1 oz every 30–60 min—of an oral electrolyte solution. After the vomiting has stopped, it is preferable to give larger volumes at 2- to 4-hr intervals. After the child has begun drinking clear liquids for 6–18 hr, he can start on a bland diet.

Moderate to Severe Dehydration

When more than 5% of body weight is lost within 24 hr because of diarrhea and vomiting, signs and symptoms of dehydration become obvious (Table 11.2). If more than 10% of body weight is lost over 24 hr, generally the patient should be admitted to a hospital, where oral rehydration is used to augment intravenous fluid replacement. Dehydration of between 5 and 10% can usually be managed on an outpatient basis under medical supervision. Orally administered fluid has been shown to correct volume depletion of up to 8% of body weight, acidosis with pH as low as 7.15, and moderate electrolyte disturbance with serum sodium as low as 119 or as high as 168 mEq/liter.[29,30]

Table 11.4 describes the composition of three oral electrolyte solutions, two of which have been field tested in rehydration centers in other countries where moderate and severe dehydration have been treated,[31–33] while the third has been used at two large hospital clinics in the United States.[28] The electrolyte and glucose compositions advocated in cholera-endemic areas are quite similar, and either solution is suitable for use.

TABLE 11.4
Oral Therapy for Rehydration of Diarrhea

Glucose[a]	Na[b]	K[b]	Cl[b]	Bicarbonate[b]	Citrate[b]	PO$_4$[b]	Reference
110	90	20	80	30	—	—	31
110	120	25	98	48	—	—	72
167	49	20	30	—	29	10	28

[a]mM/liter.
[b]mEq/liter.

Although glucose (20 g/liter) has certain advantages over sucrose (40 g/liter), either may be used. Sucrose is cheaper and more readily available.

Three factors which may impair the effectiveness of oral therapy are vomiting, comatose state, and purging rates greater than 120 ml/kg/8-hr period.[32] When one of these conditions is present, initial intravenous therapy may be necessary. In many cases, the oral solution (made up in a rehydration center or hospital) can be given to mothers to administer to children *ad libitum*, after instruction to feed as the child will accept. If fluid losses in stool cannot be matched or if vomiting does not permit feeding, the child should be brought back to the rehydration center or hospital. If children are given solutions containing high concentrations of sodium (i.e., 90 mEq/liter), they should also be given plain water as tolerated. Therapy of young children with diarrhea in this country generally does not require the use of rehydration solutions containing such high concentrations of sodium.

Oral fluid therapy will increase the stool output by as much as one-third (compared to patients receiving fluids intravenously)[31,34] since the entire solution is not absorbed; this generally is of no concern, however, since positive water–electrolyte balance can be expected. Sucrose is associated with greater stool volume output than glucose, perhaps because of the occurrence of sucrase deficiency in patients with diarrhea[35-37]; however, sucrose and glucose solutions appear to be equally effective in the oral therapy of children with cholera.[32] Despite the common occurrence of vomiting, the apparent lack of glucose-facilitated sodium and water absorption,[4] and the lower stool concentrations of sodium,[38] the higher-sodium oral fluid therapy has been used to successfully rehydrate children with RV diarrhea maintained under close supervision,[16] although solutions with a sodium content that more closely approximates the loss in stool may be preferable.[28]

Milk is withheld for at least 6 hr to prevent a delay in gastric emptying during oral rehydration and because of its lactose content. Oral treatment is directed toward preventing volume depletion, supplying water and electrolyte deficits, and meeting caloric and nutritional needs of the intestine and body in general. Breast-feeding should be continued throughout illness unless symptoms and signs of lactose intolerance develop. In most cases, milk is reintroduced within 24 hr to improve nutritional aspects (see "Initiation of a Modified Diet," below). Medical care should be sought when three sequential feedings are lost due to vomiting, a change in sensorium occurs, or significant purging persists.

Intravenous Rehydration

In any patient in whom 10% dehydration is found, intravenous fluid replacement is indicated. Fluids used in intravenous therapy of severe dehydration are listed in Table 11.5. Ringer's lactate solution is adequate and is generally available in the United States. The 5:4:1 formula developed at the Cholera Research Laboratory in Dacca, Bangladesh, is easily produced by mixing 5 g NaCl, 4 g $NaHCO_3$, and 1 g KCl with sufficient sterile distilled water to make 1 liter of fluid. An acetate solution has advantages, particularly in warm climates with inadequate storage facilities, in that it is a more stable preparation.[39]

The objective of therapy is to treat hypovolemic shock and correct electrolyte deficits as rapidly as possible. The exception to rapid correction of electrolyte deficits is seen in patients with hypernatremia, where the electrolyte abnormality should be corrected more slowly. Isotonic solutions should not be used to treat patients with hypovolemic shock. In adults, intravenous fluid infusion can be given at a rate of 2–100 ml/min (depending on state of dehydration) until a strong radial pulse is restored, followed by infusion of isotonic fluids given to replace intestinal and urinary losses. In children, a bolus of 20 ml/kg of normal saline or Ringer's lactate solution should be given over 1 hr. Although blood pressure and pulse are often used to judge fluid therapy, plasma specific gravity and measurement of left ventricular filling pressure by a determination of either central venous pressure (CVP) or pulmonary wedge pressure (PWP) are better measurements of fluid requirements and are mandatory in patients who do not respond to attempts at volume expansion.[40] If the CVP or PWP remains low or normal during fluid challenge, hypovolemia is present, and volume expansion is continued in the same manner. If the patient has not clinically improved when the CVP reaches 15 cm H_2O or the PWP reaches 18 mm Hg, then other causes of circulatory failure should be sought. Vascular overload is rare if the CVP is maintained below 15 cm H_2O or the PWP below 18 mm Hg. For each 0.001 increase in plasma specific gravity above 1.025, the patient will require approximately 4 ml of isotonic fluid/kg of body weight.[41] Successive dilution of plasma protein follows a logarithmic curve, so that to go from a specific gravity of 1.026 to 1.023 will require more fluid than to go from 1.029 to 1.026.[35] One approach to fluid therapy is to administer intravenous fluids until plasma specific gravity reaches 1.030, at which time the intravenous fluid therapy is discontinued and oral therapy is initiated. Oral therapy given concomitantly can decrease the intravenous fluid requirement by 80%.[33]

INITIATION OF A MODIFIED DIET

After the rehydration phase has been completed, a modified diet must be initiated. In any feeding mixture given during or after an episode of diarrhea, three factors need be considered: (1) renal solute load, related directly to the protein and electrolyte content of the formula, (2) osmolarity, related to the total solute concentration, and (3) specific carbohydrate content. Table 11.6 outlines the renal solute load and osmolarity of various products used for infant feeding. We will deal with the three important dietary concerns in some detail.

Renal Solute Load

Renal solute load refers to solutes that must be excreted in the urine.[42] Inherent problems with an overconcentrated formula are its low content of water and high concentration of solutes. When this kind of formula is used in infant feeding, fluid intake may become deficient, causing a diminished volume of renal water available for excretion of solutes. Functional immaturity of the infant kidney compromises renal excretory ability even further.[43] When the volume of renal water becomes inadequate for the removal of solutes, body water is utilized and dehydration results. If the problem of hypertonic dehydration is to be avoided, formulas yielding low renal solute loads should be used, especially if decreased fluid intake, increased extrarenal water losses, and/or impaired renal function are present. Except for cow's milk, and possibly Nutramigen, Pregestamil, and some soy-based formulas, the renal solute load produced by most other commercially available formulas, such as Enfamil, Similac, SMA 20, and by human milk (Table 11.6) should cause no problem in refeeding infants after an episode of diarrhea. The protein content of cow's milk is significantly higher than that of other milk-based and soy-isolated-based formulas (Table 11.7) and accounts for the high renal solute load.

TABLE 11.5
Intravenous Replacement Fluids (m Eq/liter) for Dehydration Due to Diarrhea

	Na^+	K^+	Ca^{++}	Cl^-	HCO_3^-	Acetate	Lactate	Advantage
Dacca 5:4:1 solution	133	14	—	99	48	—	—	Ease of production and reduced cost
NAMRU acetate[a]	120	10	—	100	—	30	–	Stability and reduced cost
Ringer's lactate	130	4	3	109	—	—	28	Availability
Normal saline	154	—	—	154	—	—	—	Availability
Plasmalyte	140	10	5	103	—	47	8	Availability

[a]Watten *et al.*[39]

TABLE 11.6
Renal Solute Load and Osmolarity of Commercially Available
Preparations[a]

Product	Estimated renal solute load (mosmol/liter)	Osmolarity (mosmol/liter)
Human milk	79	286
Cow's milk	221	260
Milk-based formulas		
Enfamil	105	288
Similac	108	295
SMA 20	91	300
Soy-isolate-based formulas		
Isomil	127	223
Neo-Mull-Soy	124	273
Mull-Soy	120	273
ProSobee	150	251
Nutramigen	130	443
Pregestamil	130	590
5% glucose	0	298
10% glucose	0	618
Pedialyte	80	409
Lytren	80	539

[a]Ziegler and Fomon,[42] Paxson *et al.*,[44] and Matsuda *et al.*[71]

TABLE 11.7
Concentration of Protein Per Unit of Calories in Various Foods
Commonly Fed to Infants

Formula	Protein (g/100 kcal)
Human milk	1.6
Commercially prepared formulas	
Milk-based	2.3–2.7
Soy-isolate-based	2.7–3.3
Whole cow's milk	5.0

Osmolarity

Osmolarity, which is a measure of the total carbohydrate and mineral content of the formula, increases with increasing caloric content. Paxson and associates[44] noted differences in concentration of formulas due to the variation among lots from a single manufacturer or due to alterations in the method of reconstitution. Consistently greater osmolarities were found in the resultant formula prepared from powder as compared to the same product in the ready-to-feed liquid form.[44] Formulas prepared by the use of a scoop may have an osmolarity approaching twice that of the same formula reconstituted by weight per the manufacturer's formulation. The epidemic of hypernatremia that occurred during the late 1950s and early 1960s was attributed in large part to unintentional variation in the solute load of formulas fed to infants.[45,46] Boiled skimmed milk and commercially or home-prepared oral electrolyte solutions have been responsible for a large percentage of cases of hypernatremia[47] and should not be used for feeding infants in the recovery phase of gastroenteritis.

Solutions with osmolarities as high as 500 mosmol/liter will pass from the stomach as rapidly as water.[48] It has been suggested that hyperosmolar feedings might result in mucosal damage.[49] This suggestion is based on the observations that in rats and in humans, hyperosmolar solutions containing 550 mosomol/liter of mannitol, in addition to isotonic sodium chloride at 310 mosmol/liter, caused an impairment of intestinal glucose absorption as well as injury to the tips of the jejunal and ileal microvilli.[50,51]

The standard commercially available 67 kcal/100 ml formulas such as Enfamil, Similac, and the soy-based formulas that routinely are fed to infants have osmolarity values similar to that of breast milk and pose no apparent increased risk of mucosal insult. However, the hypercaloric formulas and some special products such as Nutramigen and Pregestamil have osmolarities sufficiently high that caution must be taken when they are used in patients with diarrhea. The prudent physician will know what each formula contains, will continue to insist that the formulas be carefully prepared, and may require that liquid preparations, rather than those made from powder, be used.

Carbohydrate Activity in the Gastrointestinal Tract

In children and infants, the carbohydrate fraction of milk may lead to a worsening or reactivation of diarrhea due to disaccharidase deficiency acquired as a result of the intestinal infection. Table 11.8 outlines the classes and types of carbohydrates. With the exception of crude fiber, all of the oligosaccharides, monosaccharides, and polysaccharides are di-

TABLE 11.8
Carbohydrates

Class	Type	Digested in small intestine
Oligosaccharides	Sucrose	+
	Lactose	+
	Maltose	+
Monosaccharides	Glucose	+
	Fructose	+
	Galactose	+
Polysaccharides	Dextrins	+
	Starch	+
	Dietary crude fiber	−

gested in the small intestine. Lactose, sucrose, and maltose are disaccharides which are hydrolyzed to monosaccharides in the intestine by disaccharidase enzymes. The disaccharidases are located within the microvillus membrane of the brush border of intestinal absorptive cells throughout the entire length of the small bowel, although their concentration is greatest in the jejunum.[52]

Lactose is a disaccharide found only in milk. It is normally absorbed intact into the epithelial cell and hydrolyzed to glucose and galactose by lactase which is localized in the cellular brush border. Sucrose is a disaccharide which is readily digested to glucose and fructose. Maltose is readily changed to dextrose and absorbed. Maltose is used extensively in combination with dextrose and dextrin in preparations such as dextrimaltose, Karo syrup, and cartose. The polysaccharide dextrins are the least fermentable of sugars and are the slowest in digestion and absorption. They are always used with maltose. Preparations high in dextrins are often used in the treatment of diarrhea. Dextrose is a monosaccharide which is readily absorbed without further digestion. It is seldom used alone in infant feeding but is the carbohydrate found in rehydrating solutions such as Pedialyte and Lytren.

The activity of lactase is lowest among the intestinal discchardases.[52] This, and not the glucose–galactose transport mechanism, is a rate-limiting factor in lactose digestion.[53] The other disaccharides and oligosaccharides are rapidly hydrolyzed, with a rate-limiting step in their absorption being the monosaccharide transport system. Glucose and galactose are both transported across the absorptive cell by the same sodium-dependent transport process. Fructose, which is released by hydrolysis of sucrose, is the only other important dietary monosaccharide and appears to be transported by a carrier mechanism that is independent of both the sodium and the glucose–galactose transport mechanisms.[52]

Composition of Standard and Soy Formulas

Table 11.9 outlines the fat, carbohydrate, and protein composition of standard and soy formulas. Standard formulas are most commonly used for routine infant feeding and contain animal protein and lactose as the major source of carbohydrate. Soy formulas contain various amounts of soy, corn, or coconut oil as the fat source. The amount of water, solids and fat in human milk is similar to that of cow's milk, but human milk contains only about one-third of the protein and ash present in cow's milk. In contrast, the amount of lactose in human milk is greater than that of cow's milk.

The electrolyte content of cow's milk and evaporated milk varies according to season, breed, and different manufacturing formulations and processing techniques of evaporated milk. The sodium and potassium

TABLE 11.9
Fat, Carbohydrate, and Protein Composition of Standard, Soy, and Other Formulas

	Fat	Carbohydrate	Protein
Standard formulas			
Cow's milk	Butterfat	Lactose	Cow's milk protein
Enfamil	Soy and coconut oils	Lactose	Cow's milk protein
Evaporated milk 1:2	Butterfat	Lactose	Cow's milk protein
Human milk	Human milk fat	Lactose	Human milk protein
Similac	Coconut and soy oils	Lactose	Cow's milk protein
SMA 20	Coconut, soy, and safflower oils, oleo	Lactose	Cow's milk protein and whey
Soy formulas			
Isomil	Coconut and soy oils	Sucrose and corn syrup	Soy isolate
Mull-Soy	Soy oil	Sucrose	Soy isolate
Neo-Mull-Soy	Nonhydrogenated soy oil	Sucrose	Soy isolate supplemented with methionine
ProSobee	Soy oil	Sucrose and corn syrup solids	Soy isolate
Nursoy	Coconut, safflower, and soy oils, oleo	Sucrose and corn syrup solids	Soy isolate
Soyalac	Soy oil	Sucrose, maltose, dextrins, dextrose	Soybean solids
Others			
Nutramigen	Corn oil	Sucrose, tapioca starch, and dextrin	Casein hydrolysate
Pregestamil	Medium-chain triglycerides and corn oil	Dextrose, tapioca starch, and corn syrup solids	Casein hydrolysate
Goat's milk	Goat's milk	Lactose	Goat's milk protein

contents of all infant formulas are similar, with human milk having the lowest concentrations (Table 11.10). Serum sodium and potassium concentrations of children receiving standard and soy formulas generally are similar.

DISACCHARIDASE DEFICIENCY

Lactase deficiency occurs normally in a high percentage of non-whites. It occurs sporadically in any patient during acute intestinal infections,[54,55] which may explain protracted diarrhea after a bout of acute gastroenteritis. During infancy, enteric infection, often of viral origin, is the most common cause of secondary lactase deficiency. Since lactase levels are rate-limiting for absorption of lactose, a fall in the level of lactase is accompanied by clinical symptoms of disaccharidase intolerance: diarrhea, abdominal distention, flatulence, emesis, and perianal pain when lactose is ingested. The severity of the secondary disaccharidase deficiency depends upon the causative agent and duration of diarrhea.

A characteristic nonspecific histologic lesion develops in the proximal small intestine during the course of gastroenteritis induced by RV or Norwalk-like agents.[56] The mucosal architecture is altered, and the villi are shortened, with intestinal crypts becoming hyperplastic. Infiltration of the lamina propria with polymorphonuclear leukocytes and increased numbers of mononuclear cells occurs early. The histologic changes may resemble other nonspecific jejunal mucosal lesions such as those found in tropical sprue and intraluminal bacterial overgrowth. In patients with diarrhea due to Norwalk-like agents, malabsorption of fat and glucose may occur and persist for at least one week after infection, although clinical symptoms last only one to two days.[57,58] Decreased levels of the brush-border enzymes trehalase and alkaline phosphatase were regularly

TABLE 11.10
Approximate Electrolyte Content (mEq/liter) of Infant Formulas

Formula	Na	K	Ca	P	Cl	Total electrolyte content
Human milk	7	14	17	9	12	70
Commercially prepared formulas						
Milk-based	7–18	14–28	21–50	21–48	11–23	89–194
Soy-isolate-based	13–24	18–40	21–60	21–46	6–16	114–210
Evaporated milk 1:2	18	25	42	37	20	165
Whole cow's milk	25	36	61	53	34	219

observed during acute Norwalk illness, with decreases in the levels of sucrase and lactase being less consistent.[57,58] The disaccharidases maltase, sucrase, isomaltase, and lactase have been shown to be depressed in infantile gastroenteritis due to RV.[59,60] The severity of the histologic lesion correlates with the degree of disaccharidase depression.[59] Disaccharidase deficiency with resultant stool losses may help to explain the higher incidence of dehydration among children with viral gastroenteritis when compared to children with diarrhea due to other causes.

Unhydrolyzed disaccharides which result when intestinal disaccharidase levels become depressed, as during infectious diarrhea, increase the intraluminal solute content and, therefore, the osmotic activity of the intestinal fluid, giving rise to the following effects: (1) increased fluid load, particularly in the jejunum and ileum, due to osmotic activity of luminal contents; (2) accelerated intestinal transit because of increased intraintestinal volume; (3) fermentation of lactose and other carbohydrates to lactic acid and fatty acids, which increases the solute content and may act as a bowel irritant; and (4) inadequate absorption of the fluid load presented to the colon. Stools from children with disaccharidase deficiency have a low pH and contain reducing substances, and anal irritation may occur. The fall in lactase levels after acute gastroenteritis may result from loss of microvilli and villi due to diarrhea or from loss of the protective glycocalyx, which may function as a barrier against the hostile environment within the gut lumen and subsequent action of pancreatic proteases or lactase.[54]

The development of lactase deficiency during a diarrheal illness may require some alteration in diet. In a study by Leake and associates,[61] young infants with dehydration and acidosis initially were rehydrated intravenously, then fed sucrose- or lactose-containing formulas. The success rate of soy-based sucrose-containing formulas was 91%, in contrast to a 36% success rate with cow's-milk-based formula feedings. In children with acute diarrhea, it is recommended that lactose be reduced or eliminated from the diet early in the illness to minimize the effects of disaccharide intolerance. Relative lactose intolerance has been shown to persist for two to six weeks after an episode of diarrhea.[62] Other disaccharidases may be reduced during infection, influencing absorption of other sugars. The ability of the small-bowel mucosa to split sucrose during acute infantile diarrhea was evaluated by Chatterjee and associates.[63] Disaccharidase levels were determined in jejunal mucosal biopsy specimens obtained from children with diarrhea during the acute phase. Reduced levels of lactase were found in 75% and reduced sucrase levels in 18%. Maltase levels were adequate; however, the scarcity and cost of maltose precludes its use as a component of rehydrating formulas.

Palmer *et al.*[64] showed that sucrose was as effective as glucose in an oral electrolyte solution for severe diarrhea in patients over five years of age. Their failure rates of 13% and 15% for sucrose and glucose, respectively, were similar to those found by other workers using oral glucose–electrolyte solutions in severe diarrheal disease.[31,33,34,36] Failure of oral therapy to successfully rehydrate the patients generally reflected the rate of fluid loss and not the solution used, where patients could not keep up with fluid losses and maintain hydration by mouth due to severe diarrhea and vomiting. Moenginah and associates[65] compared glucose and sucrose solutions in children with noncholera diarrhea and had a failure rate of 12% with glucose and 19% with sucrose solutions. Sack *et al.*[16] rehydrated 57 children with diarrhea due to RV with either a sucrose or glucose solution administered orally and found no difference in the rate of rehydration. Nalin *et al.*[15] found that rehydration of children with gastroenteritis using a sucrose solution produced a slower correction of electrolyte abnormalities and a higher percentage of patients who needed more than 24 hr of therapy when compared to children rehydrated with a glucose solution. These studies indicate that sucrose can be used in the majority of patients with acute diarrhea; however, potential disadvantages of this sugar in selected patients include insufficient glucose generation to affect electrolyte fluid absorption owing to rapid intestinal transit and greater number of stools, where administration of the disaccharide may increase the already large stool loss into the small intestine due to sucrase deficiency.[35,37,66]

During mild episodes of diarrhea, refeeding can be begun with one of the standard formulas containing lactose, but if stooling increases, a change to a non-lactose-containing formula should be made. If diarrhea is not adequately controlled, a non-lactose-containing formula (usually soy-based, sucrose-containing) is begun at one-fourth strength in a volume which fulfills fluid requirements. The formula is advanced to one-half strength, then full strength, over a 24- to 48-hr period. During the diet advancement, the child is observed closely. If an increase in stool number, volume, or water content occurs, the formula is stopped and a glucose–electrolyte solution is begun, and the formula is then advanced more slowly. Recurrence of diarrhea during feeding is frequently accompanied by a fall in stool pH to below 6 and the presence of reducing substances, indicating disaccharidase deficiency.

Occasionally, an infant may not be able to tolerate a sucrose-containing formula. In these cases, either carbohydrate-free formula or Pregestamil, which contains glucose, medium-chain triglycerides, and a predigested protein, is used. A carbohydrate such as glucose or fructose must be added to carbohydrate-free formula. This carbohydrate can be added gradually until a tolerance is achieved. With chronic diarrhea, these special formulas should be given for at least one month before trying to switch to a more conventional formula. The changeover should be gradual, and if diarrhea recurs or worsens, the special formula should be continued. Disaccharidase deficiency may persist for up to one year. If protracted diarrhea necessitates parenteral hyperalimentation, continued feedings have been shown to facilitate a more rapid return of intestinal function and of some intestinal enzymes.[67]

Monosaccharide intolerance is rare and usually restricted to infancy. It is characterized by the malabsorption of all carbohydrates, including glucose. Klish and associates[68] reported that glucose malabsorption was associated with a decreased intestinal absorptive surface area, occurring during the acute phase of diarrhea and improving during convalescence. A linear correlation was observed between the ability to absorb glucose and the intestinal surface area.

Mild transient steatorrhea has been demonstrated[69] to follow seemingly insignificant episodes of diarrhea in children. This is probably of minor consequence to most otherwise healthy infants in the United States; however, it should be considered along with mild lactose intolerance in those infants manifesting slightly abnormal stools or poor weight gain subsequent to an episode of diarrhea. This finding may be of special importance in infants subjected to repeated episodes of diarrhea.

DIAGNOSIS OF CARBOHYDRATE MALABSORPTION

Lactose intolerance is suspected in children who have increased stooling with development of perianal rash due to low pH when milk is added to their diet.

The most commonly used screening test for carbohydrate malabsorption to the determination of fecal pH using Combistix, pH paper, or pH electrodes. It is important that stool not be contaminated with urine and be tested promptly for an accurate pH determination. A pH value of 5.5 or less may indicate the presence of disaccharidase breakdown products such as lactic acid or other organic acids.

Kerry and Anderson[70] described a simple test for fecal reducing substances which uses Clinitest tablets. This test is useful as a screening test to detect diarrhea that may be due to malabsorption of carbohydrates in older or newborn infants.[71] One part stool is mixed with two parts water and then centrifuged. Fifteen drops of the supernatant are placed in a clear test tube and a Clinitest tablet added. The resulting reaction is allowed to proceed undisturbed for 15 sec, after which the tube is gently agitated and the color is compared to that on the color chart provided with the Clinitest tablets. Results of the test are graded from 0 to 4+, and values of 1+ or greater in children are considered abnormal and strongly suggestive of the presence of intestinal malabsorption of carbohydrates. Heating the stool extract with hydrochloric acid before adding the Clinitest tablet enables sucrose to be detected. Paper chromatography can be used to determine the specific reducing substance present. Tolerance tests to determine the specific disaccharide or monosaccharide may be performed but generally are unnecessary. To definitely establish the diagnosis of disaccharidase deficiency, disaccharidase levels may be measured in biopsies from the small intestine.

REFERENCES

1. Talbot, N. B., Crawford, J. D., Butler, A. M. Homeostatic limits to safe parenteral fluid therapy. *N. Engl. J. Med.* **248**:1100–1108, 1953.
2. Winters, R. W. Regulation of normal water and electrolyte metabolism; Maintenance fluid therapy. In R. W. Winters (ed.), *The Body Fluids in Pediatrics: Medical, Surgical and Neonatcl Disorders of Acid–Base Status, Hydration, and Oxygenation.* Little, Brown, Boston, 1973, pp. 95–112; and 113–133.
3. McClung, H. J., Butler, D. G., Kerzner, B., *et al.* Transmissible gastroenteritis: Mucosal ion transport in acute viral enteritis. *Gastroenterology* **70**:1091–1095, 1976.
4. Davidson, G. P., Gall, D. G., Petric, M., *et al.* Human rotavirus enteritis induced in conventional piglets. *J. Clin. Invest.* **60**:1402–1409, 1977.
5. Holt, L.L E., Courtney, A. M., Fales, H. L. The chemical composition of diarrheal as compared with normal stools in infants. *Am. J. Dis. Child.* **9**:213–224, 1915.
6. Darrow, D. C. The retention of electrolyte during recovery from severe dehydration due to diarrhea. *J. Pediatr.* **28**:515–540, 1946.
7. Chung, A. W. The effect of oral feeding at different levels on the absorption of food stuffs in infantile diarrhea. *J. Pediatr.* **33**:1–13, 1948.
8. Weil, W. B., Wallace, W. M. Hypertonic dehydration in infancy. *Pediatrics* **17**:171–181, 1956.
9. Metcoff, J., Frenk, S., Gordillo, G., *et al.* Intracellular composition and homeostatic mechanisms in severe chronic infantile malnutrition: IV. Development and repair of the biochemical lesion. *Pediatrics* **20**:317–335, 1957.
10. Finberg, L.. Cheung, C. S., Fleishman, E. The significance of the concentrations of electrolytes in stool water during infantile diarrhea. *Am. J. Dis. Child* **100**:809–813, 1960.
11. Kooh, S. W., Metcoff, J. Physiologic considerations in fluid and electrolyte therapy with particular reference to diarrheal dehydration in children. *J. Pediatr.* **62**:107–131, 1963.
12. Teree, T. M., Mirabal-Font, E., Ortiz, A., *et al.* Stool losses and acidosis in diarrheal disease of infancy. *Pediatrics* **36**:704–713, 1965.
13. Mahalanabis, D., Wallace, C. K., Kallen, R. J. *et al.* Water and electrolyte losses due to cholera in infants and small children: A recovery balance study. *Pediatrics* **45**:374–385, 1970.
14. Kerzner, B., MacKenzie, C., Middleton, P., *et al.* Clinical, laboratory, epidemiological features of a recently recognized viral enteritis (abstract). *Proc. Soc. Pediatr. Res.* St. Louis, April, 1976.
15. Nalin, D. R., Levine, M. M., Mata, L., *et al.* Comparison of sucrose with glucose in oral therapy of infant diarrhoea. *Lancet* **2**:277–279, 1978.

16. Sack, D. A., Chowdhury, A. M. A. K., Eusof, A., *et al.* Oral hydration in rotavirus diarrhoea: A double blind comparison of sucrose with glucose electrolyte solution. *Lancet* **2**:280–283, 1978.

17. Crane, R. K. Na[+]-dependent transport in the intestine and other animal tissues. *Fed. Proc. Fed. Am. Soc. Exp. Biol.* **24**:1000–1006, 1965.

18. Shultz, S. G., Curran, P. F. Coupled transport of sodium and organic solutes. *Physiol. Rev.* **50**:637–718, 1970.

19. Fordtran, J. S. Stimulation of active and passive sodium absorption by sugars in the human jejunum. *J. Clin. Invest.* **55**:728–737, 1975.

20. Scanlon, J. W. Electrolyte content of commercial gelatin products and sweetened liquid mixtures in treatment of diarrhea. *Clin. Pediatr.* **9**:508–509, 1970.

21. Composition of foods. U.S. Dep. Agric., *Agric. Handb.* No. 8–1, 1976, p. 89.

22. Vaughan, V. C., III, McKay, R. J., Nelson, W. E. (eds.). *Textbook of Pediatrics.* W. B. Saunders, Philadelphia, 1975, pp. 1802–1803.

23. DeGenaro, F., Nyhan, W. L. Salt—a dangerous "antidote." *J. Pediatr.* **78**:1048–1049, 1971.

24. Coodin, F. J., Gabrielson, I. W., Addiege, J. E., Jr. Formula fatality. *Pediatrics* **47**:438–439, 1971.

25. Saunders, N., Balfe, J. W., Laski, B. Severe salt poisoning in an infant. *J. Pediatr.* **88**:258–261, 1976.

26. Oral glucose/electrolyte therapy for acute diarrhea (editorial). *Lancet* **1**:79–80, 1975.

27. Nalin, D. R., Cash, R. A. Sodium content in oral therapy for diarrhea (letter). *Lancet* **2**:957, 1976.

28. Finberg, L. The role of oral electrolyte–glucose solutions in hydration for children—international and domestic aspects. *J. Pediatr.* **96**:51–54, 1980.

29. Hirschhorn, N., Cash, R. A., Woodward, W. E., *et al.* Oral fluid therapy of Apache children with acute infectious diarrhoea. *Lancet* **2**:15–18, 1972.

30. Hirschhorn, N., McCarthy, B. J., Ranney, B., *et al. Ad libitum* oral glucose–electrolyte therapy for acute diarrhea in Apache children. *J. Pediatr.* **83**:562–570, 1973.

31. Sack, R. B., Cassells, J., Mitra, R., *et al.* The use of oral replacement solutions in the treatment of cholera and other severe diarrhoeal disorders. *Bull. W.H.O.* **43**:351–360, 1970.

32. Sack, D. A., Islam, S., Brown, K. H., *et al.* Oral therapy in children with cholera: A comparison of sucrose and glucose electrolyte solutions. *J. Pediatr.* **96**:20–25, 1980.

33. Nalin, D. R., Cash, R. A., Islam, R., *et al.* Oral maintenance therapy for cholera in adults. *Lancet* **2**:370–373, 1968.

34. Pierce, N. F., Sack, R. B., Mitra, R. C., *et al.* Replacement of water and electrolyte losses cholera by an oral glucose–electrolyte solution. *Ann. Intern. Med.* **70**:1173–1181, 1969.

35. Hirschhorn, N., Nalin, D. R. Sucrose or glucose for diarrhea. *Lancet* **2**:1230, 1977.

36. Nalin, D. R. Sucrose in oral therapy for cholera and related diarrhoeas. *Lancet* **1**:1400–1402, 1975.

37. Hirschhorn, N., Molla, A., Molla, A. M. Reversible jejunal disaccharidase deficiency in cholera and other acute diarrheal diseases. *Johns Hopkins Med. J.* **125**:291–300, 1969.

38. Tallett, S., MacKenzie, C., Middleton, P., *et al.* Clinical, laboratory, and epidemiologic features of a viral gastroenteritis in infants and children. *Pediatrics* **60**:217–222, 1977.

39. Watten, R. H., Gutman, R. A., Fresh, J. W. Comparison of acetate, lactate and bicarbonate in treating acidosis of cholera. *Lancet* **2**:512–514, 1969.

40. Love, A. H. G., Phillips, R. A. Measurement of dehydration in cholera. *J. Infect. Dis.* **119**:39–42, 1969.

41. Phillips, R. A. Water and electrolyte losses in cholera. *Fed. Proc. Fed. Am. Soc. Exp. Biol.* **23**:705–712, 1964.

42. Ziegler, E. E., Fomon, S. J., Fluid intake, renal solute load, and water balance in infancy. *J. Pediatr.* **78**:561–568, 1971.

43. Edelmann, C. M., Jr., Spitzer, A. The maturing kidney: A modern view of well-balanced infants with imblanced nephrons. *J. Pediatr.* **75**:509–519, 1969.

44. Paxson, C. L., Jr., Adcock, E. W., III, Morriss, F. H., Jr. Osmolalities of infant formulas. *Am. J. Dis. Child.* **131**:139–141, 1977.

45. Colle, E., Ayoub, E., Raile, R. Hypertonic dehydration (hypernatremia): The role of feedings high in solutes. *Pediatrics* **22**: 5–12, 1958.

46. Abrams, C. A., Phillips, L. L., Berkowitz, C., *et al.* Hazards of overconcentrated milk formula: Hypersomolality, disseminated intravascular coagulation, and gangrene. *J. Am. Med. Assoc.* **232**:1136–1140, 1975.

47. Berenberg, W., Mandell, F., Fellers, F. X. Hazards of skimmed milk, unboiled and boiled. *Pediatrics* **44**:734–737, 1969.

48. Hunt, J. N., Pathak, J. D. The osmotic effects of some simple molecules and ions on gastric emptying. *J. Physiol. (London)* **154**:254–269, 1960.

49. Book, L. S., Herbst, J. J., Atherton, S. O., *et al.* Necrotizing enterocolitis in low-birth-weight infants fed an elemental formula. *J. Pediatr.* **87**:602–605, 1975.

50. Kameda, H., Abei, T., Nasrallah, S., *et al.* Functional and histological injury to intestinal mucosa produced by hypertonicity. *Am. J. Physiol.* **214**:1090–1095, 1968.

51. Nasrallah, S. M., Coburn, W. M., Jr., Iber, F. L. The effect of hypertonic mannitol on the intestine of man. *Johns Hopkins Med. J.* **123**:134–137, 1968.

52. Gray, G. M., Carbohydrate digestion and absorption: Role of the small intestine. *N. Engl. J. Med.* **292**:1225–1230, 1975.

53. Gray, G. M., Santiago, N. A. Disaccharide absorption in normal and diseased human intestine. *Gastroenterology* **51**:489–498, 1966.

54. Alpers, D. H., Seetharam, B., Pathophysiology of diseases involving intestinal brush-border proteins. *N. Engl. J. Med.* **296**:1047–1050, 1977.

55. Ament, M. E. Malabsorption syndromes in infancy and childhood: Part II. *J. Pediatr.* **81**:867–884, 1972.

56. Schreiber, D. S., Trier, J. S., Blacklow, N. R. Recent advances in viral gastroenteritis. *Gastroenterology* **73**:174–183, 1977.

57. Blacklow, N. R., Dolin, R., Fedson, D. S., *et al.* Acute infectious nonbacterial gastroenteritis: Etiology and pathogenesis. *Ann. Intern. Med.* **76**:993–1008, 1972.

58. Schreiber, D. S., Blacklow, N. R., Trier, J. S. The mucosal lesion of the proximal small intestine in acute infectious nonbacterial gastroenteritis. *N. Engl. J. Med.* **288**:1318–1323, 1973.

59. Barnes, G. L., Townley, R. R. Duodenal mucosal damage in 31 infants with gastroenteritis. *Arch. Dis. Child.* **48**:343–349, 1973.

60. Barnes, G. L., Bishop, R. F., Townley, R. R. Microbial flora and disaccharidase depression in infantile gastroenteritis. *Acta Paediatr. Scand.* **63**:423–426, 1974.

61. Leake, R. D., Schroeder, K. C. Benton, D. A., *et al.* Soy-based formula in the treatment of infantile diarrhea. *Am. J. Dis. Child.* **127**:374–376, 1974.

62. Lifshitz, P., Coello-Ramirez, R., Gutierrez-Topete, G., *et al.* Carbohydrate intolerance in infants with diarrhea. *J. Pediatr.* **79**:760–767, 1971.

63. Chatterjee, A., Mahalanabis, D., Jalan, K. N., *et al.* Evaluation of a sucrose/electrolyte solution for oral rehydration in acute infantile diarrhea. *Lancet* **1**:1333–1335, 1977.

64. Palmer, D. L., Koster, F. T., Islam, R. A. F., *et al.* Comparison of sucrose and glucose in the oral electrolyte therapy of cholera and other severe diarrheas. *N. Engl. J. Med.* **297**:1107–1110, 1977.

65. Moenginah, P. A., Suprapto, J., Soenarto, J., *et al.* Oral sucrose therapy for diarrhea. *Lancet* **2**:323, 1975.

66. Sandle, G. I.., Lobley, R. W., Holmes, R. Oral therapy in cholera (letter). *N. Engl. J. Med.* **298**:797–798, 1978.

67. Greene, H. L., McCabe, D. R., Merenstein, G. B. Protracted diarrhea and malnutrition in infancy: Changes in intestinal morphology and disaccharidase activities during treatment with total intravenous nutrition or oral elemental diets. *J. Pediatr.* **87**:695–704, 1975.

68. Klish, W. J., Udall, J. N., Rodriguez, J. T., *et al.* Intestinal surface area in infants with acquired monosaccharide intolerance. *J. Pediatr.* **92**:566–571, 1978.

69. MacLean, W. C., Jr., Klein, G. L., Lopez de Romana, G., *et al.* Transient steatorrhea following episodes of mild diarrhea in early infancy. *J. Pediatr.* **92**:562–565, 1978.

70. Kerry, K. R., Anderson, C. M. A ward test for sugar in feces. *Lancet* **1**:981–982, 1964.

71. Matsuda, I., Kamimura, M., Oka, Y., *et al.* Osmolalities of infant formulas in Japan (letter). *Am. J. Dis. Child.* **131**:1403, 1977.

72. Nalin, D. R., Cash, R. A. Oral therapy for diarrhoea: *Lancet* **1**:1059–1960, 1977.

Index